Kathryn J. Hannah • Pamela Hussey
Margaret A. Kennedy • Marion J. Ball
Editors

Introduction to Nursing Informatics

Fourth Edition

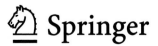 Springer

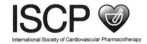

Editors

Kathryn J. Hannah, PhD, RN
Calgary
Alberta
Canada

Marion J. Ball, EdD, FACMI, AMIA
IBM Research Center for Healthcare
Management
Baltimore, MD
USA

Pamela Hussey, RN, RCN, MEd, MSc, PhD
Dublin City University
Dublin
Ireland

Margaret A. Kennedy, RN, BScN, MN,
PhD, CPHIMS-CA, PMP,
PRINCE2 Practitioner
Global Village Consulting Inc
Merigomish
Nova Scotia
Canada

ISBN 978-1-4471-2998-1   ISBN 978-1-4471-2999-8   (eBook)
DOI 10.1007/978-1-4471-2999-8
Springer London Heidelberg New York Dordrecht

Library of Congress Control Number: 2014955372

Springer is part of Springer Science+Business Media (www.springer.com)

The authors of this book share many passions and values. The strongest of these is the incomparable value of family and friends. We dedicate this new edition to our family, friends, and wonderful colleagues for their generosity of support and inspiration.

Series Preface

The Health Informatics Series is directed to healthcare professionals who are leading the transformation of health care by using information and knowledge. Launched in 1988 as "Computers in Health Care", to offer a broad range of titles: some addressed to specific professions such as nursing, medicine, and health administration; others to special areas of practice such as trauma and radiology; still other books in the series focused on interdisciplinary issues, such as the computer based patient record, electronic health records, and networked healthcare systems.

Renamed "Health Informatics" in 1998 to reflect the rapid evolution in the discipline known as health informatics, the series continues to add titles that contribute to the evolution of the field. In the series, eminent experts, serving as editors or authors, offer their accounts of innovations in health informatics. Increasingly, these accounts go beyond hardware and software to address the role of information in influencing the transformation of healthcare delivery systems around the world. The series also increasingly focuses on the users of the information and systems: the organizational, behavioral, and societal changes that accompany the diffusion of information technology in health services environments.

Developments in healthcare delivery are constant; most recently developments in proteomics and genomics are increasingly becoming relevant to clinical decision making and emerging standards of care. The data resources emerging from molecular biology are beyond the capacity of the human brain to integrate and beyond the scope of paper-based decision trees. Thus, bioinformatics has emerged as a new field in health informatics to support emerging and ongoing developments in molecular biology. Translational informatics supports acceleration, from bench to bedside, i.e. the appropriate use of molecular biology research findings and bioinformatics in clinical care of patients.

At the same time, further continual evolution of the field of health informatics is reflected in the introduction of concepts at the macro or health systems delivery level with major national initiatives in many countries related to concepts such as electronic health records (EHRs) and personal health records; public health informatics; and data analytics, eHealth and digital health with the associated data, terminology and messaging standards essential to clinical interoperability.

We have consciously retained the series title Health Informatics as the single umbrella term that encompasses both the microscopic elements of bioinformatics and the macroscopic aspects of large national health information systems. Ongoing changes to both the micro and macro perspectives on health informatics will continue to shape health services in the twenty-first century. By making full and creative use of the technology to tame data and to transform information, Health Informatics will foster the development and use of new knowledge in health care. As coeditors, we pledge to support our professional colleagues and the series readers as they share advances in the emerging and exciting field of health informatics.

Victoria, BC, Canada   Kathryn J. Hannah, PhD, RN
Dublin, Ireland   Pamela Hussey, RN, RCN, MEd, MSc, PhD
Halifax, NS, Canada   Margaret Ann Kennedy, RN, BScN, MN, PhD,
                                                CPHIMS-CA, PMP, PRINCE2 Practitioner
Baltimore, MD, USA   Marion J. Ball, EdD, FACMI, AMIA

Preface

The publication of this 4th edition of *An Introduction to Nursing Informatics* is timely. Its core purpose is to act as primer for nurses searching for basic information on the topic of nursing informatics. Interest in health informatics and its relevance to eHealth is expanding at a dynamic pace. The commitment of funding by the World Health Organization (WHO), Pan American Health Organization (PAHO), European Union (EU) and United States (USA) indicates that the integration of informatics competencies and its associated role in eHealth service delivery is a key priority. As a profession, nursing is accountable for a significant contribution to health care service provision. Contemporary nursing practice is changing and, at the same time, facing a number of critical challenges. For example, two global issues that the profession is striving to address include high staff turnover and nursing skill mix shortages. Articulating the nursing contribution to holistic care is therefore as important now as ever. Nursing informatics continues to be an essential aspect not only in providing information about the profession but also in helping nurse leaders in their quest for the expansion of nursing knowledge and theory development.

Twenty-first-century medicine offers exciting opportunities for the nursing profession to engage with and develop within. An example includes the opportunity to contribute to the design of emerging eHealth models of care. Additionally, concepts relating to health ecosystems which can be used to transform and enhance health and social care in society are seeking nurses' expertise and imagination. There is a need to ensure that resources such as electronic health records and mobile technology (mTechnology) applications are pragmatic and fit for purpose. Nurses, often described as context experts, understand the flow of health care processes and are key agents in requirements identification and evaluation of systems under development.

In this edition, the editors have collected the best available evidence to inspire and support nurses to think critically about both current and future practice. This book is presented in such a manner as to encourage the reader to pause and reflect upon key concepts presented from the perspective of their existing practice domain. Starting with the fundamental concepts of nursing practice, information management and its relationship to informatics, this edition includes a number of contributions from leading experts who have practised in the field of informatics over a number of years. Preparing nurses for engagement with initiatives relating to eHealth transformational programmes locally, regionally or nationally is supported with additional files for downloading from extras.springer.com. There is a strong emphasis on both education and continuous professional development, and the pedagogical framework used to devise the core learning activities is explained in Chapter 1. This book builds on previous editions and provides readers with a basic primer for searching information on the topic of nursing informatics. It includes online resources and tools to support the acquisition of informatics skills for future professional development. We hope you enjoy this 4th edition.

Victoria, BC, Canada   Kathryn J. Hannah, PhD, RN
Dublin, Ireland   Pamela Hussey, RN, RCN, MEd, MSc, PhD
Halifax, NS, Canada   Margaret Ann Kennedy, RN, BScN, MN, PhD,
                                                CPHIMS-CA, PMP, PRINCE2 Practitioner
Baltimore, MD, USA   Marion J. Ball, EdD, FACMI, AMIA

Contents

Part III   Administration

Part IV   Research

Part V   Education

Contributors

Marion J. Ball, EdD, FACMI, AMIA Clinical Solutions Healthlink, Inc., Baltimore, MD, USA

Anne Casey, RN, MSc, FRCN Royal College of Nursing, London, UK

Polun Chang, PhD Institute of Biomedical Informatics, National Yang-Ming University, Taipei, Taiwan, ROC

Hélène Clément, RN, BScN, MHA, CPHIMS-CA Richmond Hill, ON, Canada

Julie Doyle, BSc, PhD CASALA and the Netwell Centre, Dundalk Institute of Technology, Dundalk, County Louth, Ireland

Tracy Forbes, BComm Gevity Consulting Inc, Vancouver, BC, Canada

Joanne Foster, RN, DipAppSc-NsgEdn, BN School of Nursing, Queensland University of Technology, Kelvin Grove, QLD, Australia

Ross Fraser, CISSP, ISSAP Sextant Corporation, Toronto, ON, Canada

Kathryn J. Hannah, PhD, RN School of Nursing, University of Victoria, Victoria, BC, Canada

Christopher Henry Digital Media Engineer, Dublin, Ireland

Pamela Hussey, RN, RCN, MEd, MSc, PhD Lecturer in Health Informatics and Nursing, School of Nursing and Human Sciences, Dublin City University, Dublin, Ireland

Margaret Ann Kennedy, RN, BScN, MN, PhD, CPHIMS-CA, PMP, PRINCE2 Practitioner Atlantic Branch, Gevity Consulting Inc, Halifax, NS, Canada

Ming-Chuan Jessie Kuo, RN, MS Nursing Department, Cathay General Hospital, Taipei, Taiwan, ROC

Shaio-Jyue Lu, RN, MS Nursing Department, Taichung Veterans General Hospital, VACRS, Taichung, Taiwan, ROC

Breane Manson Lucas Cerner Corporation, Kansas City, MO, USA

Stephen P. Murray, BSc, EBU, MBA, PMP, ISP, CPHIMS Whiteshadow Inc., Charlottetown, PE, Canada

Kathryn Momtahan, RN, PhD Nursing Professional Practice, The Ottawa Hospital and the Ottawa Hospital Research Institute, Ottawa, ON, Canada

Lynn M. Nagle, RN, BN, MScN, PhD Lawrence S. Bloomberg, Faculty of Nursing, University of Toronto, Toronto, ON, Canada

Paula Mary Procter, RN, MSc, FBCS, FIMIANI Department of Nursing and Midwifery, Sheffield Hallam University, Sheffield, UK

Sally Remus, RN, BScN, MScN Doctoral Student, Arthur Labatt Family School of Nursing, Western University, London, ON, Canada

Fintan Sheerin, BNS, MA, PhD, RNID, FEANS c/o School of Nursing and Midwifery, Trinity College Dublin, Dublin, Ireland

Sally E. Schlak, BSN, MBA The TIGER Initiative Foundation, Chicago, IL, USA

Anne Spencer, BA (Hons), MSc Partners in Education Teaching and Learning (PETAL), Dublin, Ireland

Beverley Thomas, RN, Cert Ed (FE). MPH. Dip HSM NHS Wales Informatics Service, Cardiff, Wales, UK

Lorcan Walsh, B. Eng, PWD CASALA and the Netwell Centre, Dundalk Institute of Technology, Dundalk, County Louth, Ireland

Karen Witting, MS, MA, BA IBM T.J. Watson Research Center, Yorktown Heights, NY, USA

List of Electronic Supplementary Material

Extra material available from Springer Extras page (extras.springer.com)

Chapter 1

Educational Template (PDF 235 kb)
Educational Template (PPTX 263 kb)
Learning Plan (PDF 445 kb)
Learning Plan (DOCX 98 kb)
Audio 1.1 Podcast discussing the overall design of this new edition (MP3 1886 kb)
Glossary for Introduction to Nursing Informatics (XLSX 46 kb)

Chapter 2

Educational Template (PDF 108 kb)
Educational Template (PPTX 120 kb)

Chapter 3

Educational Template (PDF 110 kb)
Educational Template (PPTX 133 kb)

Chapter 4

Educational Template (PDF 7160 kb)
Educational Template (PPTX 3625 kb)
Audio 4.1 Marion Ball: Naming Nursing Informatics as Specialist Area
  (MP3 6801 kb)
Presentation 4.1 History of computing and technology (PPTX 3527 kb)

Chapter 5

Educational Template (PDF 4179 kb)
Educational Template (PPTX 1665 kb)

Chapter 6

Educational Template (PDF 98 kb)
Educational Template (PPTX 127 kb)

Chapter 7

Educational Template (PDF 103 kb)
Educational Template (PPTX 116 kb)

Chapter 8

Educational Template (PDF 89 kb)
Educational Template (PPTX 125 kb)

Chapter 9

Educational Template (PDF 98 kb)
Educational Template (PPTX 128 kb)

Chapter 10

Educational Template (PDF 97 kb)
Educational Template (PPTX 115 kb)
Video 10.1 GRASP (Grace Reynolds Application and Study of PETO). An example of a popular administrative solution used for workload management. With permission from GRASP Systems International, Inc (MP4 50378 kb)

Chapter 11

Educational Template (PDF 98 kb)
Educational Template (PPTX 114 kb)

Chapter 12

Educational Template (PDF 103 kb)
Educational Template (PPTX 123 kb)
Audio 12.1 The role of the informatics nurse by Roy Simpson, RN, C, CMAC, FNAP, FAAN, current role Vice President, Nursing Informatics, at Cerner Corporation (MP3 17564 kb)
Audio 12.2 The role of the informatics nurse by Cheryl Stephens-Lee, RN, BScN, MScNI, Clinical Applications Consultant, Markham Stouffville Hospital, Markham, Ontario, Canada (M4A 11840 kb)
Audio 12.3 The role of the informatics nurse by Suzanne Brown, RGN, RM, BNs, MScHealth Informatics, Assistant Nurse Coordinator Computer Services, Mater Misericordiae University Hospital, Information Management Services Department, Dublin, Ireland (MP3 4834 kb)
Audio 12.4 The role of the informatics nurse by Dairin Hines, RGN, RCN, BSc, HSM, MScHealth Informatics, Clinical Informatics Manager, Temple Street Children's University Hospital, ICT Department, Dublin, Ireland (MP3 4567 kb)
Audio 12.3 Transcript (PDF 300 kb)
Audio 12.4 Transcript (PDF 37 kb)

Chapter 13

Educational Template (PDF 102 kb)
Educational Template (PPTX 116 kb)

Chapter 14

Educational Template (PDF 7160 kb)
Educational Template (PPTX 3625 kb)

Chapter 19

Educational Template (PDF 89 kb)
Educational Template (PPTX 120 kb)

Chapter 20

Educational Template (PDF 97 kb)
Educational Template (PPTX 123 kb)

Chapter 21

Educational Template (PDF 90 kb)
Educational Template (PPTX 127 kb)

Part I
Introduction

Chapter 1
Introduction

Pamela Hussey and Margaret Ann Kennedy

Abstract Chapter 1 introduces the reader to the structure and content of this new edition. Designed as an ebook, this fourth edition describes how the acronym CARE originally introduced in early editions by Hannah and Ball is now adapted and used to present content in four discrete sections. Educational tools devised to support the reader are also presented in Chaps. 1, and 3 distinct learning approaches; assimilative, productive and interactive/adaptive styles are explained. Each chapter has an associated learning template that can be downloaded at the end of the resource. In Chap. 1 the structure and presentation of the learning templates is also presented.

Keywords Introduction to 4th edition structure • Supporting educational resource tools • Learning approaches explained • The CARE acronym

Key Concepts

Introduction to 4th Edition Structure
Supporting Educational Resource Tools
Learning Approaches Explained
The CARE Acronym

This 4th edition of Introduction to Nursing Informatics is designed for use with practicing nurses and students in undergraduate programmes of study. It presents the fundamental concepts of Nursing Informatics, and includes a number of contributions from leading experts who have practiced in the field of informatics over a number of years. As an ebook, the information is presented and integrated in a purposeful

---

The online version of this chapter (doi:10.1007/978-1-4471-2999-8_1) contains supplementary material, which is available to authorized users.

P. Hussey, RN, RCN, MEd, MSc, PhD (✉)
Lecturer in Health Informatics and Nursing, School of Nursing and Human Sciences, Dublin City University, Dublin, Ireland
e-mail: pamela.hussey@dcu.ie

M.A. Kennedy, RN, BScN, MN, PhD, CPHIMS-CA, PMP, PRINCE2 Practitioner
Atlantic Branch, Gevity Consulting Inc, Halifax, NS, Canada
e-mail: mkennedy@gevityinc.com

© Springer-Verlag London 2015
K.J. Hannah et al. (eds.), *Introduction to Nursing Informatics*,
Health Informatics, DOI 10.1007/978-1-4471-2999-8_1

Fig. 1.1 CARE (Connected
Health, Adminstration,
Research and Education)
diagram 1: Introduction

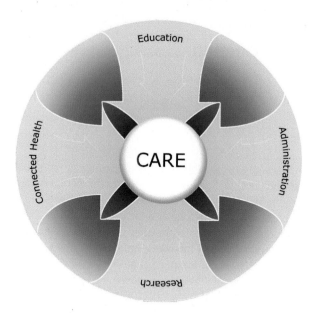

manner to encourage you to explore key concepts. We start with fundamental concepts in part one of the book, and then progress on to core concepts and practice applications in sections two through four. The content is linked with case based examples to contextualise the theory presented by authors. A content map which demonstrates the overall structure of the book is presented in Fig. 1.1 will be explained in greater detail in Chap. 2. Briefly, the word CARE is presented as an acroynm for Connected Health, Administration, Research and Education and the book is organised sections into these sub themes. Part one is included as an introductary section. A podcast discussing the overall design of this new edition is available (Audio 1.1).

Writing this fourth edition presented us with a wonderful opportunity to build on the previous established editions of an *Introduction to Nursing Informatics*. Key objectives for us were to move beyond the initial ideas within the original score. Our focus is identifying what we believe to be the contemporary issues that nurses must understand in order to achieve competency for practice within both the current and future context of healthcare. Figure 1.2 offers you an illustrative example of what has changed between this fourth edition and the last edition of An Introduction to Nursing Informatics.

It is important that you have a clear understanding of how we have approached the process of developing this new edition. Our goal is to help nursing see the relevance of Informatics and appreciate what they are learning in the context of both their own and the authors' experiences. We have therefore also included in Fig. 1.3 for an overview of the methods adopted to draft this latest edition of the text.

The associated learning activities are presented at the end of each chapter in a template and the structure of the template is explained at the end of this introductory chapter (Fig. 1.4). As an ebook, it is important that you have an opportunity to view a site map of the content in order to synthesize the material in a structured and systematic way. In each chapter, a signpost will direct you to a set of learning activities designed to assist you to meet your personal learning objectives. Drawing on years of lecturing and teaching informatics in both face to face and online programmes, we advocate this as an effective way to maximise potential learning and understanding of the topic.

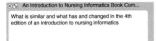

An introduction to nursing informatics book comparison

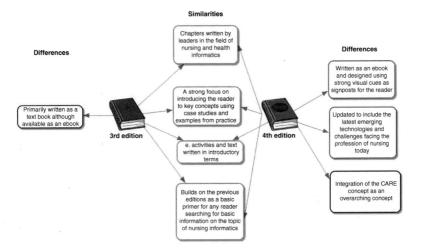

Fig. 1.2 Book comparison 3rd and 4th editions

Fig. 1.3 Approach to development of this new edition

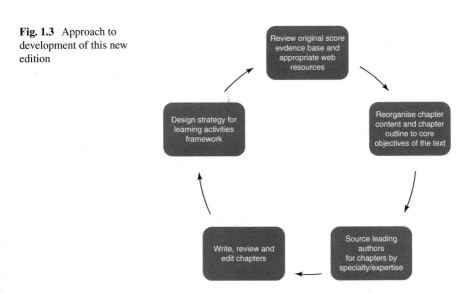

Adopting Connole's (2013) work [1], three specific activity profiles are presented to assist you to learn. The first and largest activity profile is to review the material presented in this ebook by reading, watching, accessing and thinking about the informatics material presented. This process is known as assimilative activity. The second activity is to produce, list create, construct, compose, draw or write what you read and are assimilating, this process is called a productive activity. Finally we

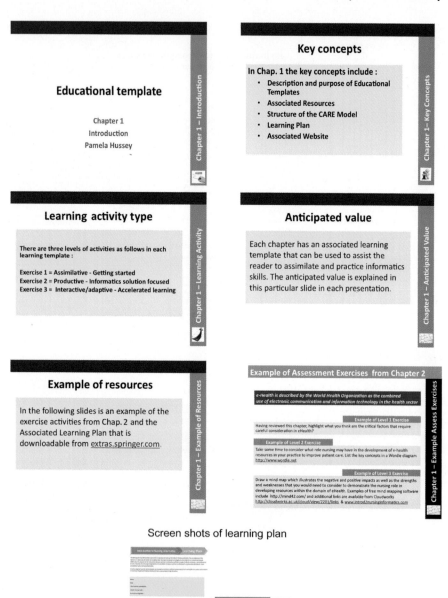

Fig. 1.4 Educational activity template

would ask you to consider completion of the assimilative and production activities by engaging with interactive or adaptive activities. Such activities involve your exploring newly acquired information by experimenting, and simulating the

Fig. 1.5 Summary diagram
of this process

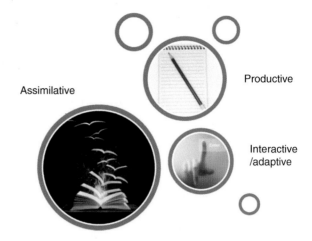

Assimilative

Productive

Interactive
/adaptive

information using design patterns with a view to you enhancing your practice. The blending of these three activities, with your practice experience in association with reading through this text offer you as a practicing nurse or informatics student, a fundamental understanding of what nursing informatics is. In this way informatics and it role can be located and understood within the profession of nursing. Figure 1.5 offers a summary diagram of this process.

Each of the learning approaches identified in Fig. 1.4 can be used by educators and trainers with different design tools to assist the student or practitioner to contextualise the material within the individual chapters. Drawing on the work of Conole in 2008 and 2013 [1, 2], specific learning activities can be used to abstract and transfer key learning material which can be cognitively processed by you and then applied to differing contexts. The following summary provides some examples of the tools that we have included within this ebook.

Summary of Learning Tools and Supporting Resources Included in This Book

Case studies are useful for developing and testing problem solving skills. They are used in this text to demonstrate a particular challenge relating to informatics within the nursing context that the student must overcome in order to achieve the desired outcome.

Rationale We have included case studies in this book to assist you to reflect on pertinent issues facing nursing today which informatics may have a direct impact on.

Design Patterns capture a recurring problem, the context in which it occurs and a possible method of solution derived from experience and backed up by theory. Design patterns often include an interactive learning pattern which is described by Conole in 2013 [1] as creating an interactive space for team work as well as interpersonal reflection. The pattern usually includes: lectures, keeping a diary, elaboration of a team project, self and or peer evaluation and summative assessment [1, p 42].

> **Rationale** Nursing as a skill based profession engages in a dual role [3] being part of a team and working independently. Design patterns will assist you to achieve key attributes for self-development on informatics tools and their overall impact upon nursing practice.

Scenarios which can offer more current and future challenges facing practitioners can be used as test cases to demonstrate the validity and utility of patterns within the informatics domain [4].

> **Rationale** Healthcare operates within a dynamic environment and the pace of progression with topical issues such as the eHealth agendas requires that the nursing profession can adopt and adapt to this changing environment. Using scenarios will assist nurses to recognise future nursing informatics requirements in their practice domain.

Visual representations such as mind maps or formalised diagrams to summarise or outline key points noted in the material reviewed.

> **Rationale** Using mind maps will assist you to generate and link core concepts assimilated in the text. The process of mind mapping may include an associated hierarchy using images lines and links as well as random associations.

Role play often linked with visual representations such as mind maps or web searches to design discuss or report on material reviewed within a chapter [4].

> **Rationale** Presents to you a learning opportunity to develop a greater awareness of the issues raised in a particular setting and can develop a more focused approach on the specific knowledge presented in a chapter. Role play demonstrates how well the learner understands the topic and provides dedicated time to apply what is learned to practice in a safe environment removed from the practice setting.

A **Reflective practitioner** exercise which encourages you to answer a question, make a judgement, or react to the material presented in the chapter. While this exercise can be completed as a stand-alone activity it is useful to complete this activity as part of a peer review exercise.

> **Rationale** The advantages of reflection in practice and on reflective practice within the profession of nursing are well documented and are recognised as a credible educational tool [5].

In addition to the learning tools in this text we have also included some support resources to accompany the text. These include a website podcasts, a glossary, and in Chap. 4 a summary PowerPoint presentation. A brief description for these supporting resources is included in the following section.

Glossary

The glossary of key terms frequently used within the domain of nursing informatics has been included. You can search the glossary independently as a resource, or alternatively click on key words within the glossary for an explanation of the terms used in this resource.

Powerpoint Presentations

The purpose of including PowerPoint presentations with some of the chapters is to offer you the key points identified in the chapter in a short summarised format.

Podcasts

In some of the chapters we have included podcasts which are available to download in MP3 format. In all instances the podcasts are short in duration.

Downloads

Available from extras.springer.com:

Educational Template (PDF 235 kb)
Educational Template (PPTX 263 kb)

Learning Plan (PDF 445 kb)
Learning Plan (DOCX 98 kb)
Audio 1.1 Podcast discussing the overall design of this new edition (MP3 1886 kb)
Glossary for Introduction to Nursing Informatics (XLSX 46 kb)

References

1. Conole G. Designing for learning in an open world, Explorations in learning sciences, instructional systems and performance technologies. 4th ed. New York: Springer; 2013.
2. Conole G. Capturing practice; the role of mediating artefacts in learning design. In: Lockyer I, Bennett S, Agostinho S, Harper B, editors. Handbook of learning designs and learning objects. Hershey: IGI Global; 2008.
3. Hovenga EJS, Kidd M, Garde S. Health informatics: an overview. 2nd ed. Amsterdam: Ios Press; 2010.
4. Mor Y, Warburton S, Winters N. Practical design principles for teaching and learning with technology: a book for sense publishers technology enhanced learning series. Available from: http://www.practicalpatternsbook.org/. Accessed 28 Feb 2013.
5. Bradbury-Jones C, Hughes SM, Murphy W, Parry L. A new way of reflecting in nursing: the Peshkin approach. Available from: http://www.ncbi.nlm.nih.gov/pubmed/19832751. J Adv Nurs. 2009;65(11):2485–93.

Chapter 2
Nursing Informatics

Margaret Ann Kennedy and Pamela Hussey

Abstract This chapter introduces the reader to the scope and practice of nursing informatics. Contextualized across the health care system from an international perspective, the authors lead readers through an exploration of information and communication technologies (ICT), concepts related to eHealth and mHealth, and emerging topics such as clinical intelligence as they inform and support professional nursing practice. An overview of nursing informatics as a specialty practice distinct from health informatics and the evolution of definitions and competencies are also presented.

Keywords Health informatics • Nursing informatics • eHealth • mHealth • Nurse role • Evidence • Information

Key Concepts
Health informatics
Nursing informatics
eHealth
mHealth
Nurse role
Evidence
Information

The online version of this chapter (doi:10.1007/978-1-4471-2999-8_2) contains supplementary material, which is available to authorized users.

M.A. Kennedy, RN, BScN, MN, PhD, CPHIMS-CA, PMP, PRINCE2 Practitioner (✉)
Atlantic Branch, Gevity Consulting Inc, Halifax, NS, Canada
e-mail: mkennedy@gevityinc.com

P. Hussey, RN, RCN, MEd, MSc, PhD
Lecturer in Health Informatics and Nursing,
School of Nursing and Human Sciences, Dublin City University, Dublin, Ireland
e-mail: pamela.hussey@dcu.ie

© Springer-Verlag London 2015
K.J. Hannah et al. (eds.), *Introduction to Nursing Informatics*,
Health Informatics, DOI 10.1007/978-1-4471-2999-8_2

Introduction

This chapter offers an introduction on the fundamental concepts in nursing informatics. By exploring the topic from differing perspectives, it provides the reader with an insight into this rapidly evolving domain. In particular, it considers the relevance of informatics for the profession of nursing, its impact on clinical practice, and how nurses in the future can contribute to the development of eHealth systems ensuring that they are fit for purpose. Topics discussed in this chapter include:

- Health informatics
- Nursing informatics
- eHealth
- mHealth
- Nurse role
- Evidence
- Information

We are in the digital age. What does this mean to us as nurses? The convergence of the telecommunications and computer industry has seen a pervasive increase in how we communicate and process information. Social network communications and sensor technologies are available for use across the age spectrum of health care [1, 2]. Information and communications technology (ICT) underpins how we now complete business transactions, educate our children and how we observe the world in which we live. In healthcare, recent advances in mobile technologies and the patient-held record see the patient as an active citizen in the management of their health. The health care process is now moving beyond standard data processing for administrative functions common to all organisations such as human resources, and financial information systems. An ever-expanding and aging population with increasing cost projections suggests that eHealth is the preferred solution and can no longer be considered as an option. In 2010 A Digital Agenda for Europe [3] was launched, as part of the 2020 EU strategy, this initiative was devised to assist digital technologies to deliver sustainable growth within Europe. In 2012 the Pan American Health Organisation launched its eHealth Strategy and Plan of Action (2012–2017) [4] to improve health services access and quality, this strategy argues the case that access to health information is a basic right for citizens, and in 2012 launched an eHealth newsletter to improve and promote co-operation amongst countries. The concept of information as a valuable commodity comparable to oil was considered at IMIA NI2012 [5]. Whether or not this is the case it is reasonable to suggest that health and health information is increasingly considered important and internationally investment in eHealth is growing. One example is the European Union Digital Agenda strategy which outlines EU policy directly relating to health [6], a second example is the EU Horizons Research Programme in ICT [7] which begins in 2014 will invest 80 Billion in ICT research between 2014 and 2020.

Fig. 2.1 The dimensions of data quality see copyright permission p.11 Source HIQA website

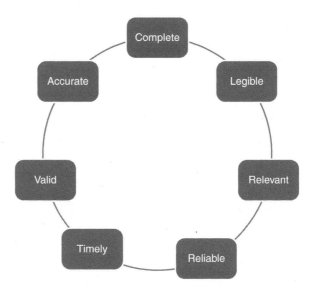

Emerging eHeath Agenda

A key driver in considering eHealth is to consider the importance of health information. Safe reliable health and social care is underpinned by access to and use of quality data. It is the cornerstone on which the health care process is built and is critical for continuing care, strategic planning and management of the services. So what are the characteristics of health information? Figure 2.1 offers one example from the Health Information and Quality Authority in Ireland who define the international dimensions of quality healthcare data.

The concepts above are defined by HIQA as follows

1. **Accurate Data** refers to how closely the data correctly captures what is was designed to capture
2. **Complete data** has all those items required to measure the intended activity or event.
3. **Legible data** is data that the intended users will find easy to read and understand.
4. **Relevant data** meets the needs of the information users
5. **Reliable data** is collected consistently over time and collects the true facts
6. **Timely data** is collected within a reasonable agreed time period after the activity that it measures and is available when it is required and as often as it is required.
7. **Valid data** is collected in accordance with any rules or definitions applicable for that type of information. These rules check for correctness and meaningfulness before the data is used [8, p. 12–18].

An emerging area topic in the area of health information management is *clinical intelligence* (CI), which is defined as the "electronic aggregation of accurate, relevant and timely clinical data into meaningful information and actionable knowledge in order to achieve optimal structures, processes, and outcomes" (Harrington [9], p. 507) Harrington compared CI to business intelligence which informs business decisions through data which is transformed to information and subsequently into knowledge. Harrington explained that CI is the same type of transformational process, with the focus on using clinical data to inform decisions. Organizations rely on CI to help them realize the value of the immense amount of data generated as a consequence of electronic health records and clinical information systems.

A key message that is consistently documented in the literature and which has a direct bearing on eHealth system implementation is that the primary data collection processes should not impose any burden on the health and social care system and should be part of the routine process of health care provision. We will return to this point in Chap. 3 on eHealth.

The collection of quality data and information for secondary use focuses very much on building evidence and demonstrating effectiveness. The international growing debate about whether the anticipated benefits and savings can be gained or indeed even measured is ongoing. One contributory factor to the success or failure directly relates to financial investments. Spending on ICT in OECD countries has been relatively small. According to the Organisation of Economic Co-operation and Development (OECD) from 1990 through to 2009, an increasing share of the gross domestic product (GDP) of OECD countries has been spent on health care provision. On average total health care spending represented just under 9 % of GDP in 2007. By 2010 this share is projected to increase to over 10 % (OECD [10], p. 28).

Examples of best practice and value for money are illustrated by the World Health Organization (WHO) Department of Data Statistics and Epidemiology. This department focuses on the generation, synthesis, analysis and use of evidence to inform their strategic planning on key goals within health and social care. For example, data is used in a cyclical process to inform research development, complete implementation programmes and then evaluate their impact with a view to informing future planning and changes in international policy. These projects include, but are not restricted to, implementation of eHealth systems to impact on the status of individual citizen's health and social well- being. All World Health Organisations Statistical Reports are available to download from here [11], Within the WHO, key drivers in strategic planning are the Millennium Development Goals (MDG) which was initially established in 2000 by the United Nations. One hundred and ninety three member states of the United Nations in association with a number of international organizations have agreed to achieve these goals by the year 2015. The eight goals are presented in Fig. 2.2.

Each goal has specific targets and dates and an informational video which tracks the progression of projects is available to view from the United Nations website here [12]. Indicators are used to evaluate the effectiveness of programmes and research in achieving the MDGs. When establishing goals, indicators are used to establish how well these goals are being met. Indicators could therefore be described as data collected for a distinct purpose. Increasingly indicators are used within the domain of healthcare as decision making tools by health care services in relation to quality of a service. The health service providers develop a series of indicators which are then measured over a specific regular time interval, for example by yearly quarter. In the United Kingdom, the National Institute for Health and Clinical

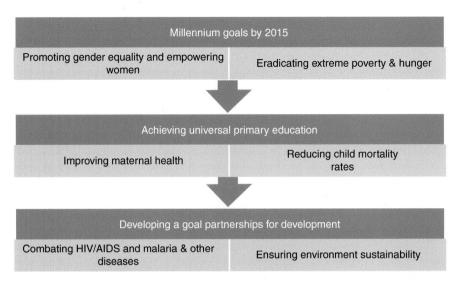

Fig. 2.2 Millennium Goals United Nations Online Resource [11]

Excellence under the Quality and Outcomes Framework have a list of indicators that can be viewed from here [13].

Nursing researchers also contribute studies to determine the nursing profession's ability to find evaluate, and use clinical evidence in their practice studies. A paper by Mills et al. [14] reported upon a cross sectional study (n = 590), which identifies five domains of influence on the nursing translation of evidence. This research, which was completed in Australia, built upon an earlier study which used a survey instrument originally developed by Gerrish et al. [15] in the United Kingdom to explore nurses' use of evidence. In the acute or secondary health service domain, modern technologies such as point of care systems, medication management systems are evaluated in terms of demonstrating effectiveness in patient outcomes [16, 17]. Likewise, in the community or primary care setting, the use of sensor technologies and the design of the smart home tailored to fit individual patient needs are also researched extensively, particularly in regard to the impact on the individual patient's health state. Such phenomena are reaching a level of maturity to indicate that they are fit for purpose [18], and increasingly multinational industries are now investing significant funds in cognitive system development with a view to transforming how organisations learn.

IBM, a multinational industry, suggests that data will grow globally at 800 % in the next 5 years and that 90 % of this data will be less than 2 years old. In their research and development department IBM is developing a cognitive system entitled *Watson* which will collect and analyse data on human behaviour. For example, how do people interact within healthcare organisations? What behaviour can be augmented to deliver evidence based responses for better patient outcomes? The Watson programme by IBM [19] is included as an exemplar and the link includes access to a short clip on how the research and development programme envisages Watson will transform Healthcare. Supporting citizens to maintain independence within their home environment by monitoring patient maintenance outcomes on health wellness indicators, such as activity, sleep and communication is also emerging as a future health informatics trend. By tailoring health promotion activities which are individualised to the patient health state, home care solutions can be more focused on maintaining independence, CASALA [20] is one example that we have opted to include in this book in Chap. 9.

The emergence of web enabled services also provides a means for viewing, reporting and presenting information from different data entry sources, for example, from clinician versus patient views. As mentioned above in the clinical intelligence discussion, policy makers, health administrators and clinicians alike can adopt more effective and efficient use of existing health resources based on the most current data available. Some examples which this data can impact include health planning-management of well-baby clinics; disease prevention; smoking cessation; staffing trends, and outcome evaluation.

Globally the role of the nurse in this digital agenda could be described as at varying stages of evolution. Nurses have always had a major communication role at the interface between the patient/client and the healthcare system. In some instances this role directly relates to information management and this approach to nursing informatics can be considered from a framework of Clinical-Administrative-Research-Education, originally identified by Ball and Hannah [21] as the CARE acronym. The notion of considering informatics from the perspective of the acronym CARE has been noted as a useful framework and a beneficial signpost for nurses engaging with informatics for the first time. Consequently, this framework is adopted in this latest edition of an Introduction to Nursing Informatics by the editors with one change- the C in care is now considered as connected health and Fig. 2.3

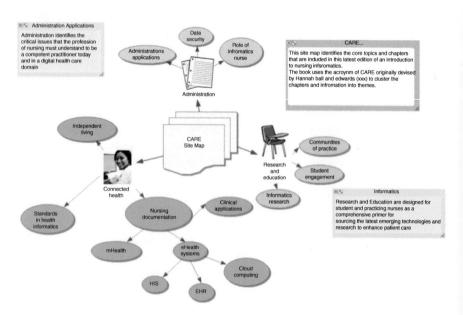

Fig. 2.3 Conceptual CARE Frame

offers a graphical representation of the CARE framework acronym which will be used in the text.

The scope of informatics is broad and in order to appreciate both the scale of the specialization and where nursing fits, it is important to first establish definitions of nursing and nursing informatics. The following section will therefore briefly summarise nursing by its definition, introduce origins and definitions of medical/health informatics and define nursing informatics.

Nursing As an Art or Science?

Virginia Henderson's [22] seminal article on the Nature of Nursing argued the case that an occupation especially a profession such as nursing that affects human life must clearly define its function. Henderson's article argued the case that attempts to identify a definition were slow to emerge and as such unfinished. In 1989, Schlotfeldt [23] described the two criteria for a profession – a social mission and a calling for examiners to assist in knowledge generation supporting practice advancement. Nursing's social mission is to "appraise and assist human beings in their quest to optimize their health status, health assets, and health potential" (Schlofedlt [23], p. 17). Nursing theory has continued to evolve and challenge the boundaries of conventional thinking. In 2010 the International Council of Nursing defined nursing as:

> Nursing encompasses autonomous and collaborative care of individuals of all ages, families, groups and communities, sick or well and in all settings. Nursing includes the promotion of health, prevention of illness, and the care of ill, disabled and dying people. Advocacy, promotion of a safe environment, research, participation in shaping health policy and in patient and health systems management, and education are also key nursing roles [24]

Earlier in 2003, a consultation report by the Royal College of Nursing in the United Kingdom defined nursing in the following manner but also stipulated six defining characteristics for the profession of nursing as follows:

> The use of clinical judgement in the provision of care to enable people to improve, maintain, or recover health, to cope with health problems, and to achieve the best possible quality of life, whatever their disease or disability, until death. Royal College of Nursing 2003 [25]

Key defining characteristics include a particular **purpose, intervention, domain and focus**, as well as a **value base** associated with a **commitment to partnership**. The full report is available to view from the Royal College of Nursing Website [25].

The implications on the above definitions of nursing on the specialty of informatics are worthy of some consideration. The ICN definition includes health systems management within its scope and RCN's defining characteristics map well on to the many roles and responsibilities that nurses engage with including but not restricted to managerial roles, as well as those activities that include both direct and indirect care interventions. It is also important to note that nursing functions include both delegated tasks and autonomous nursing activities, which all have a direct bearing on the design and use of information systems in practice. By nursing performing a dual role the focus for nursing activity can be identified both as an independent practitioner and as part of a multidisciplinary team. As nursing is one of the largest stakeholder groups in most countries engaged in direct and indirect patient care, their voice within the specialty of Health informatics needs to be a strong one.

What Is Health Informatics?

Francois Gremy of France is widely credited with coining the term *informatique medical*, which was translated into English as *medical informatics*. Early on, the term medical informatics was used to describe "those collected informational technologies which concern themselves with the patient care, medical decision making process" (Greenburg AB. Medical informatics: science or science fiction. 1975. unpublished). Another early definition, in the first issue of the *Journal of Medical Informatics*, proposed that medical informatics was "the complex processing of data by a computer to produce new kinds of information" (Anderson [26]). As our understanding of this discipline developed, Greenes and Shortliffe [27] redefined medical informatics as "the field that concerns itself with the cognitive, information processing and communication tasks of medical practice, education, and research, including the information science and the technology to support these tasks. An intrinsically interdisciplinary field . . . [with] an applied focus. . . [addressing] a number of fundamental research problems as well as planning and policy issues." Shortliffe et al. [28] also defined medical informatics as "the scientific field that deals with biomedical information, data, and knowledge—their storage, retrieval and optimal use for problem-solving and decision-making." [28]

One question consistently arose: "Does the word *medical* refer only to physicians, or does it refer to all healthcare professions?" In the first edition of this book, the premise was that *medical* referred to all healthcare professions and that a parallel definition of medical informatics might be "those collected informational technologies that concern themselves with the patient care decision-making process performed by healthcare practitioners." Thus, because nurses are healthcare practitioners who are involved in the patient care and the decision-making process that uses information captured by and extracted from the information technologies, there clearly was a place for nursing in medical informatics. Increasingly, as research was conducted and medical informatics evolved, nurses realized there was a discrete body of knowledge related to nursing and the use of informatics. During the early 1990s, other health professions began to explore the use of informatics in their disciplines. Mandil [29] coined the phrase "health informatics," which he defined as the use of information technology (including both hardware and software) in combination with information management concepts and methods to support the delivery of healthcare. Thus, health informatics has become the umbrella term encompassing medical, nursing, dental, and pharmacy informatics among others. Health informatics focuses attention on the recipient of care rather than on the discipline of the caregiver.

The term *nursing informatics* (NI) was introduced initially by Dr. Marion Ball at the 1983 International Medical Informatics Association (IMIA) Conference in Amsterdam (Hannah et al. [30]).

Nursing's Early Role in Medical Informatics

The nurse's early role in medical informatics was that of a consumer. The literature clearly shows the contributions of medical informatics to the practice of nursing and patient care (See Chap. 5).

Early developments in medical informatics and their advantages to nursing have been thoroughly documented (Hannah [31]) see also Chap. 4 of this volume). These initial developments were fragmented and generally restricted to automating existing functions or activities such as automated charting of nurses' notes, automated nursing care plans, automated patient monitoring, automated personnel time assignment, and the gathering of epidemiological and administrative statistics. Subsequently, an integrated approach to medical informatics resulted in the development and marketing of sophisticated hospital information systems that included nursing applications or modules.

As models of health services delivery have shifted toward integrated care delivery across the entire spectrum of health services, integrated information systems are developing slowly. Such enterprise systems will provide an integrated clinical record within a complex integrated healthcare organization, however for many countries such systems have yet to be realised and their core occupation is integration and management of fragmented data from across a number of silos. This is well articulated in the following quote from the OECD [10]:

> A widely recognised source of inefficiencies is the fragmentation of the care delivery process and the poor transfer of information. Health care "systems" across OECD countries are largely organised in the form of separate "silos", consisting of groups of large and small medical practices, treatment centres, hospitals, and the people and agencies that run them. At present, nothing really links these isolated structures into a system within which information is easily shared and compared [10, p. 26].

Integrated systems support evidence-based nursing practice, facilitate nurses' participation in the health care team, and document nurses' contribution to patient care outcomes. They have failed, however, to meet the challenge of providing a nationwide comprehensive, lifelong, electronic health record that integrates the information generated by all of a person's contacts with the healthcare system. Further, as Hannah et al. [30] noted, despite the escalation of technology in health care and the recognition of NI, a persistent absence of universally accepted methods for defining and coding nursing contributions to health outcomes remains, challenging the visibility of nursing contributions.

In 2010, C-HOBIC was designated as a Canadian Approved Standard (CAS) by Canada Health Infoway [32] C-HOBIC is a suite of nursing-sensitive patient outcomes and provides a mechanism to systematically record nursing contributions. C-HOBIC may be used electronically or in paper format (see Table 2.1).

By comparing C-HOBIC assessments across time, nursing contributions become evident and can be explicitly documented (Fig. 2.4). Additionally, such diagramming exposes where additional efforts are required to support patients' needs and where efforts have yielded positive results.

Table 2.1 C-HOBIC was designated as a Canadian Approved Standard (CAS) by Canada Health Infoway

Acute care and home care measures	Long-terms care and complex continuing care measures
Functional status: ADL[a] and bladder continence[a] (IADL[a] for home care)	Functional status: ADL[a] and bladder continence[a]
Symptom management: Pain[a], fatigue[a], dyspnea[a], nausea	Symptom management: Pain[a], fatigue[a], dyspnea[a], nausea
Safety outcomes : Falls[a], pressure ulcers[a]	Safety outcomes : Falls[a], pressure ulcers[a]
Therapeutic self-care	Collected on admission and quarterly/client condition changes
Collected on admission and quarterly/ client condition changes	

C-HOBIC is a suite of nursing-sensitive patient outcomes and provides a mechanism to systematically record nursing contributions. C-HOBIC may be used electronically or in paper format
[a]interRAI measures

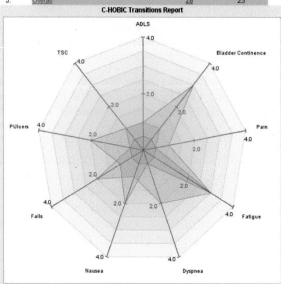

	Scale Name	Admission	Discharge
A.	ADL - Activities of Daily Living	19	11
B.	Bladder Continence	1	3
C.	Pain Scale	0	1
D.	Fatigue	3	3
E.	Dyspnea	2	0
F.	Nausea	1	2
G.	Falls	2	1
H.	Pressure Ulcers	0	2
I.	Therapeutic Self-Care (Sidani & Doran) v2	1	1
J.	Overall	28	23

C-HOBIC Transitions Report

- Discharge - Admission

Fig. 2.4 Rose diagram based on C-HOBIC assessments

Nursing Informatics: Progression of a Specialty

Nursing informatics, as originally defined (Hannah [21], p. 181) referred to the "use of information technologies in relation to those functions within the purview of nursing that are carried out by nurses when performing their duties". Today, we extend Hannah's definition to include communication or connected health. We suggest that nursing informatics relates to any use of ICT by nurses in relation to the care of patients. This includes the administration of healthcare facilities, the educational preparation of individuals to practice, and connected healthcare. Matney et al. [33] identify nurses as knowledge workers who translate data to information, information to knowledge and knowledge to wisdom. While nursing has a rich history of theoretical thinkers which explore the knowledge of nursing, some authors argue what is now required is to advance nursing knowledge to a position of practice theory. This is often articulated as a quest for a theoretical basis for the practice of the profession [34, 35]. We would argue that the contribution that informatics can make to this space is significant. Requirements within nursing include a desire to adopt, innovate and develop our informatics skills to make our contribution to the patient care process and patient outcome visible.

Figure 2.5 offers some examples of the scope of systems and agents which we consider nursing informatics would be engaged with in the primary and secondary care setting. Figures 2.6 and 2.7 offer examples of care planning and patient summary record systems used by nurses that software companies implement in the health care domain from Europe and Canada.

As the field of nursing informatics evolves, the definitions of nursing informatics have also advanced Table 2.2 presents key definitions of nursing informatics that have been considered significant to the nursing informatics agenda over the past 30 years. However in this text we support the IMIA NI definition [5] which was revised and updated in 2009 in Finland as follows:

> Nursing Informatics science and practice integrates nursing, its information and knowledge and their management with information and communication technologies to promote the health of people, families and communities world-wide IMIA NI 2009 Online Source [5]

Some of the more popular definitions are also included in Table 2.2 for discussion and consideration

While the Staggers and Thompson definition [46] built on the ANA work to propose that the goal of nursing informatics is to improve the health of populations,

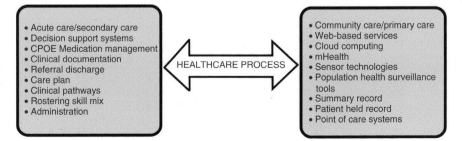

Fig. 2.5 Scope of systems used in nursing

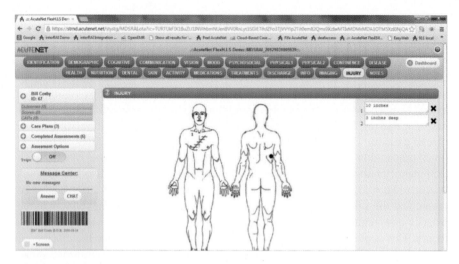

Fig. 2.6 Acute net injury assessment screen

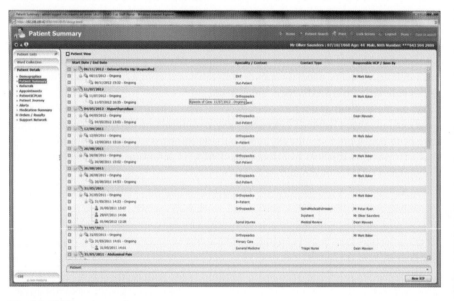

Fig. 2.7 IMS maxims patient summary

communities, families and individuals by optimizing information management and communication. This includes the use of information and communication technology in the direct provision of care, in establishing effective administrative systems, in managing and delivering educational experiences, in supporting lifelong learning, and in supporting nursing research. In 2004 a number of nurses with an interest in informatics came together and formed the TIGER (Ball et al. [47]). This acronym stands for **Technology Informatics Guiding Educational Reform** has grown in

Table 2.2 Evolution of nursing informatics definitions [5, 21, 29, 36–46]

Focus of definition	Date	Author	Definition
Information technology	1984; 1994	Ball and Hannah [21] Hannah et al. [29]	"any use of information technologies by nurses in relation to the care of their patients, the administration of health care facilities, or the educational preparation of individuals to practice the discipline is considered nursing informatics"
	1986	Saba and McCormack [36]	"systems that use computers to process nursing data into information to support all types of nursing activities"
	1989	Zeilstorff et al. [37]	Central role of technology
	1996	Saba and McCormack [38]	"use of technology and/or a computer system to collect, store, process, display, retrieve, and communicate timely data and information in and across health care facilities that administer nursing services and resources, manage the delivery of patient and nursing care, link research resources and findings to nursing practice, and apply educational resources to nursing education"
	1998	IMIA [5]	"the integration of nursing, its information, and information management with information processing and communication technology, to support the health of people world wide"
	2000	Ball et al. [39]	"all aspects of nursing—clinical practice, administration, research and education—just as computing holds the power to integrate all four aspects"
	2001	CNA [40]	"the application of computer science and information science to nursing. NI promotes the generation, management and processing of relevant data in order to use information and develop knowledge that supports nursing in all practice domains"
Conceptual	1986	Schwirian [41]	"solid foundation of nursing informatics knowledge [that] should have focus, direction, and cumulative properties"
	1989	Graves and Corcoran [42]	A combination of computer science, information science, and nursing science designed to assist in the management and processing of nursing data, information, and knowledge to support the practice of nursing and the delivery of nursing care
	1996	Turley [43]	Development of a NI model which included cognitive science, information science, and computer science

(continued)

Table 2.2 (continued)

Focus of definition	Date	Author	Definition
Role centered	1992	American Nurses Association (ANA) [44]	"specialty that integrates nursing science, computer science, and information science in identifying, collecting, processing, and managing data and information to support nursing practice, administration, education, and research and to expand nursing knowledge. The purpose of nursing informatics is to analyze information requirements; design, implement and evaluate information systems and data structures that support nursing; and identify and apply computer technologies for nursing"
	1994	ANA [45]	"specialty that integrates nursing science, computer science, and information science in identifying, collecting, processing, and managing data and information to support nursing practice, administration, education, research, and expansion of nursing knowledge. It supports the practice of all nursing specialties, in all sites and settings, whether at the basic or advanced level. The practice includes the development of applications, tools, processes, and structures that assist nurses with the management of data in taking care of patients or in supporting their practice of nursing"
	2002	Staggers and Bagley-Thompson [46]	Nursing informatics is a specialty that integrates nursing science, computer science, and information science to manage and communicate data, information, and knowledge in nursing practice. Nursing informatics facilitates the integration of data, information, and knowledge to support patients, nurses, and other providers in their decision making in all roles and settings. This support is accomplished through the use of information structures, information processes, and information technology

membership and capacity since this date and is now an internationally recognised organisation dedicated to nursing informatics education. The TIGER initiative was originally conceived by number of NI leaders including Dr Marion Ball. This innovative collaboration brings together nursing stakeholders to develop a shared vision, strategies, and specific actions for improving nursing practice, education, and the delivery of patient care through the use of health information technology. The

TIGER initiative devised 9 core topics [48] within action plan to promote nursing informatics on a global scale. These topics include but are not restricted to National Health Information Technology Agenda, Informatics competencies and leadership development.

Further information on TIGER is available from their website [48]. One major initiative that TIGER has invested time in over the past several years is their online resource. This resource will be discussed in further detail in Chap. 16.

Impact on Nursing Informatics on Nursing

Nursing informatics as a specialty practice within the nursing discipline has moved beyond merely the use of computers and increasingly reflects the impact of information and information management on the discipline of nursing. Over 10 years ago, Staggers and Thompson [46] affirmed our long-held position that nurses are "information integrators at the patient level." More recent papers by Matney Brewster, Sward, Cloynes and Staggers [33] demonstrate how the core concepts of nursing informatics data, information, knowledge and wisdom can be used as a theoretical framework to assist nurses to link theory and practice.

As the largest group of healthcare professionals, nursing has a significant role to play in the design and development of health information systems. Often labelled as knowledge workers or the glue that holds the process of health care in place, it is important that we recognise our potential and our vulnerability while considering the potential impact that nursing informatics competencies or lack of competencies may have not only on our profession but also on the clients and patients that we care for. The American Nurses Association [49] recognized nursing informatics as a nursing specialty in 2001. Hospitals and other health care organizations are now recruiting informatics nurse specialists and informatics nurse consultants to engage as part of the ICT development teams in the design and implementation of information systems. This topic will be explored further Chap. 12. According to the Irish poet W.B Yeat *Education is not the filling of a pail but the lighting of a flame* [50] In Chap. 5 we will explore how nurses can harness the potential of emerging learning technologies and Web 2.0 for use with their patients/clients and to develop their personal aptitudes to become more proficient knowledge workers. Using the CARE acronym we will discuss terms and concepts key to the advancement of nursing as a profession in this text.

Nursing Informatics Competencies

As core stakeholders in the planning, management, provision, and evaluation of patient care, nurses must adopt a proactive approach to attaining core competencies in nursing informatics. As Remus and Kennedy [51] pointed out, NI competencies are not a new requirement, noting that the American Nurses Association was one of the first nursing professional bodies to endorse NI through a formal certification program and a published NI Scope and Standards of Practice (note title case) in 2001. Numerous nursing researchers and theorists have continued to explore and build on this work, including Gonçalves et al. [52], Manos [53]; Schleyer et al. [54]; Harrington [55]; Booth [56]; Barton [57]; Staggers and Thompson [46], and Staggers et al. [58].

In 2012, the Canadian Association for Schools of Nursing published Nursing Informatics Entry to Practice competencies for Registered Nurses [59] Three competencies and specific evalaution indicators were developed within an overarching competency of "Uses information and communication technologies to support information synthesis in accordance with professional and regulatory standards in the delivery of patient/client care" (CASN [59], p. 5) (Table 2.3).

Although much of the literature speaks to basic competencies, a renewed call for NI competencies among nurse leaders is emerging. Authors including Remus and Kennedy [51], Meyer et al. [60], TIGER [48] have called for nursing leaders to develop skills in nursing informatics to support transformative leadership in nursing and healthcare.

In support of competency development, a variety of educational programs exist, ranging from university degrees, continuing education programs, and professional education initiatives such as the TIGER initiative [61].

Table 2.3 Three competencies and specific evalauton indicators were developed by the Canadian Association for Schools of Nursing within an overarching competency of "Uses information and communication technologies to support information synthesis in accordance with professional and regulatory standards in the delivery of patient/client care" (CASN [59], p. 5)

Competency	Indicators
Uses relevant information and knowledge to support the delivery of evidence-informed patient care	Performs search and critical appraisal of on-line literature and resources (e.g., scholarly articles, websites, and other appropriate resources) to support clinical judgement, and evidence-informed decision making
	Analyses, interprets, and documents pertinent nursing data and patient data using standardized nursing and other clinical terminologies (e.g., ICNP, C-HOBIC, and SNOMED- CT, etc.) to support clinical decision making and nursing practice improvements
	Assists patients and their families to access, review and evaluate information they retrieve using ICTs (i.e., current, credible, and relevant) and with leveraging ICTs to manage their health (e.g., social media sites, smart phone applications, online support groups, etc.)
	Describes the processes of data gathering, recording and retrieval, in hybrid or homogenous health records (electronic or paper), and identifies informational risks, gaps, and inconsistencies across the healthcare system
	Articulates the significance of information standards (i.e., messaging standards and standardized clinical terminologies) necessary for interoperable electronic health records across the healthcare system
	Articulates the importance of standardized nursing data to reflect nursing practice, to advance nursing knowledge, and to contribute to the value and understanding of nursing
	Critically evaluates data and information from a variety of sources (including experts, clinical applications, databases, practice guidelines, relevant websites, etc.) to inform the delivery of nursing care

(continued)

Table 2.3 (continued)

Competency	Indicators
Uses ICTs in accordance with professional and regulatory standards and workplace policies	Complies with legal and regulatory requirements, ethical standards, and organizational policies and procedures (e.g., protection of health information, privacy, and security)
	Advocates for the use of current and innovative information and communication technologies that support the delivery of safe, quality care
	Identifies and reports system process and functional issues (e.g., error messages, misdirections, device malfunctions, etc.) according to organizational policies and procedures
	Maintains effective nursing practice and patient safety during any period of system unavailability by following organizational downtime and recovery policies and procedures
	Demonstrates that professional judgement must prevail in the presence of technologies designed to support clinical assessments, interventions, and evaluation (e.g., monitoring devices, decision support tools, etc.)
	Recognizes the importance of nurses' involvement in the design, selection, implementation, and evaluation of applications and systems in health care
Uses information and communication technologies in the delivery of patient/ client care	Identifies and demonstrates appropriate use of a variety of information and communication technologies (e.g., point of care systems, EHR, EMR, capillary blood glucose, hemodynamic monitoring, telehomecare, fetal heart monitoring devices, etc.) to deliver safe nursing care to diverse populations in a variety of settings
	Uses decision support tools (e.g., clinical alerts and reminders, critical pathways, web- based clinical practice guidelines, etc.) to assist clinical judgment and safe patient care
	Uses ICTs in a manner that supports (i.e., does not interfere with) the nurse-patient relationship
	Describes the various components of health information systems (e.g., results reporting, computerized provider order entry, clinical documentation, electronic Medication Administration Records, etc.)
	Describes the various types of electronic records used across the continuum of care (e.g., EHR, EMR, PHR, etc.) and their clinical and administrative uses
	Describes the benefits of informatics to improve health systems, and the quality of interprofessional patient care

Future Implications

As ICT becomes more pervasive within our society there is a need for nursing as a profession to embrace this dynamic phenomenon and recognise it as an enabler. There is significant evidence globally to suggest that designing and implementing ICT within the healthcare domain can be not only a costly but detrimental exercise when the projects are poorly planned [62, 63]. Nurses are being held responsible and accountable for the systematic planning of holistic and humanistic nursing care for patients and their families. Nurses are also increasingly responsible for the continual review and examination of nursing practice (using innovative,

Table 2.4 Nursing must be part of future developments in ehealth systems [48] informatics with strong input regarding such decisions

What information do nurses require to make clinical judgements and decisions relating to patient care?
What information do caregivers from other health professions require from nursing?
To what extent can nursing informatics support improvements in the quality of care received by patients
How can the financial and emotional costs of care to patients be reduced using nursing informatics?
What is the impact of nursing interventions on client or patient outcomes?

continuous quality improvement approaches), as well as applying the evidence base to finding creative solutions for patient care problems and the development of new models for the delivery of nursing care. Increasingly, nurses will practice in primary care adopting eHealth solutions which include web based services for community-based programs. Key solutions include providing health promotion and early recognition of case surveillance and prevention of illness. Adopting technology enhanced learning resources, the nurse's role as patient educator will extend to virtual sessions with patients and clients. Nurse Gudrun [64] is included here as one working example of such an approach. Nurses will also learn to engage with third generation cognitive systems; researchers in Asia are now publishing development work on the android nurse which is available to view in YouTube (Super Realistic Robot Nurse [50]). This topic will be explored further in Chap. 19 in nursing informatics future trends.

Nurses still must assess, plan, carry out, and evaluate patient care, but advances in the use of information management, information processes, and communication technology will continue to create a more scientific, complex approach to the nursing care process. Nurses will require more sophisticated informatics competencies to practice in a digital society and will be better equipped by their education and preparation to have a more inquiring and investigative approach to patient care. Evidence-based nursing practice is the yardstick by which our profession will be measured. As information systems assume more routine clerical functions, nurses will have more time for direct patient care. Accordingly, nursing must be part of future developments in ehealth systems [63] informatics with strong input regarding such decisions as listed in Table 2.4.

Summary

The role of the nurse will intensify and diversify with the widespread integration of computer technology and information science into healthcare agencies and institutions. Redefinition, refinement, and modification of the practice of nursing will intensify the nurse's role in the delivery of patient care. At the same time, nurses will have greater diversity by virtue of practice opportunities in the nursing informatics field. Nursing's contributions can and will influence the evolution of healthcare informatics. Nursing will also be influenced by informatics, resulting in a better understanding of our knowledge and a closer link of that knowledge to nursing practice [43]. As a profession, nursing must anticipate the expansion and development of nursing informatics. Leadership and direction must be provided to ensure that nursing informatics expands and improves the quality of healthcare received by patients within the collaborative interdisciplinary venue of health informatics.

Downloads

Available from extras.springer.com:

Educational Template (PDF 108 kb)
Educational Template (PPTX 120 kb)

References

1. Winston E, Medlin BD, Romaniello BA. An ePatient's enduser community: the value added of social network communications. Comput Hum Behav. 2012;28:951–7.
2. Alemdar H, Ersoy C. Wireless sensor networks for healthcare: a survey. Comput Netw. 2010;54:2688–710.
3. A digital agenda for Europe. Available at: https://ec.europa.eu/digital-agenda/Accessed. 17 Nov 2012.
4. Pan American Health Organisation eHealth Strategy and Plan of Action (2012–2017). Available at: http://new.paho.org/ict4health/. Accessed 17 Nov 2012.
5. International Medical Informatics Association Nursing Interest Group (IMIA NI). Available at: http://imianews.wordpress.com/tag/imia-ni/. Accessed 17 Nov 2012.
6. European Union Digital Agenda for Europe Strategy. Available at: https://ec.europa.eu/digital-agenda/en/digital-life/health. Accessed 17 Nov 2012, Accessed 12 Nov 2012.
7. Horizons ICT Research Programme 2014–2020. Available from: https://ec.europa.eu/digital-agenda/en/information-and-communication-technologies-horizon-2020. Accessed 2 Dec 2012.
8. HIQA Data Quality. Available from: http://www.hiqa.ie/category/publication-category/health-information. Accessed 30 Nov 2012.
9. Harrington L. Clinical intelligence. J Nurs Adm. 2011;41(12):507–9.
10. Organisation of Economic Co-operative Development Improving Health Care Efficiency the role of ICT eBook 2010. Available from: http://ec.europa.eu/health/eu_world/docs/oecd_ict_en.pdf. Accessed 2 Dec 2012.
11. World Health Organisation, Global health observatory. Available from: http://www.who.int/gho/publications/world_health_statistics/en/index.html. Accessed 1 Dec 2012.
12. United Nations Millennium Goals Development. Available from: http://www.un.org/millenniumgoals/bkgd.shtml. Accessed 1 Dec 2012, Accessed 3 Dec 2012.
13. NICE Quality Outcomes and Indicators Framework. Available from: http://www.nice.org.uk/aboutnice/qof/indicators.jsp. Accessed 2 Dec 2012.
14. Mills J, Field J, Cant R. Factors affecting evidence translation for general practice nurses. Int J Nurs Pract. 2011;17:455–63.
15. Gerrish K, Ashworth P, Lacey A, et al. Factors influencing the development of evidence based practice; a research tool. J Adv Nurs. 2007;57:328–38.
16. Chaudhry B, Wang J, Wu S, Maglione M, Mojica W, Roth E, Morton SC, Shekelle PG. Systematic review: impact of health information technology on quality, efficiency, and costs of medical care. Ann Intern Med. 2006;144(10):742–52.

17. Shekelle PG, Goldzweig CL. Costs and benefits of health information technology: an updated systematic review. London: Health Foundation on behalf of the Southern California Evidence-based Practice Centre, RAND Corporation; 2009.
18. Gilman E, Davidyuk O, Su X, Reikki J. Towards interactive smart spaces. J Ambient Intell Smart Environ. 2013;5(1):5–22.
19. IBM website. Available from: http://www-03.ibm.com/innovation/us/watson/. Accessed 3 Dec 2012.
20. Centre for Affective Solutions for Ambient Living Awareness CASALA. Available from: http://www.casala.ie/. Accessed 13 Dec 2012.
21. Ball MJ, Hannah KJ. Using computers in nursing. Reston: Reston Publishing; 1984.
22. Henderson V. The nature of nursing. Am J Nurs. 1964;64(8):62–8.
23. Schlodfeldt R. Structuring nursing knowledge: a priority for creating nursing's future. In: Cody W, editor. Philosophical and theoretical perspectives for advancing nursing practice. 5th ed. Burlington: Jones and Bartlett; 1989. p. 15–21.
24. International Council of Nurses. Available from: http://www.icn.ch/. Accessed 14 Dec 2012.
25. Royal College of Nursing Defining Nursing Report Online Resource Available from: http://www.rcn.org.uk/__data/assets/pdf_file/0008/78569/001998.pdf. Accessed 3 Dec 2012.
26. Anderson J. Editorial. J Med Inform. 1976;1:1.
27. Greenes RA, Shortliffe EH. Medical informatics: an emerging academic discipline and institutional priority. J Am Med Assoc. 1990;263(8):1114–20.
28. Shortliffe EH, Perreault LE, Wiederhold G, Fagan LM, editors. Medical informatics: computer applications in healthcare and biomedicine. 2nd ed. New York: Springer; 2001. p. 21.
29. Mandil S. Health informatics: new solutions to old challenges. World health 2 (Aug/Sept):5.1989.
30. Hannah KJ, Ball M, Edwards MJA. Introduction to nursing informatics. 3rd ed. New York: Springer; 2006.
31. Hannah KJ. The computer and nursing practice. Nurs Outlook. 1976;24(9):555–8.
32. Canada Health Infoway. Canadian Health Outcomes for Better Information and Care. 2014. Available from: https://www.infoway-inforoute.ca/index.php/programs-services/standards-collaborative/pan-canadian-standards/canadian-outcomes-for-better-information-and-care-c-hobic. Accessed 21 Jan 2014.
33. Matney S, Brewster P, Sward K, Cloynes K, Staggers N. Philosophical approaches to nursing informatics data- information-knowledge-wisdom framework. Adv Nurs Sci. 2010;34(1):6–18.
34. Reed PG, Crawford Shearer NB. Nursing knowledge and theory innovation advancing the science of practice. New York: Springer; 2011.
35. McQueen DV. Critical Issues in theory for health promotion. In: McQueen DV, Kickbusch I, editors. Health an modernity the role of theory in health promotion. New York: Springer; 2007. p. 21–42.
36. Saba VK, McCormick KA. Essentials of computers for nurses. Philadelphia: Lippincott; 1986.
37. Zielstorff R, Abraham L, Werley H, Saba VK, Schwirian P. Guidelines for adopting innovations in computer-based information systems for nursing. Comput Nurs. 1989;7(5):203–8.
38. Saba VK, McCormick KA, editors. Essentials of computers for nurses. New York: McGraw-Hill; 1996.
39. Ball MJ, Hannah KJ, Newbold SK, Douglas JV, editors. Nursing informatics: where caring and technology meet. 3rd ed. New York: Springer; 2000.
40. Canadian Nurses Association. What is nursing informatics and why is it so important? Nurs Now. 2001; 11. Retrieved 10 Mar 2014 from: http://www.cna-aiic.ca/sitecore%20modules/web/~/media/cna/page%20content/pdf%20en/2013/07/26/10/53/nursinginformaticssept_2001_e.pdf#search=%22what%20is%20nursing%20informatics%20why%20is%20it%20so%20important%3f%22.
41. Schwirian P. The NI pyramid: a model for research in nursing informatics. Comput Nurs. 1986;4(3):134–6.
42. Graves JR, Corcoran S. The study of nursing informatics. Image J Nurs Sch. 1989;21:227–31.
43. Turley JP. Developing informatics as a discipline. In: Gerdin U, Tallberg M, Wainwright P, editors. Nursing informatics: the impact of nursing knowledge on healthcare informatics. Amsterdam: Ios Press; 1997. p. 69–74.

44. American Nurses Association Council on Computer Applications in Nursing. Report on the designation of nursing informatics as a nursing specialty. Congress of Nursing Practice unpublished report. Washington, DC: American Nurses Association; 1992.
45. American Nurses Association. The scope of practice for nursing informatics. Washington, DC: American Nurses Pub.; 1994.
46. Staggers N, Bagley Thompson C. The evolution of definitions for nursing informatics: a review and analysis. J Am Med Inform Assoc. 2002;9:255–61.
47. Ball M, Douglas J, Hinton Walker P. Nursing Informatics Where caring and technology meet. 4th ed. New York: Springer; 2011.
48. Technology Informatics Guiding Education Reform TIGER. Available from: http://www.tiger-summit.com/. Accessed 14 Dec 2012.
49. American Nursing Association. Scope and standards of nursing informatics practice. Washington, DC: ANA; 2001.
50. Canadian Association of Schools of Nursing. Yeats WB. Available from Brainy Quote.com. BrainyQuote.comWebsite: http://www.brainyquote.com/quotes/quotes/w/williambut101244.html. Accessed 14 Dec 2012.
51. Remus S, Kennedy MA. Innovation in transformative nursing leadership: nursing informatics competencies and roles. Can J Nurs Leadersh. 2012;25(4):14–26.
52. Goncalves L, Wolff L, Staggers N, Peres AM. "Nursing informatics competencies: an analysis of the latest research". In: Proceedings NI2012: 11th international congress on nursing informatics. Montreal; 2012. pp. 127–131. Retrieved on 8 Sept 2012 from: http://proceedings.amia.org/29tj28/29tj28/1.
53. Manos D. A New title is emerging in healthcare: the Chief Nursing Informatics Officer (CNIO)-CNIO role on the rise. HIMSS Healthc IT News MedTech Media. 2012;9(3):1, 4–5. Retrieved from: www.HealthcareITNews.com.
54. Harrington L. The role of nurse informaticists in the emerging field of clinical intelligence. In: Proceedings NI2012: 11th international congress on nursing informatics. Montreal; 2012. pp. 162–165. Retrieved from: http://proceedings.amia.org/29tjln/29tjln/1.
55. Booth RG. Educating the future eHealth professional nurse. Int J Nurs Educ Scholarsh. 2006;3(1):1–10.
56. Barton AJ. Cultivating informatics competencies in a community of practice. Nurs Adm Q. 2005;29(4):323–8.
57. Staggers N, Gassert CA, Curran C. A delphi study to determine informatics competencies for nurses at four levels of practice. Nurs Res. 2002;51(8):383–90.
58. Staggers N, Gassert CA, Curran C. Informatics competencies for nurses at four levels of practice. J Nurs Educ. 2001;40(7):303–16.
59. Canadian Association of Schools of Nursing. Nursing informatics competencies: entry to practice competencies for registered nurses. Ottawa: Canadian Association of Schools of Nursing; 2012.
60. Meyer RM, VanDeVelde-Coke S, Velji K. Leadership for health system transformation: what's needed in Canada? Brief for the Canadian Nurses Association's National Expert Commission on The Health of our Nation – the Future of Our Health System. Can J Nurs Leadersh. 2011;24(4):21–30.
61. TIGER. Evidence and informatics transforming nursing: TIGER summit summary report. 2006. Retrieved from: http://tigersummit.com/uploads/TIGER_Final_Summit_Report.pdf.
62. Greenhalgh T, Potts HWW, Wong G, Bark P, Swinglehurst D. Tensions and paradoxes in electronic patient record research: a systematic literature review using the meta-narrative method. Milbank Q. 2009;87(4):729–88.
63. Greenhalgh T, Stramer K, Bratan T, Byrne E, Russell J, Potts W. Adoption and non-adoption of a shared electronic summary in England: a mixed methods case study. Br Med J. 2010;340:c 3111.
64. Gudrun Online Resource IT in Future Health and Social Care – Nurse Gudrun's Full-Scale Lab in Blekinge Available from: http://www.youtube.com/watch?v=KYZ0ODLF46Q. Accessed 14 Dec 2012.

Part II
Connected Health

Chapter 3
E-Health a Global Priority

Pamela Hussey and Margaret Ann Kennedy

Abstract Key motivation for the effective deployment of eHealth within health and social care will be the educational resources that can guide the thinking, planning and implementation of emerging eHealth tools within society. Understanding how eHealth can integrate with existing healthcare practices is important and in this chapter, eHealth as a global priority is discussed from a number of perspectives. The International evidence base and global policy is reviewed to provoke the reader to consider eHealth from a practical perspective and the implications of eHealth on the nursing profession.

Keywords eHealth Systems • eHealth definition • National models for health care information Care flow illustration • Mobile Technology cloud computing • eHealth systems implications for nursing

Key Concepts

eHealth Systems
eHealth definition
National models for health care information – Care flow illustration
Mobile Technology cloud computing

Introduction

This chapter will introduce the reader to the topic of eHealth systems and will assist nurses to contextualise eHealth technologies within the scope of professional practice (Fig. 3.1). The subject area is a diverse and rapidly expanding one, and some of

---

The online version of this chapter (doi:10.1007/978-1-4471-2999-8_3) contains supplementary material, which is available to authorized users.

P. Hussey, RN, RCN, MEd, MSc, PhD (✉)
Lecturer in Health Informatics and Nursing, School of Nursing and Human Sciences,
Dublin City University, Dublin, Ireland
e-mail: pamela.hussey@dcu.ie

M.A. Kennedy, RN, BScN, MN, PhD, CPHIMS-CA, PMP, PRINCE2 Practitioner
Atlantic Branch, Gevity Consulting Inc, Halifax, NS, Canada
e-mail: mkennedy@gevityinc.com

© Springer-Verlag London 2015
K.J. Hannah et al. (eds.), *Introduction to Nursing Informatics*,
Health Informatics, DOI 10.1007/978-1-4471-2999-8_3

Fig. 3.1 CARE graphic 2: connected health

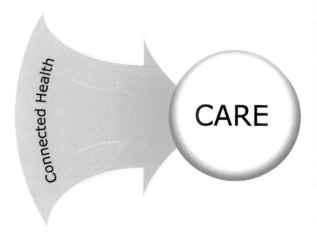

the most topical, pertinent issues from the literature base are purposefully presented to provoke the reader's consideration of eHealth systems within practice. It is also important for you to consider the direct or indirect effects eHealth systems on the individual nurse's practice in the future. As a means of background information, a number of case studies are presented which provides an overview of how nursing practice can engage in the eHealth development space, and these case studies are further elaborated upon in Chaps. 15, 16, 17 and 18. A meta- narrative analysis of eHealth systems completed in 2011 is included to offer the reader some insight into the emerging research evidence within eHealth and identifies areas that are important for the nursing profession to be aware. Such references are important for the nursing profession to engage with and contribute to for sense making of eHealth system design in the future.

Considering health as a distinct concept is useful when reviewing eHealth, as it may be argued that shifting the focus from care and onto health will have a direct impact upon how healthcare processes will be planned and delivered in the future. Ongoing changes to how health is perceived and healthcare is delivered are at different stages of advancement internationally and are attributable not only the technological revolution, but also to the increasing demand for system efficiency and productivity. Technology although a significant factor, is under debate on whether it complicates or simplifies the health care process.

In 1948 the World Health Organisation defined health as a state of complete physical, mental and social wellbeing, and not merely the absence of disease and infirmity [1]. Since 1986 at the First International Conference on Health Promotion [2], the World Health Organisation reports that health is a resource for everyday life and not just an objective for living. Important dimensions in the quality of life of individuals include a number of contributory factors not only on the physical state of citizens, but also on the state of their mental and social well-being. Health maintenance and promotion activity are increasingly perceived as enabling processes that can assist with maintaining or enhancing independence [3]. It is important for individual citizens to possess increasing control over, and maintenance of their health. Although this is a well-documented argument, 25 years after this initial WHO conference, our populations are in a state of health decline. In western society there is an increasing risk with populations being overweight or obese. An interesting study completed in Ireland (2012) revealed that over a third of direct healthcare costs are associated with individuals being overweight or obese. This all island study noted that 1.64 billion Euros was the estimated annual cost to the economy, 35 % of which was a direct healthcare cost which posed a significant threat to the individual's health state while also creating a major challenge for health service provision. The full report which was sponsored by the Health and Safe Food All Ireland Website is available to view from here [4]. For a global perspective on risk indicators and disease prevalence additional data relating smoking and obesity are available to view by country from the US Global Health Policy Site [3]. Likewise facing soaring costs in the United State, the Harvard School of Public Health cited a 2012 statistic estimating that more than $190 billion was spent in 2005 on obesity and obesity-related expenses, which reflected a doubling of previous cost estimates [5]

Some individuals debate that the general approach within health care is outdated and what is now required is to capitalise on emerging mobile technologies to strategically position the patient at the centre of their own respective health care. In 2009, globally there were 3.5 billion wireless devices in use; as these devices continue to grow in number, the Internet will increasingly serve as the interface between people moving around the world and the physical world that surrounds them [6, p. 1]. This concept is illustrated well by Victor Strecher. He outlines his innovative health promotion strategy and the associated mhealth software in a summary presentation which is available to view from here [7].

Control is acknowledged as an important factor in the eHealth debate, and one which will have a direct impact upon the scope of the profession of nursing in the future. A key message that needs to be transmitted, received and understood in eHealth systems is patient involvement. The notion of patient centeredness and "nothing about me without me" is one which is increasingly being adopted by patient advocacy groups worldwide [8].

eHealth Definition

The World Health Organisation defines eHealth as *eHealth is the use of information and communication technologies (ICT) for health.* WHO offers examples that include *treating patients, conducting research, educating the health workforce, tracking diseases and monitoring public health* [9].

The eHealth unit is located within the Department of Knowledge Management and Sharing within the WHO, and is located in the development cluster of Innovation, Information, Evidence and Research. The eHealth unit engages on a global, regional, and at a country level, promoting the update and use of information and communication technologies in health development. The centre has a number of global projects divided by regions e.g. the Region of the Americas, the Eastern Mediterranean Region, and the Western Pacific Region. The WHO eHealth website directs the viewer to some examples of their collaboration centres globally [10].

In 2005, the Fifty-eighth World Health Assembly issued WHA58.28 resolution. This resolution was based on the eHealth Report of the time, indicating that eHealth is a cost-effective and secure use of information and communications technologies [11]. This resolution urged member states to draw up long term strategic plans for developing and implementing eHealth services in areas such as health care services, health surveillance, health literature education knowledge and research. They also advocated developing the ICT infrastructure to support equitable, affordable and universal access to all citizens and partners, to reduce costs, and enable eHealth initiatives to be successful. This resolution also directed the Director General to provide support to Member States to promote the development, application and management of national standards of health information; and to collect and collate available information on standards with a view to establishing national standardized health information systems in order to facilitate easy and effective exchange of information among Member States.

Some eHealth services that have been launched since the WHA 58.28 Resolution and were previously mentioned in Chap. 1, including a Digital Agenda for Europe [12], as part of the 2020 EU strategy and the eHealth Strategy and Plan of Action (2012–2017) [13]. This strategic plan of action which was launched by the Pan American Health Organisation (PAHO) aims to improve health services access and quality [14]. In the case of both the European and the PAHO documents, the web sites argue the case that access to health information is a basic right for citizens. Because of the scale and dynamic nature of eHealth initiatives, it is difficult to establish an inclusive framework for all elements of eHealth clusters; however Table 3.1 from the PAHO eHealth Strategy (2012–2017) identifies the components to be included in eHealth. Each of these components will be expanded upon in the following sections.

Electronic Medical Records and Electronic Health Records

Globally eHealth systems such as Electronic Medical Record (EMR) or Electronic Health Record (EHR) are seen as key enablers in the organisation and delivery of health services. The benefits and motivators for EHR are well documented [15, 16] and debated [17, 18]. Despite this being the case, literature on the topic suggest that the promise of delivery can often encounter a series of false starts. Failed programmes are common and even 'successful' initiatives are plagued by delays, escalation of costs, scope creep, and technical problems [19, p. 11]. In the domain of nursing, similar evidence is emerging from both the acute sector for electronic nursing documentation [20] and from the home sector in studies evaluating medical decision support system using mHealth [21]. Tschannen et al. [22] review the impact of computerised physician order entry systems (CPOE) on nursing workflow using

Table 3.1 PAHO strategy action plan [14]

Electronic Medical Records	A real-time longitudinal electronic record of an individual patient's health information which can assist health professionals with
Electronic Health Record	decision making and treatment
Telehealth including telemedicine	The delivery of health services using ICTs, specifically where distance is a barrier to health care
mHealth including health through the use of mobile devices	A term for medical and public health practice supported by mobile devices such as mobile phones, patient monitoring devices, and other wireless devices
eLearning including distance education or learning	The use of ICTs for learning. It can be used to improve the quality of education, increase access and to make new and innovative forms of education available to more people
Continuing education in ICT	The provision of courses or programmes (not necessarily accredited) for health professionals that helps them to develop ICT skills for application in health. Includes e-publication, open access, digital literacy and the use of social networks
Standardisation and interoperability	The term "interoperability" refers to Communication between different technologies and software applications for the efficient, accurate, and sound sharing and use of data. This requires the use of standards – that is, rules, regulations, guidelines, or definitions with technical specification to make the integrated management of health systems viable at all Levels

observational analysis. Findings indicate frequent barriers to nursing workflow included systems issues (inefficient medication reconciliation processes and long order sets requiring more time to determine medication dosage), less interactions between the healthcare team, and greater use of informal communication modes being adopted. Recommendations for nursing workflow improvement in this study include medication reconciliation, order duplication, strategies to improve communication and evaluation of the impact of CPOE on practice standards [22, p. 34].

The core message is simple; the actual process of implementation of eHealth systems in the domain of healthcare is a more complex process than was originally perceived. There is still much to learn about how software implementation can have a direct bearing on nursing practice and patient care. One standardised approach to observational data measurement has been devised in New South Wales in Australia. The tool entitled Work Observation Method by Activity Time (WOMBAT) was presented in NI2012 [23]. Initial testing of WOMBAT in Canada and Australia reports that it offers a standardised tool which measures tasks completed in context by clinicians. It provides system developers key information on clinical workflow activity, and as a consequence can draw specific conclusions for future eHealth system design [23, 24]. Key factors mentioned for successful implementation include: early engagement with nurses on detailed analysis of workflow, development of careflow patterns prior to system design, development and implementations. Such practices lead to the design of clinically appropriate systems which can demonstrate realisable benefits for front line staff such as nursing. While one may argue that is not an unreasonable request, it has been identified that such practice is not always seen as a priority.

Early work by Pratt et al. [25] argues the case that those who engage at the clinical interface with electronic health records must reap appropriate rewards. Often such resources are implemented with a focus on collecting data for secondary use rather than clinical use. This in turn then leads to frustration for clinicians entering data on eHealth systems that offer no obvious contribution to the care of their patients. Similarly, when clinicians find there is a disconnect in the use of the information systems design (poorly designed systems) with their clinical working processes, they devise methods to work around the complexity of the information system [26, 27]. Briefly stated nurses adopt a strategy for working around the software misfit, in order to solve the problems that the poorly designed software fails to address [26, p. 51]. Brown and Braden emphasize that work-arounds can also be associated with unsafe practice in relation to patient safety, In order to address the issue of patient safety and work-arounds through a process of observation they identify two types of work-arounds:

1. Intuitive work-arounds which may occur instantaneously.
2. Problem solving work-arounds whereby nurses consider new approaches that they communicate with colleagues on to remedy the problem [26, p. 54].

Because of the sheer scale of debate in the literature relating to the topic of Electronic Health Records (EHR), Greenhalgh et al. in 2009 [28], undertook a systematic review of EHRs using a meta-narrative method. The purpose of this review was to gain a deeper understanding of how EHRs, and their associated study findings, are conceptualized in the literature base. Building on earlier work completed by Greenhalgh [29, 30], this review explores the key tensions emanating from the evidence base, in regard to electronic patient records, and presents a summary of their findings under seven core topics. These seven topics are summarised in Table 3.2. Greenhalgh suggests that electronic patient records require human input to contextualise knowledge and while secondary data relating to audit research and billing may be made more efficient by the electronic patient record, primary clinical work may be made less efficient. To this end, paper records may offer a unique degree of ecological flexibility, and that smaller EPR systems may sometimes be more efficient and effective than larger national or enterprise systems [28, p. 279].

Recognising the extent of research completed in the field of eHealth, Potts et al. [19] sourced 20 systematic reviews which included hundreds of primary studies and created a framework to illustrate the manner in which eHealth systems are designed and implemented.

In this review, two categories Computer Supported Co-*operative Work* and *Critical Sociology* appear to have a strong association with the nursing contribution to eHealth systems development design and implementation. They describe nursing contribution as subtle territory and hidden work and they report on nurses work as largely unpredictable, close to the patient and difficult to codify and bridging the gap between the formal and informal, the social and technical [19, p. 28].

This review document is available online to view from here. In this document, Table 8 [19, p. 157] in the appendices offers a summary overview of the philosophical basis of the different approaches to the review with associated explanations,

Table 3.2 Meta-narrative analysis by category [30, p. 749–760]

The EPR	As a container
The EPR user	As an information processor or member of socio technical network
Organisational context	The setting in which the EPR is implemented or the EPR in use
Clinical work	Decision making or situated practice
The process of change	The logic of determinism or the logic of opposition
Implementation success	Objectively defined or socially negotiated
Complexity and Scale	The bigger the better or small is beautiful

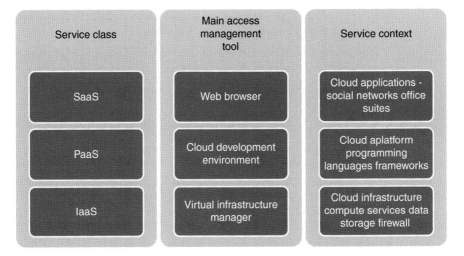

Fig 3.2 Summary of meta narrative [19]

while Table 9 [19, p. 159] gives a summary explanation of the nine meta-narratives that are identified on the development of Electronic records in organisations. Figure 3.2 is included here as a summary of the meta-narratives and the philosophical viewpoints from which the report can be considered.

Telehealth

Telehealth can be defined as the provision of personalised healthcare over a distance. It includes three distinct components; (1) the patient provides data such as video or clinical data in relation to their illness, (2) the information is transferred electronically to a second location to a healthcare professional who then, (3) uses their clinical skills and judgment to provide personalised tailored feedback to the individual [31]. There are a number of terms which are often used interchangeably when it comes to Telehealth. For example, Telemedicine is often used as an umbrella term that encompasses any medical interventions that are completed from a distance. More recently online health or eHealth are additional terms that are also used. Telehealth resources in Europe include the European Health Telematics Association [32]. Other nations also hosting centralized telehealth groups include Canada, Britain, the USA, and Australia.

Telehealth is generally considered part of an integrated home care package to assist individuals who endure chronic illness to maintain an independence lifestyle. While the benefits are considered significant, many conceptual, legal, organisational and educational challenges remain. The epSOS project is one example of flexible access to pharmacy prescriptions that can be accommodated across the European Union. The title epSOS acronym relates to European Patient using Smart Open Services. This large scale European project includes 23 countries and includes a promotional video which is available to view on the epSOS homepage the link is here [32]. In this edition Chap. 9 offers an overview of eHealth and Telemedicine capabilities. This chapter illustrates how sensor technologies are in use in the home environment and how they interface with caregivers and service providers to deliver timely interventions. Chapter 9 explores how applications are using connected television, tablets and mobile devices to assist individuals to maintain an independent lifestyle. As this is an emerging and dynamic field some studies relating to nursing are now considered.

Early work by Wotten in 2001 found that the first randomised control trial of home telenursing showed evidence of being cost effective. In this review the authors identify the use of decision support tools for video links for nurse practitioners, dealing with minor injuries as being a cost effective initiative [33]. Additional studies completed in 2011 by Hwang and Park on Nursing Informatics Competencies found that telehealth was not an area that Korean nurses competencies were high on. The analysis found that more than two thirds of the nurses surveyed considered their informatics competencies to be below average and scored lowest on competencies relating to telehealth [34, p. 173].

A systematic review published in 2012 by Tan and Lai was completed which evaluates the use of telemedicine technology to support families of new-born infants receiving intensive care. The review concluded that there was insufficient evidence to support or contest the use of telemedicine [35, p. 2]. On review of the literature for additional studies on generalised applications of nursing related eHealth projects the findings are generally positive, although it would appear additional research in designing and planning of eHealth solutions within nursing is now required [36–38].

mHealth

mHealth or mobile health refers to mobile technology and, as is the case with telehealth, the domain is one which is dynamic and emerging. mHealth is defined by the National Institute of Health as the use of mobile and wireless devices to improve health outcomes healthcare services and health research (NIH). The US Department of Health and Human Services offers a short video on what they believe mHealth is [39].

Key attributes mentioned suggest that mHealth has the potential to be an inclusive technology which can cross social boundaries and reach marginalised communities. Key areas that individuals see mHealth having a strong impact on include health promotion activities in countries particularly developing countries and underserved areas of developed countries. Furthermore, in 2010, Barra and Sazzo [40] concluded that mHealth enabled nurses engaged in the study to assess, intervene, and manage nursing care in a safe and secure manner and was noted to be practical in its application at the bedside.

Cloud Computing

It is difficult to consider mHealth without referring to cloud computing. Cloud computing is often described as an umbrella term that refers to a category of sophisticated on-demand computing services. Such services were initially offered by commercial providers such as Amazon, Microsoft or Google and the computing infrastructure is viewed as a cloud. This cloud infrastructure can be securely accessed by businesses or individuals across applications from anywhere in the world on demand [41, p. 3].

Cloud computing is defined by the National Institute of Standards and Technology in the United States as outlined in the box below.

> *A model for enabling ubiquitous, convenient, on-demand network access to a shared pool of configurable computing resources (e.g., networks, servers, storage, applications, and services) that can be rapidly provisioned and released with minimal management effort or service provider interaction.*

> *National Institute of Standards and Technology, 2011, p. 6* [41]

The general principle of cloud computing is to offer computing, storage and software as a service. The National Institute of Standards and Technology present a suite of characteristics, and deployment models on cloud computing services which are summarised in the following section.

Cloud computing can be considered to include five specific characteristics

1. *An on demand self-service;* a consumer can provide computing capabilities for example network storage as required automatically without needing human interaction with each of the service providers.
2. *Broad network access;* capabilities are available over the network and accessed through standard mechanisms for example mobile phones laptops and PDA's.

3. *Resource pooling;* the providers computing resources are pooled to serve multiple consumers using a multi-tenant model there is a sense of location independence in that the customer has no control or knowledge over the exact location of the provided resources.
4. *Rapid elasticity;* capabilities can be rapidly and elastically provisioned to quickly scale from a consumer perspective the capabilities available for provision often appear unlimited.
5. *Measured Service;* the resource of cloud systems can be monitored controlled and reported upon providing transparency for both the provider and the consumer.

As is the case with cloud computing characteristics, the National Institute of Standards and Technology identify four deployment models. A private cloud operated solely for an organisation, a community cloud which is shared by several organisations with a view to supporting a specific community. A public cloud which offers a cloud infrastructure to the general public or a large industry who is selling cloud services, a hybrid cloud which is a composition of two or more of the above cloud services [42, p. 7].

There are a number of differing layers and type of clouds in existence. Figure 3.3, which is adopted from Voorsluys et al. [41], is presented here as a summary overview. It is entitled the Cloud Computing Stack and the associated terms within this stack are explained further in the following section.

Figure 3.3 describes the different service models for cloud computing which are available. Briefly these include the notion of *cloud software as a service* (CaaS), the consumer uses applications running on a cloud server operated by the provider for example a social network like Facebook or Google Docs. The provision of a *cloud platform as a service* (PaaS), the consumer deploys on to the cloud infrastructure consumer created or acquired applications. *Cloud infrastructure as a service* (IaaS), the consumer deploys software which can include an operating system and applications. In each of the preceding service models the control and management of the software networks and operating systems is managed by the provider. As a practicing nurse, the reader may be accessing all three types of service models and it is useful to understand the distinction between the three models.

Additional information is available on Cloud computing from a recently published Canadian Government Report entitled A Canadian Best Practices Guide to Implementing Cloud services in the Canadian Public Sector. This report is available to view from here [43].

One example of a public cloud which offers a cloud infrastructure to the general public is Google. This leading industry software includes a suite of cloud based resources for individuals to use and is freely available. The suite of resources includes Google docs, GMail, and the Google You+; a recent addition to Google suite is *Google Circle* which invites users to network with friends share images and videos [44]. Some simple examples on how Cloud computing operates in Google are available to view from YouTube [45].

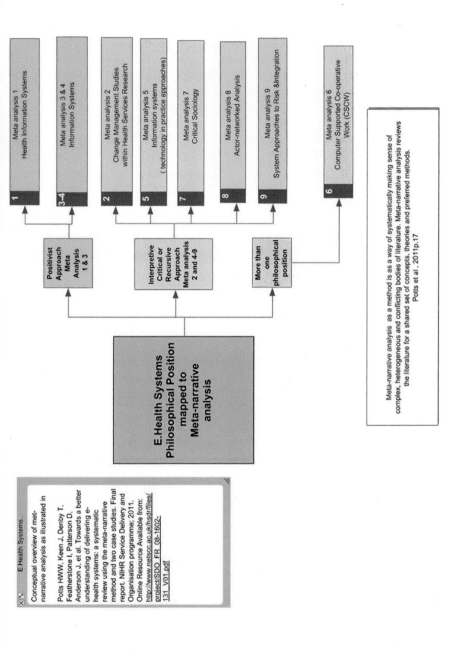

Fig. 3.3 Cloud computing Stack 1 (With permission from Voorsluys et al. [41])

eLearning and Continuing Education

The range of eLearning resources are expanding rapidly, including those which are freely available to view or download online on the World Wide Web from highly respected sources or sponsors. Coursera offers 206 online courses to 1,918443 citizens worldwide on a number of topics from computing to humanities, economics, and finance [46]. The courses are offered by leading professors and academics from universities such as Princeton [47] and Standford [48], with modules varying in duration from 4 weeks to 12 weeks, the duration varies primarily depending on the topic selected for study. Other available courses include TEDED [49] which offers 11, 398 flip classroom sessions on topics relating to science and the humanities. TED also uses videos to engage the viewer and can create lessons from "scratch" based on any video in YouTube.

Chapter 21 of this book will explore the way Communities of Practice are evolving to share knowledge and increase our understanding on a wide range of topics relating to health sciences. One of the more popular communities in this space is Cloudworks [50]. Developed with the Open University in the United Kingdom this resource offers a space for individuals to share find and discuss learning and teaching ideas and experiences.

From a health promotion perspective, using information and communications technology to increase access, and offer information to the wider community on health and health related matters is also gaining traction. For example, the Health Hub offers citizens the most up to date statistical data on core health issues in society; its introductory educational programme and suite of resources are available to view from here [51]. Likewise for nursing and nursing research, up to date statistical data by location is available from the health atlas which can found on the health well [52] and evidence based clinical guidelines are available to view from the National Institute of Clinical Excellence NICE [53].

The text boxes below include links to the more popular resources available for evidence-based research and some of the key questions identified by Greenhalgh in her book on *How to Read a Paper the basics of evidence based medicine* [54]. In most online search engines, or databases the resources will have an online tutorial. Viewing the tutorials is strongly recommended before using the resources. Searching the databases incorrectly is one of the main reasons why searches do not yield the anticipated benefits.

> - Cochrane database of systematic reviews (CDSR, http://www.thecochranelibrary.com/view/0/AboutTheCochraneLibrary.html)
> - Database of abstracts of reviews and effects (DARE, http://onlinelibrary.wiley.com/o/cochrane/cochrane_cldare_articles_fs.html)   listed   in Cochrane as other reviews includes HTA's
> - BMJ Point of Care (http://group.bmj.com/products/evidence-centre/bmj-point-of-care-1)

- Turning research into practice TRIP (http://www.tripdatabase.com/) a federated search engine
- Web of Science (http://wokinfo.com/) including science citation index and social science citation to include citation chaining
- PubMed (http://www.ncbi.nlm.nih.gov/pubmed) use the related articles function, for citation chaining
- Medline (http://www.nlm.nih.gov/bsd/pmresources.html) Centre of evidence based medicine
- Centre for Evidence Based Medicine Oxford CEBD (http://www.cebm. net/index.aspx?o=1025)

Greenhalgh, 2010, How to Read a Paper [53, p. 221–229].

From a Quantitative Perspective

1. What was the research question or hypothesis and why was the study was needed?
2. What was the research design and is it describing a primary or a secondary research study?
3. Was the research design appropriate to the research question in the study?

From a Qualitative Perspective

1. Does the paper describe an important clinical problem or does it address an issue via a clearly formulated question?
2. Was the qualitative approach used appropriately?
3. How were the subjects and the settings selected?
4. What was the researcher's perspective and has this been taken into account?
5. What methods did the researcher use for collecting data – and are they described in enough detail within the paper?
6. What methods did the researcher use to analyse the data and what quality control measures were implemented in the data analysis process?
7. Are the results credible and if so are they clinically important?
8. What conclusions are drawn and are they justified by the results presented?
9. Are the findings of the study transferable to other settings?

Greenhalgh, 2010, How to Read a Paper [53, p. 221–229].

Standardization and Interoperability

The topic of standards will be discussed in detail in Chap. 7. In Chap. 5, where the primary focus is on computer software and hardware networks in regard to communications is reviewed from a case based example to demonstrate how nursing knowledge can be created using mobile applications on medication management. Standards and interoperability play a key role in achieving this objective, and they are increasingly being seen as central to the delivery of eHealth Systems internationally [55]. There is no doubt that on review of the evidence, the process of developing and delivering eHealth system which is fit for purpose is a complex process [56]. See CIHI (Canadian Institute for Health Information) for example [56].

In Chap. 21 a case study entitled PARTNERS, reports on a nursing informatics study completed in Ireland in 2010, which explores this complex topic. The purpose of this study was to develop, with nurses, a shared assessment tool for older persons for use across and between six differing health service providers. The term PARTNERS was adopted as an acronym for *Participatory Action Research To develop Nursing Electronic Resources*. The study examined the complex process of patient referral across acute, primary and continuing care sectors as well as ongoing assessment data collection processes on individual patients over an extended time interval.

COACH, Canada's Health Informatics Association defines informatics as the "intersection between clinical, IM/IT [Information Management/Information Technology] and management practices to achieve better health" [57, p. 24]. In keeping with COACH's definition, COACH provides a variety of professional development services in Canada, including hosting the annual national eHealth conference, coordinating a variety of interprofessonal forums including telehealth, supports emerging informatics professionals through a dedicated program, conducts national industry reports, and leads the development of national guidelines and best practices in eHealth – such as Privacy and Security, and eSafety. COACH continues to support health information management in Canada by engaging clinicians and informaticians at the practicing level, the administrative level, and the executive and strategic levels.

Summary

This chapter presented a broad introduction to the topic of eHealth. It approached the topic from a number of perspectives: Electronic Medical/Health Records, Telehealth incorporating telemedicine, mobile health including the use of mobile devices, standardisation and interoperability. A number of these topics will be revisited within the following chapters in more detail as eHealth is such a broad subject the purpose of this chapter was to introduce the reader to the topic.

Downloads

Available from extras.springer.com:

Educational Template (PDF 110 kb)
Educational Template (PPTX 133 kb)

References

1. World Health Organisation Report of the Interim Commission to the First World Health Assembly: Part I: Activities. June 1948. Available from WHO Historical Collection 1948. http://www.who.int/library/collections/historical/en/index3.html. Accessed 14 Apr 2013.
2. World Health Organisation Health Promotion Global Conferences on Health Promotion. Available from: http://www.who.int/healthpromotion/conferences/previous/ottawa/en/index. html. Accessed 12 Dec 2012.
3. Perry JI, Dee A, Staines A, McVeigh T, Sweeny M. The cost of overweight and obesity on the island of Ireland Safe Food Ireland. Available from: http://www.safefood.eu/SafeFood/media/ SafeFoodLibrary/Documents/Publications/Research%20Reports/Final-Exec-Summary-The-Economic-Cost-of-Obesity.pdf. Accessed 13 Dec 2012.
4. United States Global Health Policy Statistics. Available from: http://www.globalhealthfacts. org/data/topic/map.aspx?ind=51&fmt=53&by=Data&order=a. Accessed 13 Dec 2012.
5. Harvard School of Public Health. Paying the price for those extra pounds. 2012. Available from: http://www.hsph.harvard.edu/obesity-prevention-source/obesity-consequences/economic/.
6. Raychaudhuri D, Gerla M. Emerging wireless technologies and the future of mobile internet. Los Angeles: Cambridge University Press; 2011. p. 1.
7. Victor Strecher On Purpose: Lessons in Life and Health from the Frog and the Dung Beetle Published 8 Nov 2012. 7th annual symposium on Mental Health. Available from: http://www. youtube.com/watch?v=_qCmiIQ7g3o=_qCmiIQ7g3o. Accessed 13 Dec 2012.
8. Berwick D. What patient centered should mean: confessions of an extremist health affairs. Available from: http://content.healthaffairs.org/content/28/4/w555.full. Accessed 14 Dec 2012.
9. World Health Organisation eHealth at WHO Website. Available from: http://www.who.int/ ehealth/about/en/index.html. Accessed 13 Dec 2012.
10. Regenstrief Medical Centre Indiana Network for Patient Care. Available from: http://www. regenstrief.org/medinformatics/inpc. Accessed 14 Dec 2012.
11. The Fifty Eight World Health Assembly World Health Organisation Resolution WHA 58.28. Available from: http://apps.who.int/gb/ebwha/pdf_files/WHA58-REC1/english/A58_2005_ REC1-en.pdf. Accessed 12 Apr 2013.
12. A Digital Agenda for Europe. Available at: https://ec.europa.eu/digital-agenda/Accessed. 17 Nov 2012.
13. European Health Telematics Association. Available from: http://www.ehtel.org. Accessed 14 Dec 2012.
14. Pan American Health Organisation eHealth Strategy and Plan of Action (2012–2017). Available at: http://new.paho.org/ict4health/. Accessed 17 Nov 2012.
15. Greenhalgh T, Stramer K, Bratan T, Byrne E, Russell J, Potts W. Adoption and non-adoption of a shared electronic summary in England: a mixed methods case study. Br Med J. 2010;340:c 3111.
16. Gunson J, Chawngthu L. Health economics and informatics: the gap-fit of current healthcare and parse practice. Nurs Sci Q. 2012;25(2):176–81.

17. Chunn VM. Characteristics associated with electronic health records adoption: practitioner application. J Healthc Manag. 2011;56(3):197–8.
18. Miller RH, West CE. The value of electronic health records in community health centers: policy implications. Health Aff. 2007;26(1):206–14.
19. Potts HWW, Keen J, Denby T, Featherstone I, Patterson D, Anderson J, et al. Towards a better understanding of delivering e-health systems: a systematic review using the meta-narrative method and two case studies. Final report. NIHR Service Delivery and Organisation programme; 2011. http://discovery.ucl.ac.uk/1305749/.
20. Kelley TF, Brandon DH, Docherty SL. Electronic nursing documentation as a strategy to improve quality of patient care. J Nurs Scholarsh. 2011;2011(43):154–62. doi:10.1111/j.1547-5069.2011.01397.x.
21. Johansson PE, Petersson GI, Nilsson GC. Personal digital assistant with a barcode reader-A medical decision support system for nurses in home care. Int J Med Inform. 2010;79(4):232–42.
22. Tschannen D, Talsma A, Reinemeyer N, Belt C, Schoville R. Nursing medication administration and workflow using computerized physician order entry. Comput Inform Nurs. 2011;29(7):401–10.
23. Westbrook JI, Creswick NJ, Duffield C, Li L, Dunsmuir WTM. Changes in nurses work associated with computerised information systems: opportunities for international comparative studies using the revised Work Observation Method By Activity Timing (Wombat) NI 2012 International Congress on Nursing Informatics Montreal Canada June. pp. 459–451.
24. Ballerman M, Shaw N, Mayes D, Gibney R, Westbrook J. Validation of the Work Observational Method By Activity Timing (WOMBAT) method of conducting time –motion observations in critical care setting: an observational study. BMC Med Inform Decis Mak. 2011;11:32. doi:10.1186/1472-6947-11-32.
25. Pratt W, Reddy MC, McDonald DW, Tarczy-Hornoch P, Gennari JH. Incorporating ideas from computer-supported cooperative work. J Biomed Inform. 2004;37(2):128–37.
26. Brown J, Braden C. Definition and relational specification of work-around International Congress on Nursing Informatics Montreal Canada. Montreal Canada; 23–26 June 2012.
27. Debono D, Greenfield D, Black D, Braithwaite J. Workarounds: straddling or widening gaps in the safe delivery of healthcare? Australian Institute of Health Innovation. Presented at The Seventh Biennial Conference in Organisational Behaviour in Health Care. Birmingham, 11–14 Apr 2011.
28. Greenhalgh T, Potts HWW, Wong G, Bark P, Swinglehurst D. Tensions and paradoxes in electronic patient record research: a systematic literature review using the meta-narrative method. Milbank Q. 2009;87(4):729–88.
29. Greenhalgh T, Robert G, Macfarlane F, Bate P, Kyriakidou O. Diffusion of innovations in service organizations: systematic review and recommendations. Milbank Q. 2004;82(4):581–629.
30. Greenhalgh T, Robert G, Macfarlane F, Bate P, Kyriakidou O, Peacock R. Storylines of research in diffusion of innovation: a meta-narrative approach to systematic review. Soc Sci Med. 2005;61(2):417–30.
31. McLean S, Protti D, Sheikh A. Telehealthcare for long term conditions. Br Med J. 2011;342. doi: http://dx.doi.org/10.1136/bmj.d120(Published.
32. European Patient Smart Open Services EpSOS. Available from: http://www.epsos.eu/. Accessed 14 Dec 2012.
33. Wootton R. Recent advances: telemedicine. Br Med J. 2001;323:557–60.
34. Hwang J, Park H. Factors associated with nurses' informatics competency… Reprinted from Hwang J-I, Park H-A. Factors associated with nurses' informatics competency. Cin Comput Inform Nurs. 2011;29(4):256–62. CIN: Computers, Informatics, Nursing, 29(10), pp.TC169-75.
35. Tan K, Lai NM. Telemedicine for the support of parents of high-risk newborn infants. Cochrane Database of Syst Rev. 2012;(6):CD006818. doi: 10.1002/14651858.CD006818.pub2.
36. Mougiakakou S, Kyriacou E, Perakis K, Papadopoulos H, Androulidakis A, Konnis G, Tranfaglia R, Pecchia L, Bracale U, Pattichis C, Koutsouris D. A feasibility study for the

provision of electronic healthcare tools and services in areas of Greece, Cyprus and Italy. Biomed Eng Online. 2011;10:49.
37. Nijland N, van Gemert-Pijnen JEWC, Kelders SM, Brandenburg BJ, Seydel ER. Factors influencing the use of a web-based application for supporting the self-care of patients with type 2 diabetes: a longitudinal study. J Med Internet Res. 2011;13(3):e71.
38. Gustafson D, Wise M, Bhattacharya A, Pulvermacher A, Shanovich K, Phillips B, Lehman E, Chinchilli V, Hawkins R, Kim J. The effects of combining web-based eHealth with telephone nurse case management for pediatric asthma control: a randomized controlled trial. J Med Internet Res. 2012;14(4):41–59.
39. Federal mHealth Co-ordination Team US Department of Health and Human Services Video Report What is mHealth. Available from: http://www.hrsa.gov/healthit/mhealth.html. Accessed 14 Dec 2012.
40. Barra D, Dal Sasso G. Mobile bedside technology: computerized nursing processes in intensive care unit from ICNP 1.0 [Portuguese]. Texto Contexto Enferm [serial online]. 2010;19(1):54–63.
41. Voorsluys W, Broberg J, Buyya R. Introduction to cloud computing. In: Buyya R, Broberg J, Goscinski A, editors. Cloud computing principles and paradigms. Hoboken: Wiley; 2011.
42. Mell P, Grance T. The National institute science technology definition of cloud computing recommendations of the National Institute of Standards and Technology Special Publication 800–145 (Draft). Available from: http://predeveloper.att.com/home/learn/enablingtechnologies/The_NIST_Definition_of_Cloud_Computing.pdf. Accessed 28 Nov 2012.
43. Canadian Cloud Information Cloud Best Practices Network The Canadian Government Cloud Computing Best Practice. Available from: http://canadacloud.files.wordpress.com/2012/01/govcloudcanada.pdfAccessed. 14 Dec 2012.
44. Breckenridge S. What is Google Docs 5th April 2011. Available from YouTube on: http://www.youtube.com/watch?v=EXrNfcbYnIc. Accessed 14 Dec 2012.
45. Epipheo Studios What is Google Chrome OS 18th November 2009. Available from YouTube on: http://www.youtube.com/watch?v=0QRO3gKj3qw. Accessed 13 Dec 2012.
46. Coursera Corporate Coursera Catalogue. Available from: https://www.coursera.org/. Accessed 13 Nov 2012.
47. Princeton University Coursera. Available from: https://www.coursera.org/#princeton. Accessed 13 Nov 2012.
48. Standford University Coursera. Available from: http://online.stanford.edu/courses. Accessed 15 Nov 2012.
49. Technology Entertainment Design TED. TEDED Available from: http://ed.ted.com/. Accessed 2 Nov 2012.
50. Cloudworks. Available from: http://cloudworks.ac.uk/. Accessed 2 Sep 2012.
51. The Health Hub. Available from: https://www.healthatlasireland.ie/. Accessed 3 Oct 2012.
52. The Institute of Public Health Well. Available from: http://www.thehealthwell.info/search-results/health-atlas. Accessed 14 Oct 2012.
53. National Institute of Health and Clinical Excellence NHS. Available from: http://www.nice.org.uk/. Accessed 30 Sep 2012.
54. Greenhalgh T. How to read a paper – the basics of evidence based medicine. 4th ed. London: Wiley Blackwell BMJ Books; 2010.
55. Nelson R. Major theories supporting health care informatics. In: Englebardt S, Nelson R, editors. Health care informatics: an interdisciplinary approach. St. Louis: Mosby; 2002. p. 3–27.
56. Canadian Institute for Health Information (CIHI). http://www.cihi.ca/CIHI-ext-portal/internet/EN/subtheme/standards+and+data+submission/standards/cihi010688.
57. COACH. Canada's Health Informatics Association. http://www.coachorg.com.

Additional Reading

58. Electronic Healthcare Records Systems, Int J Microgr Opt Technol. 2008;26(6):2–5.
59. Gasser L. The integration of computing and routine work. ACM Trans Office Inform Syst. 1986;4:257–70.
60. Greenhalgh T, Stramer K, Bratan T, Byrne E, Russell J, Potts W. Adoption and non-adoption of a shared electronic summary in England: a mixed methods case study. Br Med J. 2010;340:c3111.
61. Halbesleben JR, Wakefield DS, Wakefield BJ. Work-arounds in health care settings: literature review and research agenda. Health Care Manage Rev. 2008;33:2–12.
62. Kenneth T, Ming LN. 2012. Telemedicine for the support of parents of high-risk newborn infants. Cochrane Database Syst Rev. 13;6:CD006818. Available from: http://www.pubfacts.com/author/Kenneth+Tan. Accessed 13 Jun 2012.
63. Mell P, Grance T. The NIST definition of cloud computing recommendations of the National Institute of Standards and Technology Special Publication 800–145 (Draft). Available from: http://predeveloper.att.com/home/learn/enablingtechnologies/The_NIST_Definition_of_Cloud_Computing.pdf. Accessed 28 Nov 2012.
64. Raychaudhuri D, Gerla M. Emerging wireless technologies and the future of mobile internet. Los Angeles: Cambridge University Press; 2011.
65. World Health Organisation (WHO). WHA58.28 Resolution on ehealth. 2005. http://www.who.int/healthacademy/media/WHA58-28-en.pdf.

Chapter 4
History of Computing and Technology

Pamela Hussey, Margaret Ann Kennedy, and Anne Spencer

> *To understand a science it is necessary to know its history.*
> *Auguste Comte 1798–1857 Positive Philosophy*

Abstract Chapter 4 discusses early work in the development of both computers and technology. It presents the pioneers of nursing informatics describing some of the projects that they have engaged with over the past 50 years. History of Computing and Technology also includes a presentation linking to additional reference material depicting key milestones on the history of computing from 1939 to 1994.

Keywords Historical Milestones in Technology • Historical Milestones in Computing • Nursing pioneers and computer use

Key Concepts

Historical Milestones in Technology
Historical Milestones in Computing
Nursing pioneers and computer use

Introduction

Described in the early literature as a primary vehicle of communication, and forming the core of modern information technology, the digital computer is recognised by the electronic engineering community as the most important technology

---

The online version of this chapter (doi:10.1007/978-1-4471-2999-8_4) contains supplementary material, which is available to authorized users.

P. Hussey, RN, RCN, MEd, MSc, PhD
Lecturer in Health Informatics and Nursing, School of Nursing and Human Sciences,
Dublin City University, Dublin, Ireland
e-mail: pamela.hussey@dcu.ie

M.A. Kennedy, RN, BScN, MN, PhD, CPHIMS-CA, PMP, PRINCE2 Practitioner (✉)
Atlantic Branch, Gevity Consulting Inc, Halifax, NS, Canada
e-mail: mkennedy@gevityinc.com

A. Spencer, BA (Hons), MSc
Partners in Education Teaching and Learning (PETAL), Dublin, Ireland
e-mail: aspencer@petal.ie

© Springer-Verlag London 2015
K.J. Hannah et al. (eds.), *Introduction to Nursing Informatics*,
Health Informatics, DOI 10.1007/978-1-4471-2999-8_4

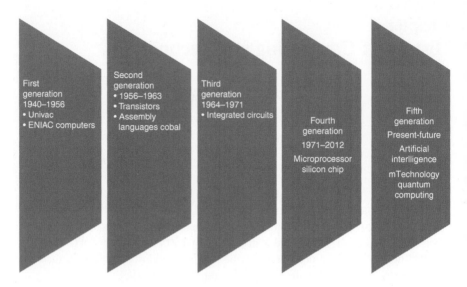

Fig. 4.1 Summary of generation computing historical timeline [3]

invented in the second half of the twentieth century [1, p. 113, 2]. Since the 1950s, the computer has replaced traditional methods of counting and record keeping, offering industry practical alternatives for handling information such as data processing. This chapter summarises the early work on the development of technology that contributes to the history of computing. It includes a review of the associated theories, which over the passage of time have culminated in to the history of informatics, subsequently emerging as the foundation or corner stone for modern culture in society today. This chapter also recognises the pioneers who participated in the development of the informatics domain. It summarises some of the key projects and programmes to which nurses contributed over the years. It demonstrates the journey from initial conception of how nurses engaged with technology to more recent times where nursing informatics has emerged as an independent specialist area.

Computing can be classified into five generations of development with each generation characterised by major technical developments that changed the way computers operated in society [3]. In this chapter we will review the early generations of computing and technology, and present a timeline of the progression of computer and technology development as illustrated in Fig. 4.1. The five generations of computing timeline date from the 1940s through to the present day. It illustrates the five generations and locates society currently at various levels of advancement between generations four and five of the figure. The progression from one generation to another is characterized by the way in which computers have been integrated in society.

Examples of recent advances from fourth to fifth generation computing as applied within the health domain are discussed in Chap. 3 in eHealth and in

Chap. 9 where the authors discuss mobile computing, telehealth and independent living.

Tracing and reviewing some of the more significant events over time which have had a direct impact on the computing industry and, as a consequence, on the development of nursing informatics is summarised in the following section. The topic is extensive and challenging to summarise in its entirety. We have therefore opted to include some online resources to support various sections where appropriate and selected what we believe to be the significant milestones for the reader to view, which is available for download (Presentation 4.1).

A clear historical vantage point is presented from which to view informatics, and the impact that it has on the nursing profession. Readers are encouraged to view the following links which graphically demonstrate some of the major paradigm shifts that have occurred in the computing industry. The first resource is the Times Photos [4] which has some excellent images that illustrate the computers in a short presentation from 1946 to the present time. The second resource is the The Computer History Museum [5] which explores the timeline of computing history from 1939 to 1994, in a comprehensive manner, and is available to browse both by year and by category. These online resources also summarise generations one to three of the computing paradigm on computing devices. What follows in the proceeding sections are some of the key milestones which have been summarised.

Historical Milestones of Computing

The Computer Society divides the history of computer development into three periods which they estimate were approximately 20 years in duration. There were: the formative years dating from 1946 to the mid-60s; the growth period from the mid-60s to the late 80s prior to the internet becoming a main communication distribution network, and the most recent 20 years with the coming of the age of the Internet [2].

Historical Milestones in Nursing

There are many perspectives about how nursing groups related to informatics have been initiated, grown over time and progressed through various stages of evolution to a state of maturity and performance.

One early but influential pioneer within the profession of nursing was Florence Nightingale. She considered information a key resource for the management of health and argued the case for standardized clinical records. She sought to source information so that more detailed analysis on patient outcomes could be achieved in the longer term. Her frustration at the time (1863) is conveyed below [6, p. 175].

There is a growing conviction that in all hospitals, even those which are best conducted, there is a great and unnecessary waste of life....In attempting to arrive at the truth, I have applied everywhere for information, but in scarcely an instance have I been able to find hospital records fit for any purpose or comparison. If they could be obtained, they would enable us to decide many other questions besides the ones that eluded to ....If wisely used, these improved statistics would tell us more of the relative value of particular operations and modes of treatment than we have any means of obtaining at present. They would enable us, besides, to ascertain the influence of the hospital...... upon the general course of operations and diseases passing through its wards; and the truth thus ascertained would enable us to save life and suffering, and to improve the treatment and management of the sick....

Florence Nightingale 1863 Notes on Hospitals cited in Longman and Green 1863, p. 175–6 [6]

While the vision for information and communication technology was yet to be realised, it is evident from her quote that a key requirement for safe, effective practice was reliable data. She articulated a need for data which could be analysed statistically in order to improve the health care processes at the time. The data that she did collect she also mapped to graphical representations of care. Sadly this need persists even today as the evidence base demonstrates the ongoing debate within modern nursing research on how nursing can best record their specific contribution to the healthcare process and patient outcome. This was addressed in Chap. 2.

Application of the Tuckman model of group development to the historical evolution of nursing informatics offers us an example to view the transformation of process and concept, and refinement of both self-image and impact beyond the immediate group of nursing informatics as an advocate to the entire profession of nursing. This notion was initially introduced and discussed in Chap. 2. Table 4.1 maps Tuchman's Group Formation Framework [7] to Scholes et al. historical timeline [8].

The papers submitted to conferences over this time were analysed and presented by trend to reflect the scientific and site attractions at the conference from the seventies through to the nineties. For the 1981 conference, the Medical Informatics European Conference (MIE) received an increasing volume of papers on language classification and retrieval, with over 34 % of the papers relating to this topic. Likewise, other large trends at MIE in 1991 related to Decision Making and Artificial Intelligence (AI). However the IMIA-NI congresses which began in 1982 also had some interesting trends and Fig. 4.2 is offered as a summary of the most popular categories with a timeline.

Table 4.1 Tuckman & Scholes et al. mapping to stages of group development [8]

Stage of development linkage to NI	Description
Forming	This is the initial stage of team or group development, characterized by members trying to find common ground and interests in pursuit of a shared goal. Meetings tend to be specifically goal directed and members act on an independent basis. Team members start to get acquainted and develop relationships that will support later stages of the group evolution
Nursing submissions to informatics conferences were limited, small numbers of contributions to the Medinfo Conferences in 1974 (5 papers) and in 1977 (2 papers). MIE conference 1978 (3 papers)	
Storming	Increased clarity emerges during this second phase about the topics to be addressed by the group. Different ideas will be promoted by group members and this is where the storming occurs as options are debated and decisions are made. Group members need increasing clarity on the group roles, accountabilities, and leadership and may develop bylaws of Terms of Reference
Example 1980s MIE	
Papers demonstrating interests in nursing related activity particularly in regard to nursing contribution to information systems and databases. MIE nursing papers submitted in 1984 (13 papers), Medinfo Conference 1983 (387 papers). Nursing informatics as a speciality identified by Marion Ball 1983	
Norming	This phase is where the group comes to a consensus on their overall goal and works toward a plan of action. Options for group activities are identified and members can work effectively independently, interdependently or in groups. Bylaws or Terms of Reference would be actively used effectively to guide group functions and relationships. Some members may have to abandon their own ideas in favor of the group's priority in order to enable the team function in a coherent and cohesive manner
Example IMIA-NI Special interest group formalised 1990s	
Development of Nursing Language Classification and Retrieval e.g. Minimum Datasets Development e.g. Health Information: Nursing Components (Canadian Nursing Minimum Dataset)	
Nursing Interventions Classification 1992	
MIE nursing papers 1996 (125 papers) Medinfo 1995 (318 papers)	
Performing	Not every team will reach this level of development. This stage is characterized by a well-defined and motivated group being able to function as a coordinated system to accomplish approved objectives. Consensus is not always unanimous and disagreement can be effectively used to support the growth of the group. If major changes occur within the group, it is possible for the group to return to earlier stages such as storming and norming
National groups developed to lobby and integrate into existing national organisations such as ISO TC 215 and CEN TC 251. Nursing informaticians contributing to the development of health informatics standards internationally. Nursing categorical structure for representing nursing diagnosis and nursing actions in terminological system developed internationally ISO 18104	
Adjourning	In this stage, the goal has been accomplished and the group no longer needs to exist or the group is shut down by an eternal mechanism. The group can complete and archive files, adjourn and disband. Occasionally, the group will identify a new goal that infuses new life into the group and hey will continue on
As nursing informatics is still an evolving specialist area, this phase within Tuckman's model is not applicable	

Fig. 4.2 IMIA congress
submissions [8, p. 88]

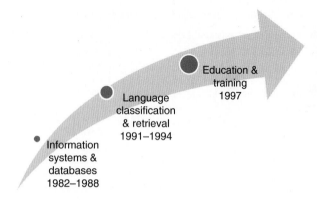

The Emergence Technology in Healthcare

For decades, healthcare has lagged behind a broad range of sectors, including government and industry, in the evaluation and adoption of technology. A variety of factors contributed to this delay in adoption. One reason was that first- and second-generation computers were not well suited for the complexity of data processing needs of hospitals.

When focusing on the use of computers in healthcare, computers traditionally gained entry through the accounting area, where most hospital computer systems still have their roots. Patient care was noted to require continuous and instantaneous response in contrast to the fiscal methodology where timing is less critical. To achieve successful utilization of computers in healthcare, both needs must be addressed. The evolution of technology itself can be viewed in Fig. 4.3 with associated links. This figure illustrates the steady progression of innovation in technology, with the notable acceleration in the 1970s. Nursing and health care have been able to capitalize on this acceleration of technology to support professional practice and improved patient outcomes. Figure 4.3 and Audio 1.1 present the evolution of technology in general, with the progression of technology in healthcare highlighted on the lower axis.

From the millennium onwards, the evolution of technology continued to progress at a rapid pace resulting in cheaper, more powerful, smaller and efficient computers. These developments led to the computers and devices that are in use in society today and they are explored further in Chap. 3.

Within the domain of health informatics the Gartner Group illustrated in 2003 the stages of the EHR lifecycle in terms of capability and integration. This work was adapted by Nagle and Catford in 2008, who linked the evolutionary model to reflect the migration from foundational systems such as infrastructure and imaging to interactive systems such as clinical documentation and order entry [9, p. 85]. This generational lifecycle is illustrated in Fig. 4.4.

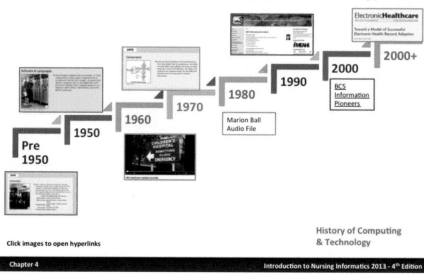

Fig. 4.3   Timeline highlights in technological evolution and adoption 1 [4–10]

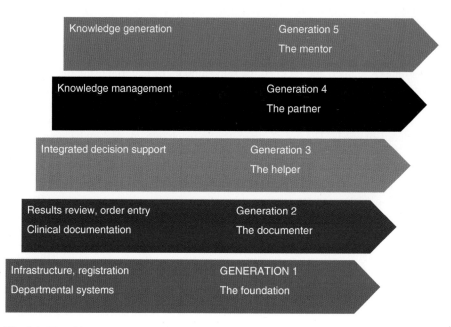

Fig. 4.4   EHR lifecycle [9]

Nursing Pioneers and Computer Use

Dating back to the 1960s, the nursing contribution to early developments in health informatics is evident in the literature of the time. Nursing contributions extended across a wide variety of areas such as nursing records, measurement of care, patient monitoring, nurse education and computer assisted learning [10].

Who were these nurses that pioneered nursing informatics? In what capacity were they involved in informatics programmes? They suggested that nurses who engaged in informatics developments of the time often joined physician-led projects, often held less academic and more applied education than their co-workers, and that they varied in age and experience from senior nurse managers and teachers to newly qualified nurses [8, p. 9].

In the sections on Nursing Education, Nursing Administration, Nursing Care and Nursing Research, we will introduce some of champions of the time and note that in many instances the nurses were poorly paid, had inadequate study leave, and in many cases left the profession of nursing to pursue careers as systems analysts or to join software companies as part of a technical support team. These sections are also supported by a presentation, which is available for download (Presentation 4.1).

Nursing Education

The seminal work in the use of computers in nursing education was conducted by Maryann Drost Bitzer. During the early 1960s, Bitzer wrote a simulation program that was used to teach obstetric nursing. It was the first simulation exercise in nursing and one of the first in the healthcare field. Bitzer's 1963 master's thesis found that students learned and retained the same amount of material using the computer simulation in one-third the time it would take using the classic lecture method [11]. During the 1970s many individual nursing faculties, schools, and units developed and evaluated computer-assisted instruction (CAI) lessons to meet specific institutional student needs. The use of computers to teach nursing content became a focal point of informatics activity in nursing education. Judith Ronald of the School of Nursing, State University of New York at Buffalo developed courseware that served as a model and inspiration for courses which were developed later in other faculties. Preparation of nurses to use informatics in nursing practice was also emerging as important. During the 1980s, leaders at other Schools of Nursing that co-ordinated nursing informatics courses included Diane Skiba at Boston College, Virginia Saba at Georgetown University, and Christine Henney of the University of Dundee.

Nursing Administration

A number of nursing administration initiatives were implemented in the 1970s and 1980s. Marilyn Plomann of the Hospital Research and Educational Trust (an affiliate of the American Hospital Association) in Chicago was actively involved for many years in the design, development, and demonstration of a planning, budgeting, and control system (PB CS) for use by hospital managers. In the late 1970s the Journal of Nursing Administration also began to feature a monthly column on computer applications in nursing [11].

In Glasgow (Scotland), Catherine Cunningham was actively involved in the development of nurse-manpower planning projects on microcomputers. Similarly, Elly Pluyter-Wenting (from 1976 to 1983 in Leiden, Holland), Christine Henney (from 1974 to 1983 in Dundee, Scotland), Phyllis Giovanetti (from 1978 to present, Professor Emerita, Edmonton, Canada), and Elizabeth Butler (from 1973 to 1983 in London, England) have been instrumental in developing and implementing nurse scheduling and staffing systems for hospitals in their areas.

In the public health area of nursing practice, Virginia Saba (formerly nurse consultant to the Division of Nursing, Bureau of Health Manpower, Health Resources Administration, Public Health Service, Department of Health and Human Services) was instrumental in promoting the use of management information systems for public health nursing services. The objective of all these projects has been to use computers to provide management information to help in decision-making by nurse administrators.

Nursing Care

Much research on the development of computer applications for use in patient care was conducted during the 1960s. Projects were designed to provide justification for the initial costs of automation and to show improved patient care. Hospital administrators became aware of the possibilities of automating healthcare activities other than business office procedures. Equipment became more refined and sophisticated. Healthcare professionals began to develop patient care applications, and the manufacturers recognized the sales potential in the healthcare market. Nurse pioneers who have contributed to the use of computers in patient care activities have been active on both sides of the Atlantic. Some of the key individuals are listed in Table 4.2.

As presented in Table 4.2, nurses recognized the potential for improving nursing practice and the quality of patient care through nursing informatics. These applications facilitate charting, care planning, patient monitoring, interdepartmental scheduling, and communication with the hospital's other computers. The informatics nursing role has since expanded. In more recent times, nurses have formed computer and nursing informatics interest groups (see Appendix 1) to provide a forum through which information about computers and information systems is communicated worldwide.

Nursing Research

Early nursing research addressed key questions of nursing knowledge representation and decision support. A key obstacle at the time was the absence of a definition and model of nursing data and information in a standardised computable format [12, p. 200].

Table 4.2 Summary of nursing pioneers 1967–1982

Maureen Scholes	United Kingdom CNO 1967	The London Hospital Real-Time Computer Project
Elizabeth Butler	United Kingdom KingsHospital London 1970–1973	Engaged in developing and implementing the computerized nursing care plan system for the Professional Medical Unit
Christine Henney	Scotland Ninewells Hospital 1974	Design and implementation of a real-time nursing system
James Crooks		
Carol Ostrowski	United States Medical Center	The development of Problem Oriented Medical Information System (PROMIS)
Donna Gane McNeill	Hospital of Vermont 1969–1979	Carol Ostrowski served as director of audit for the PROMIS system
Margo Cook	United States El Camino Hospital California 1970	Cook as nursing implementation co-ordinator on the team developed and implemented the Medical Information System
Joy Brown	Canada York Central Hospital Ontario 1982	Brown and Wright, as systems coordinators were actively involved in designing, coding, and implementing the computerized patient care system
Marjorie Wright		
Harriet Werley	USA 1960–1983	From the 1960s onwards worked with the American Nurses Association on communication and decision making in nursing. Developed NMDS 1983 with Norma Lang
Marion Ball	USA 1983	Identified Nursing informatics as a specialist area in 1983 Founder of the TIGER Initiative
Kathryn Hannah	Canada 1983	Defined nursing informatics in 1983
		Established IMIA-NI initial meeting in IMIA Tokyo. 1980 health Informatics Advisor, Canadian Nurses Association 2005 to present, Executive Lead, C-HOBIC 2007-present
June Clark & Norma Lang	USA & Wales 1992	On nursing language *If we cannot name it, we cannot control it finance it research it or put it into public policy,* Leading author ICNP ®, ICN

Scholes et al. [8] completed an analysis of the early scientific papers submitted to conferences from 1960s to 1997 and present a comprehensive overview of the material by grouping under a number of themes illustrated in Fig. 4.5.

Communicating Nursing Developments

Kathryn Hannah, of the University of Calgary, was the first nurse elected to the Board of Directors of the Canadian Organization for the Advancement of Computers in Health (COACH). In that capacity, with the assistance of David Shires of Dalhousie University (and at that time program chairman for the International

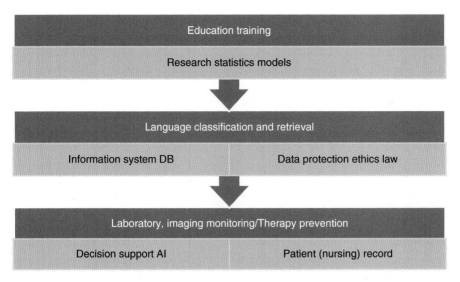

Fig. 4.5 Summary categories of classification (Adapted from Scholes Tallberg et al. [8, p. 89]

Medical Informatics Association, IMIA), Hannah was instrumental in establishing the first separate nursing section at an International Medical Informatics Association (IMIA) meeting, (Medinfo'80, Tokyo). Previously, nursing presentations at this international conference had been integrated within other sections. In 1982, based on the success of this Tokyo workshop, which Hannah also chaired, a contingent of British nurses led by Maureen Scholes mounted an International Open Forum and Working Conference on "The Impact of Computers on Nursing." The international symposium on the impact of computers on nursing was convened in London, England, in the fall of 1982, followed immediately by an IMIA-sponsored working conference.

One outcome of the working conference was a book that documented the developments related to nursing uses of computers from their beginning until 1982. The second outcome was a consensus that nurses needed a structure within an international organization to promote future regular international exchanges of ideas related to the use of computers in nursing and healthcare. Consequently, in the spring of 1983, a proposal to establish a permanent nursing working group (Group 8) was approved by the General Assembly of IMIA. In August 1983, the inaugural meeting of the IMIA Working Group on Nursing Informatics (Group 8) was held in Amsterdam. In 1992, the working group recommended a change of bylaws and began its transformation to a nursing informatics society within the IMIA. This society continues the organization of a biennial symposia for exchange of ideas about nursing informatics, dissemination of new ideas about nursing informatics through its publications, provision of leadership in the development of nursing informatics internationally, and promotion of awareness and education of nurses about nursing informatics.

In the United States in 1981, Virginia Saba was instrumental in establishing a nursing presence at the Symposium on Computer Applications in Medical Care (SCAMC). This annual symposium, although not a professional organization, provided opportunities for nurses in the United States to share their experiences. In 1982 the American Association for Medical Systems and Informatics (AAMSI) established a Nursing Professional Specialty Group. This group, which was chaired by Carol Ostrowski, provided the benefits of a national professional organization as a focal point for discussion, exchange of ideas, and leadership for nurses involved in the use of computers. Subsequently, AAMSI merged with SCAMC to become the American Medical Informatics Association (AMIA). This organization continues to have a highly active nursing professional specialty group.

Summary

Despite their wide utilization, computers are historically young and did not come into prominence until 1944 when the IBM-Harvard project called Mark I was completed. Reviewing the recent history of computing and technology the developments are presented as five generations with each generation being characterized by a major technological development [3]. During the 1950s, computers entered the healthcare professions. They were primarily used for the purposes of tabulating patient charges, calculating payrolls, controlling inventory, and analyzing medical statistics. Simultaneously, advances in the uses of computers in educational environments were initiated during the 1960s. The major focus during this decade was on showing the efficacy of computers as teaching methods. Subsequent refinement of computer technology, development of the silicon chip in 1976, development of the Internet, and the World Wide Web have made personal computers ubiquitous both in health care and society at large.

A few farsighted individuals throughout the decades, including Werley, Saba, Ball, Hannah, and Lang, recognized and pioneered the possibilities of automating selected nursing activities and records. However, little action was taken because of the inflexibility and slowness of the equipment, the general disinterest of the manufacturers in the healthcare market, and the lack of knowledge concerning such equipment among hospital management, hospital administrators, and nursing management.

During the 1970s, many projects were designed to compare student learning via computer with learning via traditional teaching methods, and the personal microcomputer emerged. Major contributions by nurses to developments leading to the use of computers in nursing were also discussed but many nurses have provided leadership both in terms of knowledge generation and application to nursing informatics. The future demands that computer technology be integrated into the clinical practice environment, education, and research domains of the nursing profession. One key principle is evident over the historical time line, the ultimate goal has always been to provide the best possible care for the patient.

Downloads

Available from extras.springer.com:

Educational Template (PDF 7160 kb)
Educational Template (PPTX 3625 kb)
Audio 4.1 Marion Ball: Naming Nursing Informatics as Specialist Area. (MP3 6801 kb)
Presentation 4.1 History of computing and technology (PPTX 3527 kb)

References

1. Mahoney M. The history of computing in the history of technology. Ann Hist Comput. 1988;
   10:113–25.
2. King WK, Land SK. A historical perspective of the IEEE computer society six decades of
   growth with the technology it represents IEEE computer society. Kobe, Japan. 2009.
3. Webopedia The Five Generations of Computers. Available from: http://www.webopedia.com/
   DidYouKnow/Hardware_Software/2002/FiveGenerations.asp. Accessed 20 Mar 2013.
4. Time Magazine A Brief History of the Computer. Available from: http://www.time.com/time/
   photogallery/0,29307,1956593,00.html. Accessed 21 Nov 2012.
5. The Computer History Museum 2006 Timeline of Computer History. Available from:
   http://www.computerhistory.org/timeline/. Accessed 22 Nov 2012.
6. Nightingale F. N Notes on hospitals. 3rd ed. Enlarged and rewritten. London: Longman Green,
   Longman, Roberts, and Green, 1863, pp. 175–6.
7. Tuckmans Stages of Group Development 1953. Available from: http://en.wikipedia.org/wiki/
   Tuckman's_stages_of_group_development. Accessed 13 Dec 2012.
8. Scholes M. Tallberg M. Pluyter-Wenting E. International nursing informatics: a history of the
   first forty years 1960–2000 British Computer Society. Swinford. 2000
9. Nagle LM, Catford P. Electronic healthcare towards a model of successful electronic health
   record adoption. Healthc Q. 2008;11(3):2.
10. Collen MF. A history of medical informatics in the United States 1950–1990. Washington,
    DC: American Medical Informatics Association; 1995. p. 242–51. ISBN 0-9647743-0-5.
11. Bitzer MD. Self-directed inquiry in clinical nursing instruction by Means ofPLATO Simulated
    Laboratory. Report R-184, Co-ordinated Science Laboratory. Urbana: University of Illinois; 1963.
12. Ozbolt JG, Saba VK. A brief history of nursing informatics in the United States of America.
    Nurs Outlook. 2008;56:199–205.

Chapter 5
The Mechanics of Computing

Christopher Henry, Pamela Hussey, and Margaret Ann Kennedy

*We don't know where we get our ideas from. What we do know
is that we do not get them from our laptops .... John Cleese*

Abstract In this short chapter an overview of technology currently in use in health care is discussed. Both hardware and software are explained offering the reader a high level summary of critical components used in conventional computing. Comparisons between computer functionality and human activity such as riding a bike or driving on a motorway are described. Cloud computing is introduced and the example of how mobile technology applications on medication management can be used is illustrated.

Keywords Hardware • Software • ICT • Cloud computing • Architecture

Key Concepts
Hardware
Software
ICT
Cloud Computing
Mobile Applications

The online version of this chapter (doi:10.1007/978-1-4471-2999-8_5) contains supplementary material, which is available to authorized users.

C. Henry (✉)
Digital Media Engineer, Dublin, Ireland
e-mail: chrispathenry@gmail.com

P. Hussey, RN, RCN, MEd, MSc, PhD
Lecturer in Health Informatics and Nursing, School of Nursing and Human Sciences,
Dublin City University, Dublin, Ireland
e-mail: pamela.hussey@dcu.ie

M.A. Kennedy, RN, BScN, MN, PhD, CPHIMS-CA, PMP, PRINCE2 Practitioner
Atlantic Branch, Gevity Consulting Inc, Halifax, NS, Canada
e-mail: mkennedy@gevityinc.com

© Springer-Verlag London 2015
K.J. Hannah et al. (eds.), *Introduction to Nursing Informatics*,
Health Informatics, DOI 10.1007/978-1-4471-2999-8_5

Introduction

Society is increasingly technologically knowledgeable and yet increasingly dependent. Rather than relying on information committed to memory, our brains "outsource" information to repositories accessed through smart phones and computers. Consider how many phone numbers people memorize compared to a number of years ago? The availability and power of technology impacts our behavior; it influences how we write, read, and what we choose to remember. As a healthcare professional, it is crucial to have an appreciation of the latest technologies and a basic understanding of how they operate. This understanding is needed as technological breakthroughs are constantly being uncovered in the pursuit of improved patient outcomes, and to improve the care delivery process for clinicians.

This chapter presents an overview of some of the latest technologies that exist today and provides a brief explanation as to how they operate. It also offers some insight into the emerging paradigm in communications technology mTechnology and offers one example of how mobile applications can be used in healthcare.

This chapter will focus on the fundamentals of computing technologies and will offer some examples on how computing technologies operate in society today. It will also explore some of the more recent technologies and explains how they can support eHealth solutions to assist health care professionals and individual patients in their daily practice and lives.

What Is a "Computer"

The vast array of twenty-first century technological advances have made it difficult to use the term "computer" to convey the conventional desktop or laptop models. Today, computers exist in almost every part of day-to-day life, from the fuel management system in a car, the program selection unit in a washing machine, the digital temperature control gauge in a refrigerator, to a Smartphone. In this sense, technology and computers are considered ubiquitous, since they are a part of everyday life activities, and so common that the majority of people no longer consider them to be out of the ordinary.

Despite the many different appearances and occurrences of computers, they are all composed of two elements – hardware and software. The hardware of a computer can be defined as being the physical components that create the computer and the software can be defined as being the stored set of instructions that allow computers to do what they do. While the overall complexity of computers today may initially seem daunting, it is important to remember that every computer is based on Boolean logic. The term Boolean relates to mathematical algebra and can be associated with variable values. Simply stated Boolean values offer a true and false variable often denoted as either 1 or 0 (on or off) in the field of computer science. This simple true/false or on/off logic, forms the platform upon which all computer functionality is built. In order to achieve this Boolean functionality, computer manufacturers use electronic components called Transistors.

A transistor can be described as being a semi-conductor device, which essentially amplifies and switches electronic signals and power. Transistors build upon the differentiation between off and on Boolean logic to create complex processes that integrate together to achieve the final communications and processing tool, that is the end-users computer.

Hardware

Hardware consists of the physical elements of a computer. Essentially, hardware can be defined as being the physical computer itself. A conventional computer model's hardware would consist of a Central Processing Unit (CPU), a monitor, a mouse and a keyboard. These components are the "seen" elements of a computer. The term hardware also covers the unseen or internal elements of a computer such as the computer's motherboard, ram, graphics card, harddrive. Table 5.1 lists some hardware components and briefly explains their function.

Random Access Memory (RAM)

The term, memory, in computing has a lot of confusion surrounding it. People often automatically equate memory with storage, which although technically correct, uses the word memory out of context. Memory, as part of a computer's specifications, does not relate solely to the amount of storage capacity a computer has. Memory on a computer is not about how many movies, songs or photos it can hold.

Table 5.1 Components of computer hardware

Component	Description
Monitor	Computers screen, used for viewing output from a computer
Mouse	Input device used to obtain motion based input from the user
Trackpad	Similar to a mouse but obtains data directly from users touch
Keyboard	Input device used to obtain static predefined symbol input
CPU (Central Processing Unit)	Processes tasks given to it by the computers operating system (explained later)
RAM (Random Access Memory)	RAM is used as temporary storage space for task data that is being processed
ROM (Read Only Memory)	ROM is a type of computer memory used mainly to store core computing software
Hard Drive	Is used to store data that will persist after the computer has powered off
Graphics Card	Used to compute the image values to be displayed on a graphical output
Bus	A network architecture in which a set of clients are connected via a shared communications structure in the single cable called a bus
Cache	A collection of data duplicating original values stored elsewhere on a computer
Persistent data	Information that continues to be stored even after power is no longer applied to it

Fig. 5.1 RAM functionality

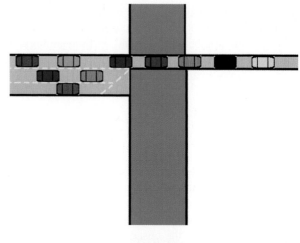

Fig. 5.2 RAM functionality

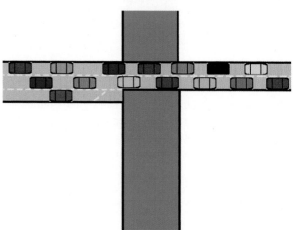

Computers require a minimum amount of "memory" or working capacity in order to process information and execute the various programs in use. Thus, the term memory relates both to how much storage memory (See section on ROM below) and also how much random access memory (RAM) a computer has available to engage in processing information.

RAM can be thought of as the platform on which tasks are processed by the machines processor. The processing unit runs the program by fetching the instructions from RAM evaluating the programs in sequence and executing them. In a way, it can be compared to a bridge on a highway where cars are tasks, the motorway's speed limit is the processor's speed and the lanes on the motorway are the processor's speed capability. When traffic converges onto the bridge, if the bridge doesn't have enough lanes or capacity to deal with the amount of cars (tasks) that the highway is capable of processing then there is going to be a traffic jam. This process is demonstrated in Figs. 5.1 and 5.2.

Adding another lane (RAM memory bank) to the bridge will significantly increase the amount of traffic crossing the river. The processor speed still has a major contribution to the overall processing of tasks. There is no point in having a four-lane bridge on a small highway that has a speed limit of 30 km/h as most of these lanes would be left idle.

ROM (Read Only Memory)

When discussing RAM, we considered real-time processing of tasks and how RAM integrates into a computer. The downfall of RAM is that its memory is not persistent through a cut-off of power. As RAM is only capable of storing memory when power is supplied to it, another type of memory is also needed to create a conventional computer. As it would be very inefficient to constantly apply power to the computer to store information that is infrequently accessed and not likely to be modified. Persistent data is needed in computing to store the start-up instructions of a computer, i.e. "boot" the computer. ROM differs from RAM in that its stored data persists even after power is no longer applied to it. Thus, ROM is ideal for use as the computer's booting memory. ROM is also the type of memory used in hard-drives to store data such as movies, music and documents. The higher the ROM capacity, the greater is the storage capability available in a computer.

Operating Systems (OS)

The computer's operating system is the fundamental set of instructions that drives the operation of the computer. It manages all of the computer's hardware and ties it to the computers software. Technically speaking, the computer's operating system is software, but it is the main software that interprets all other software.

There are two main types of Personal Computer (PC) operating systems. These are Win and Unix systems. These types of systems are the basis for the Windows and Macintosh (Mac) operating systems, with the Windows operating system being developed by Microsoft and the Mac operating system being developed by Apple.

As illustrated in the diagram below, the operating system for a computer can be interpreted as sitting between the hardware and application software for a computer (Fig. 5.3).

The Apple or "Mac" overall layout, functionality and file structure is different to that of a conventional windows (Microsoft) personal computer. This is not because of the hardware that is used in producing the different machines; it is because of the operating system that they are using.

The operating system in an Apple Mac uses different system architecture than a traditional windows machine and therefore, has different capabilities and ways of doing things. In order to get a better understanding of a computer's hardware specification, Table 5.2 outlines some perspective, relative to computing technology in 2013.

Fig. 5.3 An overview of basic computing architecture

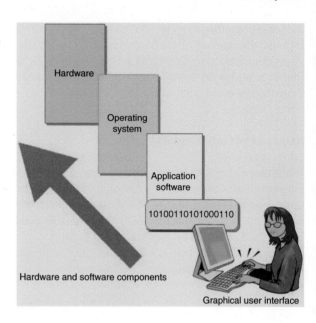

Table 5.2 Computer components specification

Specification detail	Low	Medium	High
Processor	1 GHz	2.0 GHz	3 GHz
Memory	500 MB	4 GB	16 GB
Hard Drive	128 GB	750 GB	2 TB
Graphics Video Card	Graphics cards vary depending make and model. In order to get a better understanding of a particular model, searching through reviews will provide some great insight		
Sound Card	Sound card quality tends to be consistent through computer manufacturers. Like graphics cards, it would be best to find reviews online		
Disk Drive	Disk Drive specifications on average are very similar for most computers. The only distinction between most would be different capabilities such as the ability to burn DVD's		
Screen	Screen specifications have a lot of different contributing factors. These include screen size, resolution capabilities and display technology i.e. LCD, HD		

LCD Liquid-crystal-display, *HD* High definition, *GB* gigabyte, *TB* Terabyte, *GHz* gigahertz, *MB* megabyte, *DVD* digital video disk

Networks

The topic of networks is a broad and comprehensive subject that has changed dramatically over the past 10 years as we move from third to fourth generation computing. Briefly, a network is comprised of two or more nodes that can transfer data between each other. These nodes can be classified as any entity capable of

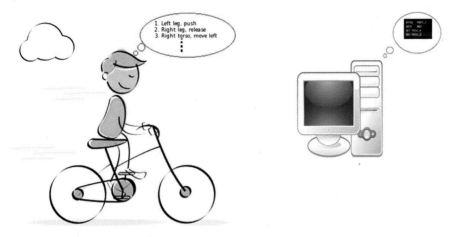

Fig. 5.4 Computer functionality

interpreting the data that it receives. In computing terms, the node will mainly refer to some form of computational device. The computational device can refer to a large spectrum of entities. On a large scale, it can refer to a server but if we reduce our spectrum, we can technically define a computer itself as being a network.

Computers are comprised of multiple pieces of hardware communicating with each other through internal networks managed by the computer's operating system. This concept of sharing data between small components to create a computer can be expanded to sharing data between computers to create a larger network such as an in-office emailing system or chat network. This concept of communication gave rise to what we know today as the Internet. The Internet is not a physical entity, it's a term used to describe the global exchange of data between computers and servers worldwide. This exchange of data is most commonly facilitated by a network protocol known as Hyper Text Transfer Protocol (http). Additional detail relating to networks can be sourced from the www3 Schools resource [1].

Software

Computer software can be defined as the stored procedures that control the internal workings of a computer. The role of software can be illustrated in the example of riding a bicycle (Fig. 5.4). In order for a person to ride a bike, their brain has a set of instructions to make the overall process possible. The rider's brain has a stored set of instructions to keep their legs peddling while maintaining balance with their overall body positioning and movement. This is exactly what software is: in order to run a program (a game for example) on a computer, the computer has a stored set of instructions to display images on the screen and to compute the physics required to make the game realistic.

Emerging Technologies for eHealth Solutions

As computing advances towards fifth generation computing, services such as cloud computing and services orientated architecture come to the forefront. The Software Section briefly outlines some of the elements that are required to deliver the fifth generation computing paradigm.

Service Orientated Architecture (SOA) and Web Services

Service oriented architecture (SOA) can be described as a dynamic framework, which establishes a set of protocols to deliver integrated services across different health care providers.

The framework comprises of a set of methods for specifying and standardizing services, and includes dynamic model for detailing interactions between and among these services. SOA emerged from the progression of delivering web-based services to advance integration and access of health data across and between service providers. Briefly, web services can glue together applications running on different messaging platforms and enable information from one application to be used by others. Web services software has grown to include a rich set of specifications and standards to facilitate interoperability across and between services. These include the ability to describe, compose, package, and transport messages and ensure that security in service access is accomplished [2]. Clinicians will see SOA in action when clinical records using information from diverse sources (laboratory, radiology, primary care providers, hospital information systems, etc.) can be viewed with a single sign on an integrated record of health information.

Despite the rapid progression of web services within the business and financial industry, its growth within the healthcare industry has been slower than in other service industries. A key reason for this directly relates to the limited uptake of health informatics standards in the healthcare industry. In addition healthcare information is considered to be sensitive data, therefore for successful implementation of shared or integrated records a robust security and data privacy platform from which healthcare service professionals can access and transfer patient records is essential. This topic will be discussed in detail in Chap. 11.

Cloud Computing

Demand for persistent and accessible data storage has contributed to the genesis of virtual storage platforms. The technologies which focus on the delivery of a virtual system, such as cloud computing aim to facilitate access to large amounts of computing power by aggregating resources and offering a single system view to the user. This view is however usually at a cost, and is based on a business model for the "on demand" delivery of computing power [3, p. 3].

The utility service for cloud computing includes the processing of information, the storage of information and the associated data and software resource requirements [4]. As a relatively new phenomenon a number of definitions exist on what cloud computing is. A short definition by Buyya is included in the box below and additional information on cloud computing is available to view in Chap. 3 [5].

> *Cloud is a parallel and distributed computing system consisting of a collection of inter-connected and virtualized computers that are dynamically provisioned and presented as one or more unified computing resources based on a service level agreement (SLA) established through negotiation between the service and consumers* [5]

Wireless Technologies and the Mobile Internet

Wireless technologies are a means of transferring data from one entity to another without the use of a cable or wire. This means of communication typically relies on radio waves with specific frequencies [6]. The mobile internet is a term used to describe internet access using Smartphones or other mobile technologies. The most common type of this communication today is known as mobile broadband, which relies on encrypted radio waves resonating at high frequencies. The progression of fifth generation technologies in society is having a direct impact on not only how we communicate, but also how we observe the physical space in which we live. By combining the power of cloud computing, search engines, and databases, individuals will have immediate access to information using mobile technology anytime and anywhere [7, p. 10].

Within the domain of healthcare, mobile technology and sensors are considered significant tools for future healthcare provision, enabling remote monitoring and improved access to health information for both clinicians and consumers. Chapter 3 describes case examples of how these technologies are being used in healthcare.

Due the low cost of deployment associated with wireless devices, wireless networks will continue to be an attractive option for connecting to the Internet of the future. Such new perspectives also present a number of challenges.

As wireless networks become more integrated into the design of future eHealth systems, questions arise as to how secure the network infrastructures can or will be. Traditional healthcare systems that functioned in isolation will not be able to provide wider access for mobile and eHealth resources and new security protocols will need to considered [8, p. 242]. This topic is explored further from a health care perspective in Chap. 9.

A Mobile Application Within Health Care

One simple example of technology in health care is the case of medication management [9]. This is particularly relevant for elderly patients who may rely on their memory, or the use of weekly pillbox storage devices to abide by their medication schedule. Often such approaches are not totally reliable or dependable, as memory deterioration can impede upon the ability to adhere to medication schedules [10].

A practical example is to use Smartphone applications with embedded alarm systems that include functionality for scheduling medications as prescribed. The mobile application (app) can remind elderly people of the time and description of the medication that they will need to take.

The Medication Manager Project Android application illustrated in Fig. 5.5 offers some assistance to patients with their medication management regime. This Android application provides key functionality for community health nurses to take a photo of the medication for the elderly person, provide a description on specific instructions on self-administration, potential diet restrictions, as well as an explanation of purpose of the drug and its potential for drug interactions. It is facilitates

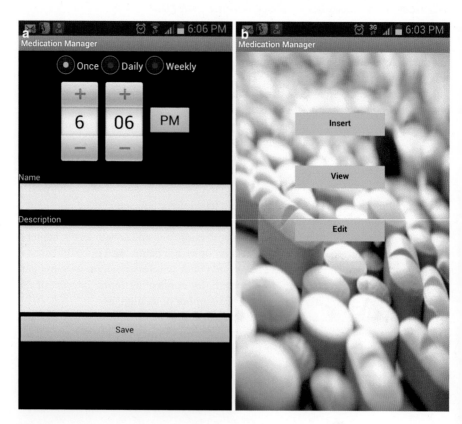

Fig. 5.5 (**a, b**) Examples of android application

scheduling of time, frequency for drug administration and prompts the user to take their medication as scheduled. The Medication Manager Project also facilitates an alarm and text messaging service so that if the medication schedule or dosage has changed, it can alert the appropriate parties to update their records accordingly.

Conclusion

This chapter presented the basic components of computers for current computing, while exploring some of the emerging technologies of fifth generation computing [11]. We have considered how technology is changing our behaviour. The pace of development in ICT over the past 30 years has been rapid and as we currently exist in a digital world, it is difficult to estimate just how mtechnology will impact on future healthcare provision. Current mTechnology such as android phones offer a resource for outsourcing information and designing new ways to read and write. Chapter 9 will revisit fifth generation computing and introduce the latest developments within ICT that health care has to offer. This chapter concludes on a cautionary note with a short clip by John Cleese on creativity [12] which relates to the opening quote. Outsourcing some of our memory to smart phones and laptops should leave time for reflection; create a space for creativity, and the development of some smart ideas to enhance individual care. It would appear that in many instances this is not the case as the short clip demonstrates. A core function of nursing informatics may then be to create time to consider just how technologies can be harnessed to offer additional time to enhance care.

Downloads

Available from extras.springer.com:

Educational Template (PDF 4179 kb)
Educational Template (PPTX 1665 kb)

References

1. WWW3 Schools. Available from: http://www.w3schools.com/. Accessed 12 Mar 2013.
2. Kreger H. Fulfilling the Web services promise. Commun ACM. 2003;46(6):29.
3. Voorsluys W, Broberg J, Buyya R. Introduction to cloud computing. In: Buyya R, Broberg J, Goscinski A, editors. Cloud computing principles and paradigms. Hoboken: Wiley; 2011. p. 3–41.
4. Foster I. The grid: computing without bounds. Sci Am. 2003;288(4):78–85.
5. Buyya R, Yeo CS, Venugopal J, Broberg J, Brandic I. Cloud computing and the emerging IT platforms: vision, hype and reality for delivering computing as the fifth utility. Future Generat Comput Syst. 2009;25:599–616.

6. Marshall B, Wilson TV. How WIFI works. Available from: http://computer.howstuffworks.com/wireless-network1.htm. Accessed 11 Dec 2012.
7. Raychaudhuri D, Gerla M. Emerging wireless technologies and the future of mobile internet. Los Angeles: Cambridge University Press; 2011. p. 1.
8. Trappe W, Baliga A, Poovendran R. Opening up the last frontiers for securing the future wireless internet. In: Raychaudhuri D, Gerla M, editors. Emerging wireless technologies and the future mobile internet, vol. 9. New York: Cambridge University Press; 2011. p. 242–79.
9. Medication Manager Project. Available from: https://play.google.com/store/apps/details?id=com.henrych2.medicationmanager&feature=search_result#?t=W251bGwsMSwyLDEsImNvbS5oZW5yeWNoMi5tZWRpY2F0aW9ubWFuYWdlciJd. Accessed 10 June 2013.
10. Stille CS, Bender CM, Dunbar-Jacob J, Sereika S, Ryan CM. The impact of cognitive function on medication management: Three studies. Health Psychol. 2010;29(1):50–5.
11. Shekelle PG, Goldzweig CL. Costs and benefits of health information technology: an updated systematic review. London: Health Foundation on behalf of the Southern California Evidence-based Practice Centre, RAND Corporation; 2009.
12. Cleese John on Creativity Dr Shock 8th September 2010. Available from: http://www.shockmd.com/2010/09/08/john-cleese-on-creativity/.

Chapter 6
Health Information Exchange: Integrating the Healthcare Enterprise (IHE)

Karen Witting

Abstract The effective and accurate exchange of information within and between healthcare organizations is dependent on the use of health information standards by all participants in the collection, use, and exchange of information. Numerous Standards Development Organizations (SDOs) create and maintain a variety of health information standards, all of which are intended to support interoperability. Integrating the Healthcare Enterprise (IHE) supports interoperability though the inclusion of key health information standards in profiles that are developed through a collaborative process directed toward priority health information needs.

Keywords IHE profile • Cross-enterprise document sharing (XDS) • Standards • Health document sharing • Health information exchange

Key Concepts

IHE Profile
Cross-Enterprise Document Sharing (XDS)
Standards, Health Document Sharing
Health Information Exchange

Introduction

As noted in Chap. 2, the variety of individual systems that comprise the Enterprise Health Information System are varied and include Lab, Radiology, Medication Management, Clinical Documentation, Scheduling, and others. Although some health care organizations have very good integration of systems and information flows freely between the various points in the system, this is not always the case.

The online version of this chapter (doi:10.1007/978-1-4471-2999-8_6) contains supplementary material, which is available to authorized users.

K. Witting, MS, MA, BA
IBM T.J. Watson Research Center, Yorktown Heights, NY, USA
e-mail: wittingkk@gmail.com

Many organizations experience issues related to interoperability – which can range from incompatible document formats between systems, preventing health information from being correctly understood, to a complete lack of access at various points in the healthcare system. These challenges are even more prevalent when information must flow across organizations, across regions, and across countries. It is critical that clinicians and administrators have appropriate access to information regardless of their location across the health care system, whether they are located within a single organization or part of the larger healthcare community. Increasingly, efforts are underway to proactively support the flow of information. Health information standards are being used to structure the communication of healthcare information so that it available in a complete and accurate manner.

Standards are important because they provide a way to ensure that computer systems can communicate in a known, understandable language. Systems need to talk to each other for many reasons and the medical community is becoming increasingly dependent on the integration across health systems. Basic understanding of the importance and role of standards will help health information specialists build systems that integrate and communicate most effectively.

This chapter presents a method for applying standards to the challenges of sharing health information within and across organizations. This method is used in many parts of the world and is significant in its breadth and scope of adoption. But there are other approaches adopted throughout the world, some unique to a particular country and others that also are used by more than one region. The goal of this chapter is to present one approach, from IHE (Integrating the Healthcare Enterprise), as an example of the typical challenges solved through the use of standards.

Health Information Standards

Health information standards come from many organizations, most of which are public, non-profit standards development organizations (SDO), which focus on developing specifications that define standards. Some of these SDO organizations are healthcare specific. For example Health Level 7 (HL7) (http://www.hl7.org/) develops specifications for exchange, integration, sharing and retrieval of electronic health information. HL7 has many different working groups, each focused on a different aspect of electronic health information exchange, including Clinical Decision Support, Health Care Devices, Orders and Observation and Structured Documents. The Structured Documents work group supports a general electronic document structure, Clinical Document Architecture (CDA), which is a common format for structuring the content of electronic healthcare documents. A CDA document can contain a wide range of clinical information including lab results, patient summaries and discharge summaries. CDA supports the interoperable exchange of clinical data by specifying how the clinical data are formatted within an electronic structure.

Other healthcare SDOs focus on more specific aspects of the healthcare system. For example the Digital Imaging and Communications in Medicine (DICOM) standard (http://medical.nema.org/) is focused on medical imaging and the exchange of images and related data. Logical Observation Identifiers Names and Codes (LOINC®) (http://loinc.org/) defines a code system for identifying laboratory and clinical results.

Still other SDOs are focused on general-purpose uses and develop standards that are used across multiple industries, including healthcare. For example, OASIS (Organization for the Advancement of Structured Information Standards) develops general electronic information exchange standards. The World Wide Web Consortium (W3C) focuses on standards for the Web.

All these standards bodies bring a wide variety of approaches to the problem of health information exchange. Some standards are very broad, allowing for a wide variety of approaches when applying the standard to problems. Some are very narrow, solving only a small part of the overall problem. These standards are plentiful, and any particular healthcare information exchange problem can usually be addressed by a variety of combinations of standards.

The Integrating the Healthcare Enterprise (IHE) (http://www.ihe.net) standards organization addresses the need for health information sharing by providing a collaborative environment where healthcare stakeholders can agree on, develop, and test standards-based approaches to solving information flow problems within healthcare situations or scenarios. IHE builds upon the wealth of existing standards to solve common healthcare information exchange problems by identifying which standards to apply to specific information exchange problems, and exactly how those standards are used for that scenario. In doing this, IHE makes use of standards from many organizations, including HL7, DICOM, OASIS and W3C.

In order to identify which healthcare scenario or health information flow problems to address and how the standards are applied, IHE brings together healthcare professionals, industry partners and many other healthcare information technology stakeholders from across the world in an annually recurring process. First, stakeholders propose new areas for IHE to focus on by submitting descriptions of healthcare information sharing use cases. These use cases outline a common information sharing problem, for example using patient demographics to request a patient's identifier (e.g., health card number) from a Master Patient Index (MPI). The stakeholders select the most urgent proposals for development into an IHE profile.

Next, technical experts develop an IHE profile.

The IHE Technical Frameworks General Introduction (http://ihe.net/uploadedFiles/Documents/Templates/IHE_TF_GenIntro_Rev1.0_2014-07-01.pdf) states:

> IHE Profiles are implementable specifications describing how to use established standards to meet specific healthcare needs. They offer a common language that healthcare professionals and vendors can use to discuss the needs of healthcare providers and the integration capabilities of Health Information Technology (HIT) systems in precise terms backed by detailed specifications.
>
> IHE profiles define the behavior of actors, which are information systems or components of information systems that produce, manage, or act on health information. Actors exchange information through standards-based messages called transactions.

An IHE profile is a specification that includes a documented use case, selected standard(s), and details of use of that standard to address the use case. For example the Patient Demographic Query (PDQ) profile addresses the need to search an MPI using patient demographics. The selected standard comes from the Health Level 7 (HL7) organization and the profile specification describes precisely how to use the standard to search for a patient identity.

Once developed, an IHE profile is implemented by industry vendors in Health Information Technology (HIT) systems. These implementations are tested at IHE Connectathons (http://www.ihe.net/connectathon), which are testing events, planned and supervised by IHE, and held in many parts of the world. Two of the largest IHE Connectathons are the North American Connectathon and the European Connectathon. These events each draw hundreds of HIT systems together in one place where conformance to IHE profiles is tested by running use cases which require cross-system integration. The results of this testing are published at http://connectathon-results.ihe.net/.

Privacy and security are enabled and enforced through many approaches including policy, physical environment, procedures, organizational, departmental, functional, and information technology. IHE addresses Privacy and Security by assessing each profile for risks and managing those risks through mitigations. IHE provides profiles that support privacy and security audit logging, user and system identification and authentication, access control, encryption, data integrity, digital signatures, and privacy consent management. Further discussion of security and privacy issues in exchanging health information is in Chap. 11.

Communities for Health Information Exchange (HIE)

Across the world there is a need for communities to organize themselves for the purposes of the safe and effective exchange of health information. This principle of organization is foundational to most systems of cross-organization exchange and is particularly important to IHE's approach to this challenge. These communities for Health Information Exchange (HIE) develop shared processes and procedures, agreements about security requirements, privacy policies and consent requirements, and more. Today, there are many communities already in production and many more are being planned. The size, nature and scope of communities varies widely but can be characterized by a number of different aspects.

First, some communities are geographically focused while others are not. What often comes to mind when speaking of a community is a regional organization that facilitates information exchange across multiple organizations that are relatively close in proximity. Major metropolitan areas tend to be the focus of these communities, but often a regional community encompasses several rural locales. On the opposite extreme of the geographic aspect of communities is the network of United States Veterans Hospitals. The United States Department of Veterans Affairs (VA) hospitals are spread across the entire USA and beyond, yet significant efforts have been spent on being able to exchange data among these geographically separated care centers.

A second characteristic by which to categorize communities is the organizational structure of the community. In some cases, the community consists of a single hospital and several out-patient clinics that have a referral relationship with the hospital. In other cases, a network of competing hospitals, laboratories and private clinics may collaborate to form a community.

A community may be a single organization, like the USA Veterans Administration, a complex community of many organizations, or a more simple organization like a single small hospital or facility. Cross-community describes an environment where multiple communities, be they simple, small, complex or large, interact without any understanding of or access to the internal structure of any of the other participants. A large federation of communities is exemplified by the multi-national exchange "European Patients – Smart Open Service" (epSOS).

A third means to describe communities is related to the scope of shared content. Some communities have very limited exchange functionality. For instance, a community may focus entirely on electronic lab result delivery or e-prescribing. Most communities define a moderate scope to their exchange activities that might include results delivery, electronic referrals, and perhaps some sharing of encounter-based information (e.g., dictations). More advanced communities leverage their network to include even larger scopes (perhaps including the sharing of documents with the patient's Personal Health Record, exchange of clinical summaries, regional patient centric workflows, etc.). No two communities are alike in terms of the set of exchange activities that they facilitate.

Finally, a fourth aspect of a community is the size, scope and political jurisdiction(s) that regulate it. The simplest community uses an adhoc arrangement to push documents from one organization to another. National and sub-national jurisdictions have significant effects on the organization and operations of a community.

Despite all the variance among communities, each has the same ultimate goal: to increase the authorized exchange of patient health information across organizations so that clinicians can make more informed decisions about the care that they provide. This ultimate goal provides the reason why the community exists, it is their affinity.

The Integrating the Healthcare Enterprise (IHE) standards profiling organization has developed a collection of profiles which can be leveraged by healthcare communities for the purposes of the exchange of health information. Collectively, these profiles are referred to as the Health Document Sharing profiles. These profiles are designed to address specific aspects of exchanging healthcare information by exchanging documents within and across communities. Each profile addresses part of the broad set of challenges involved in health information exchange. The profiles, however, do not attempt to address governance and policy choices that significantly affect how the profile is adapted in a particular community.

This chapter will describe a set of building blocks defined by IHE for health document sharing. Each environment will use some set of those building blocks to enable the architecture desired by the community or communities participating.

IHE Principles for Health Document Sharing

IHE defines a set of profiles, called IHE Health Document Sharing profiles, which support interoperable exchange of health documents. These profiles define mechanisms for sharing documents within and across communities and make use of several key principles that resolve many of the common challenges in Health Information Exchange. These principles are foundational to IHE's approach to effective health document sharing.

General Standards Development Organization Principles

IHE is a Standards Development Organization (SDO) and follows several general principles that are typical in a SDO.

- Standards typically focus on the communications between systems and not the implementation within systems. IHE describes communications between systems by defining transactions, which are technically specific and detailed enough to ensure interoperability among implementing systems. The internal implementation of the systems is not prescribed by IHE. For example, for patient demographic matching, IHE specified the format of the query and response, but not the algorithm or method used for the demographic matching. This allows freedom for implementations to address scalability, creative functionality, reliability, and other value-add.
- Standards strive to support a wide variety of governance and policies. Because IHE supports adoption of its profiles around the world it is rarely possible to define policies that are applicable in all countries. For this reason IHE profiles are designed with a variety of governance and policies in mind and are therefore applicable to a wide variety of environments. Since IHE profiles are designed to be policy neutral and support a broad set of governance, before they can be deployed there are many governance and policy issues that the communities must agree on. Examples of governance and policy issues include: roles and responsibilities, privacy, signature requirements, authorization, when to publish, what to publish, administrative roles, configuration, service level agreements, clinical pathways, long-term availability, etc.

Use of Documents

IHE's approach to health information exchange is through Health Document Sharing, where a complete set of health information is packaged in a document and exchanged between parties. There are other approaches which are used, the most common of which is sending messages containing fragments of health data.

Table 6.1 Distinction between messages and documents

Health Document	Persistent	Complete	Ownership	Legally authenticated
Health Message	Transient	Context may be implied	In flight	Authenticity implied by context

A Health Document is a complete set of information, documenting a clinical event, status or activity, which is expected to be stored, managed and used over long periods of time. Its technical form usually stays the same as it moves from system to system. Examples of documents include assessments, reports (eg., post operative reports), consultations, and diagnotics documents.

A Health Message, on the other hand, is less likely to be a complete set of information, but represents a single unit of information at a moment in time, which only makes sense within the environment that transmits the message . Messages are typically not saved in the same technical form as they are sent, although their contents may be saved within systems or documents for later use. Examples of messages are patient registration, lab order, observation and alarm.

HL7 characterizes a document (http://www.hl7.org/implement/standards/product_brief.cfm?product_id=7) by the following properties:

- *Persistence* – Documents exist for long periods of time and are assumed to be saved for future reference. The content of the document does not change from one moment to another. A document represents information stored at a single point in time.
- *Wholeness* – A document is a whole unit of information. Parts of the document may be created or edited separately but the entire document is still to be treated as a whole unit.
- *Stewardship* –A document is maintained over its lifetime by a Health Information custodian, either an organization or a person entrusted with its care.
- *Context* – A clinical document contains all necessary information to establish the complete clinical context for its contents. For example, a document will identify the associated patient, the provider who took action, the purpose of the document, and so on. By contrast, a message may assume this contextual information is implied by the environment in which the message was sent.
- *Potential for authentication* – A clinical document is a compilation of information that is intended to be legally authenticated. This compilation may be related to a single event (such as an examination or surgical event) or may be a synthesis of multiple types of information (such as may be contained in a heath history or consultation report).

The distinction between messages and documents can get blurry at times, as messages sometimes can be persisted and can contain all necessary context (Table 6.1). In fact, messages can be converted to documents and can carry documents within their content. But documents are expected to be persistent, relevant over time and having the same meaning regardless of environment. And messages need not be any of those things.

IHE Document Sharing supports documents containing any type of clinical information, for example diagnostic imaging reports, referral reports or health summary reports. This flexibility allows the method of exchanging information to be independent of the type of information being exchanged and is referred to as content neutral or content agnostic. IHE Document Sharing is also flexible in terms of how the clinical information is represented in electronic form. This is called the format of the document. The simplest document format is a text document that contains only the words used to express the clinical information. Another very common format is PDF (Portable Document Format), which adds graphical formatting to the information which can then be consistently displayed by many systems. The preferred formats include more structured information, like the HL7 Clinical Document Architecture (CDA) standard. CDA encodes the clinical information in a standardized way, which allows both computer systems and humans to interpret and act on the clinical content. By contrast, textual and PDF formats require human interpretation in order to understand the content.

IHE and other organizations have profiles that define document content and format for specific, commonly occurring cases. For example, the IHE Laboratory domain has defined a content profile to support sharing laboratory reports. Likewise, the IHE Patient Care Coordination (PCC) domain has defined various content profiles including a Medical Summary content profile and an Emergency Department Referral content profile. In each of these cases, it is useful for IHE to profile (define) both the transport and the content of the documents so that true interoperability can more easily be achieved throughout the healthcare continuum.

Value of Metadata

Another key principle leveraged by IHE Document Sharing is the use of metadata. Metadata are data that provides information about one or more aspects of the document. IHE defines a collection of specific metadata attributes that accompany every document shared through an IHE profile. Example attributes are patient identifier, patient demographics, author, confidentiality, creation time, service time, healthcare facility, and practice setting. The values are collected prior to sending a document and can be used upon receipt of a document to administer and route the document in an appropriate way. By providing a standard set of metadata attributes a receiving system can manage the document without requiring access to the detailed clinical information contained within the document. The metadata aid in the document's identity, discovery, routing, security, provenance, privacy, authenticity and electronic pre-processing. The set of metadata are defined to facilitate interoperability, so that receiving systems can manage, route and administer documents without having to interpret the contents of the document.

Document Sharing Governance

IHE enables interoperable sharing of documents but assumes this sharing occurs under a document sharing governance structure agreed to by all parties involved. The governance structure addresses all policy issues necessary to enable document sharing – content format and coding, and other operational characteristics. The IHE profiles are designed to be neutral, or agnostic, to governance and policy, while also being designed to support and enforce those governance and policy choices. The governance model may apply only within a small group, such as a hospital and small physician's office, or may apply at a large level, like an entire nation. In fact, sometimes temporary or informal governance (e.g. via phone call) based on understanding of existing laws or customs is used for exchange among participants. Typically, in order to allow for effective and efficient interactions, the governance structure is formalized through some legal mechanism. Overlapping governance is common, where one set of agreements exist in the region and a different set of agreements exist across the nation, yet most organizations will eventually want to exchange documents regionally, nationally and internationally.

In addition to general governance agreements, a document sharing community should address the following issues:

- **Format of document content**: To enable interoperable transfer of documents the receiving side must understand the format and structure generated by the sending side. Typically there is an agreement on a set of document formats, which must or may be supported. This could include unstructured content like PDF or text documents, or a more structured format like CDA or a specific implementation guide applied to CDA for a particular purpose. The key is to ensure that whatever type of content is shared, the receiving system is able to interpret the content in an appropriate way, either through human review or machine processing.
- **Coding within documents**: Structured documents often include coded data derived from a coding system. Agreeing on which coding systems to use for specific data is often covered by an implementation guide for the structured document. Agreeing to an implementation guide, or a general guideline for coding systems to use, is necessary to ensure that every receiver of the document has the same understanding of its clinical content.
- **Coding of metadata**: Metadata are pieces of information that provide facts about one or more aspects of the document. In the case of IHE-defined document exchange, specific metadata are coded within the structure of the content being exchanged. Some of that metadata have values chosen from a coding system defined by the governance of the sharing community. Because IHE profiles can be applied in many parts of the world where coding systems are different, IHE has not specified which code sets to use and this decision must be made among the systems exchanging documents.

Locating Sharing Partners

One of the challenges of sharing health information is finding the right places to send and search for information. This ability to discover sharing partners can be accomplished in many different ways and a clear preference is not yet apparent. In some environments, a directory or local service is provided which supports a search for electronic locations. This search could be by healthcare provider name, organization name or some other aspect of a healthcare facility that sufficiently identifies the other party for sharing of healthcare information. In some environments, the search for this information may be more difficult, requiring manual means, including phone calls and other actions to determine the appropriate electronic address. More sophisticated mechanisms are appearing which support searching by patient, meaning a search for which electronic partner has information about a particular patient.

IHE provides some building blocks to be applied to these problems. The Healthcare Provider Directory (HPD, http://wiki.ihe.net/index.php?title=Current_ Published_ITI_Educational_Materials#Healthcare_Provider_Directories)   profile supports a directory of individual and organizational providers. For locating sources of information about a particular patient, IHE supports the Patient Specific Health Data Locator found in the Cross-Community Patient Discovery (XCPD, http://wiki. ihe.net/index.php?title=Current_Published_ITI_Educational_Materials#Cross-Community:_Peer-to-Peer_sharing_of_healthcare_information) specification.

Document Sharing Models

There are several different approaches to organizing systems of health information exchange. IHE enables three common approaches through a set of profiles, which support interoperable exchange of health documents. These approaches, called Document Sharing Models, share the principles outlined above. Because the principles across the models are the same, it is relatively simple to implement more than one model in order to accomplish multiple objectives.

The key actors in health information exchange are:

- Document Source Actors – those applications or modules that create the document to be shared.
- Document Consumer Actors – those applications or modules that receive or retrieve the document to act on it (i.e., present it to the user, import it into the receiving system, etc.).

The value of the Document Sharing profiles is that they enable effective sharing of data among multiple, disparate systems in a way that minimizes the burden that data sharing imposes on those systems. These profiles may be categorized according to three different data sharing models:

- Direct Push – in this model, clinical content in the form of documents and metadata is sent directly to a known recipient, or published on media for delivery. Document Sources send content directly to Document Consumers.
- Centralized Discovery and Retrieve – in this model, a centralized locator is used to enable document sharing. Document Sources publish the location of documents to the locator. Document Consumers search the locator to discover document locations and pull a copy of the document.
- Federated Discovery and Retrieve – in this model, a collection of peer entities are enabled to query each other to locate documents of interest, followed by retrieval of specific documents. Document Consumers pull directly from Document Sources which are found through manual means or a directory.

The three models are designed to support different types of information exchange use cases. Direct Push is best used in simple scenarios like patient referral, where the receiving provider is known to the sending provider or sending lab order results when the ordering provider is known to the lab. The Direct Push model can be relatively simple but it cannot satisfy all use cases because it relies on the source of documents knowing where documents will be needed. The Discovery models can also handle use cases like:

- Treatment of a new condition where prior conditions may be relevant
- Open Referral, where the patient is allowed to choose the specialist
- Highly mobile patient
- Emergency
- Patient with many medical conditions
- Patient with complex condition

The IHE profiles addressing these models are:

- Direct Push – Cross-Enterprise Document Reliable Interchange (XDR) and Cross-Enterprise Document Media Interchange (XDM, http://wiki.ihe.net/index. php?title=Current_Published_ITI_Educational_Materials#Point-to-Point_ Transmission_of_Documents)
- Centralized Discovery and Retrieve – Cross-Enterprise Document Sharing (XDS, http://wiki.ihe.net/index.php?title=Current_Published_ITI_Educational_ Materials#Publication_and_Discovery)
- Federated Discovery and Retrieve – Cross-Community Access (XCA, http://wiki.ihe.net/index.php?title=Current_Published_ITI_Educational_ Materials#Cross-Community:_Peer-to-Peer_sharing_of_healthcare_information)

Figure 6.1 shows the flow of data for each of these models. Figure 6.2 shows this as a continuum from a simple point-to-point push model on the bottom middle to a highly scaled multi-community federated discovery on the top left. Across the bottom are the use-cases we have been discussing and coming from the right are the IHE profiles that address these use-cases.

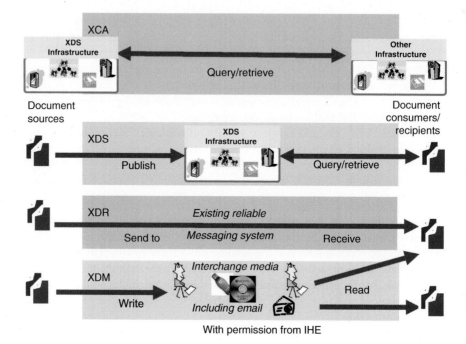

Fig. 6.1 Document sharing models

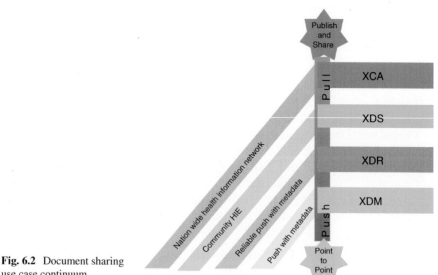

Fig. 6.2 Document sharing
use case continuum

Patient Identity Management

The Document Sharing defined by IHE is patient centric, meaning that a patient is associated with each document shared. When data related to an individual patient is exchanged among healthcare information systems, it is critical to ensure that the participating systems are referring to the same patient. This requirement can be accomplished in several different ways.

One possible way to manage patient identification is to have each transaction carry enough demographic data to ensure that the partner is able to match the patient through demographic matching with locally held characteristics. The challenge of attaching "enough" demographic data is a difficult problem. It includes issues around demographics changing over time (name changes) and other aspects of demographics matching rules. There is also concern around privacy when unnecessarily transporting patient demographics.

Thus IHE recommends that the identification of the patient be done through patient identifiers in a common or accepted patient identification domain. Prior to the exchange of healthcare information, the partners agree on a commonly known patient identifier to refer to the patient. This requirement, however, is often difficult and the IHE patient identity management profiles serve the purpose of enabling this aspect of Document Sharing. Some regions and nations have enabled the use of a unique patient identifier that is widely available but many places still need profiles that aid in patient identifier discovery.

Patient Identity Cross-Reference (PIX)

Most health information systems assign to each patient an identifier (usually a string of letters and/or numbers) that is unique to the patient within only that information system. Thus, Gene Contin may be identified as P-176 at the office of his Primary Care Physician (PCP) and S-443 at his specialist's clinic.

IHE utilizes the concept of Patient Identifier Domains, which define a domain of patient identifiers, like identifiers assigned within a PCP office, assigned by a single authority and an identifier for each assigning authority. For example, the PCP office identifier is unique within the assigning authority for the PCP. If the PCP's system wants to communicate with the specialist's system about Gene Contin, both systems must be able to know that P-176 assigned by the PCP offices is equivalent to S-443 assigned by the specialist's office, both with birthdate of 2/27/62, and that neither of those identifiers is equivalent to Gene Contin with an ID of H-15098 at a local Hospital whose birthdate is 9/17/95. This is known as a cross-reference that links the two patient identifiers for Gene Contin (Fig. 6.3).

The PIX profile is IHE's answer to the difficulty of managing an individual patient's multiple Identifiers. A Patient ID Manager system receives patient demographic data, including identifiers, from multiple patient identity domains, such as

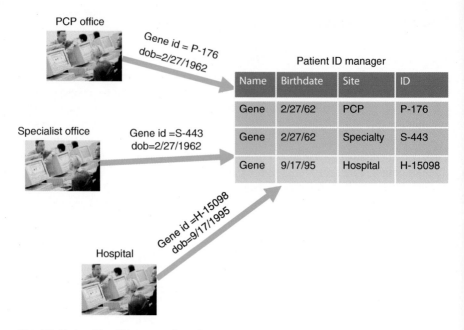

Fig. 6.3 Patient identifier cross-referencing

the PCP and specialist offices, and uses the demographics to create a cross-referencing table, which associates identities with matching demographics and does not associate identities found not to match.

Patient Demographics Query (PDQ)

Demographics (information describing the patient in general) are used to help identify the patient. As an example, consider the search for Leslie Ramaley. With information on dates of birth and sex, information about Leslie Ramaley, a male born on March-5-1972, can be distinguished from that of Leslie Ramaley, a female born on June-17-1978. To help information systems improve their management of patient demographic information and matching of patients across systems, IHE defines a profile called patient demographics query (PDQ). This profile supports the ability to send a limited set of patient demographic data and return a list of potentially matching patients.

A typical use of PDQ is to discover the patient's previously assigned patient identifier. Imagine that Justin McCarthy heads to the local public health department for a vaccination. The public health department's clinical system wishes to send Justin's immunization record to the regional HIE system. The public health department can use PDQ to find matches for Justin and will receive Justin's patient identifiers as part of the demographics returned. With the knowledge of Justin's appropriate patient identifier, the public health department can now publish his immunization record to the HIE community via the XDS profile.

Cross-Community Patient Discovery (XCPD)

PIX and PDQ assume a centralized model, where all patient demographic information is collected in one IT system and a single query request returns a list of patients which match the input demographics, each patient on this list associated with one of the participating systems. A similar profile, Cross-Community Patient Discovery (XCPD) also uses demographic matching to support patient identification. However, the difference is that XCPD allows for a non-centralized search for matching patients. Instead of sending just one query to a centralized system and receiving a list of matching results, the initiator sends many query requests to many systems (such as hospital system, state HIE system, lab system) and then must collect each of those responses into one consolidated answer. This is a more complicated and less efficient approach, so a centralized system is recommended whenever feasible. Most often PDQ and PIX are used within a regional area and XCPD is used across those regional areas, for when the population is too large or risk averse to accumulate all demographic patient information into a single system, for example large countries like the United States or China.

International Health Information Exchange Approaches

Health information exchange is increasingly the focus of governments and communities around the world. Many areas have adopted some portion of the IHE document sharing profiles, or have considered doing so. Each year many countries advance their understanding and approach to Health Information Exchange. This section discusses a couple of countries and their status as of 2013.

United States

In the United States the approaches to solving health information exchange continue to evolve. Federal laws encourage some level of health information exchange, and further federal government action is expected. But there is significant flexibility in terms of how standards are applied to the problem and, at the federal level, this is considered advantageous. There are many advocates, distributed across the federal, state and private levels, each having a point of view about what standards and approaches are best for accomplishing health information exchange. Because of this disparity of views, and despite increasing focus, the United States environment continues to be a fragmented one. Several organizations and public/private consortiums have formed and are independently making progress. Cooperation across these groups is growing, with sharing and integration across the groups becoming more and more common. This method of integrating multiple ground-up approaches is appropriate for the United States, which values independence over top-down management. As the market for health information exchange develops, the best approach is expected to be adopted based on the existence of a significant level of deployment of that approach. Federal government action is focused on recognizing this approach only after significant adoption is identified.

A few of the largest organizations and consortium at work in the United States are:

- The Direct Project http://directproject.org/
- eHealth Exchange http://healthewayinc.org/index.php/exchange
- HIE Interoperability Workgroup www.interopwg.org

The Direct Project formed in 2010 and brought together many stakeholders to address a highly constrained, simple use case for direct push between known parties. Many of the challenges addressed by IHE were deemed out of scope by the Direct Project, such as patient identification, consent and authentication. The Direct Project chose encrypted email as its method of transport and allowed any content to be carried in this way. The Direct Project supports pilot implementations of this transport and has wide adoption across the United States.

An alternate view of health information exchange has existed since 2008 and relies heavily on the IHE Document Sharing profiles described in this chapter. Support for this approach, originally held by the federal government and called the Nationwide Health Information Network (NwHIN) Exchange, was transferred in 2012 to a public/provide partnership called the eHealth Exchange. The eHealth Exchange brings together federal agencies, like the Department of Veterans Affairs (VA) and Social Security Administration (SSA), with non-federal organizations like Kaiser-Permanente and MedVirginia, to select standards and support their use for health information exchange. Selected standards, which have been described earlier in this chapter, include XDR, XCA, and XCPD.

These two approaches to health information exchange, the Direct Project and eHealth Exchange, are considered applicable to different kinds of technical and political environments. But exchange across the two environments is also necessary and important. As part of the Direct Project this need was addressed through an interoperability guide called "XDR and XDM for Direct Messaging" (http://wiki.directproject.org/XDR+and+XDM+for+Direct+Messaging). This guide explains how to convert from Direct messages to standards adopted by the eHealth Exchange, and vice versa.

The HIE Interoperability Workgroup, launched in 2011, is a coalition of 15 States (and growing) and many Vendors organizations. It leverages existing standards to support interoperability between software platforms. Since the participating states represent 50 % of the United States population, this workgroup has significant impact on the adoption of standards in the United States. This coalition works closely with the eHealth Exchange and has adopted the work of The Direct Project.

These three groups provide the most common approaches of applying standards to the needs of United States Health Information Exchange. But other approaches exist, including proprietary ones designed by vendor and provider organizations.

France

France, as compared to the United States, has a more centralized and harmonized approach to health information exchange. The French government agency, ASIP Santé (http://esante.gouv.fr/en/asip-sante), has developed a blueprint for all health information exchange with the French national Electronic Health Record (EHR) system. This system is called Dossier Medical Personnel (DMP) (http://www.dmp.gouv.fr/) and it enables patients to access their own data and to define access rights to their data for providers. Use of the ASIP Santé blueprint is also recommended for local, non-DMP related, health information exchange. The blueprint is well aligned with IHE, using most of the profiles described in this chapter. In particular, the XDS profile is foundational and all shared content is published using the XDS profile and available for authorized access. The IHE security and privacy profiles are also used to address risks and help to ensure that documents are shared in a safe, secure manner with only those authorized to receive them.

One of the most significant challenges experienced in France was the completion of, agreement on, and testing of the blueprint by the all the stakeholders. This has taken 3 years for the current version, which is now implemented in the DMP, and required significant detailed understanding and communication by the ASIP Santé agency. Despite the challenges, the value of having a single blueprint for a national and centralized health document sharing facility is self-evident. Once vendors have adopted the blueprint for connecting their products to the national health document sharing infrastructure, it becomes quickly pervasive since all systems are built on the same blueprint.

Further Reading

This introduction to Health Information Exchange is based upon an IHE IT Infrastructure White Paper titled "Health Information Exchange: Enabling Document Sharing Using IHE Profiles" (http://www.ihe.net/Technical_Framework/upload/IHE_ITI_White-Paper_Enabling-doc-sharing-through-IHE-Profiles_Rev1-0_2012-01-24.pdf). In addition to the introductory material used as a basis for this chapter, the White Paper includes much more depth and detail and is recommended follow-on reading. For additional details please refer to:

1. IHE IT Infrastructure Educational slides and webinars (http://wiki.ihe.net/index. php?title=Current_Published_ITI_Educational_Materials)
2. IHE IT Infrastructure Technical Framework and supplements (http://www.ihe. net/Technical_Framework/index.cfm#IT)
3. A white paper that covers deployment planning for an exchange "Template for XDS Affinity Domain Deployment Planning" from IHE IT Infrastructure White Papers. (http://www.ihe.net/Technical_Framework/index.cfm#IT)

Downloads

Available from extras.springer.com:

Educational Template (PDF 98 kb)
Educational Template (PPTX 127 kb)

Acknowledgements This chapter is based upon an IHE (Integrating the Healthcare Enterprise) white paper titled Health Information Exchange: Enabling Document Sharing Using IHE Profiles (http://www.ihe.net/Technical_Framework/upload/IHE_ITI_White-Paper_Enabling-doc-sharing-through-IHE-Profiles_Rev1-0_2012-01-24.pdf). Many thanks to the all the members of the IHE IT Infrastructure Planning Committee, who contributed countless hours to the paper, as well as the leaders of IHE for granting permission for the content of the white paper to be used as a basis for this chapter. As this original content was transformed into content appropriate for this book, many people contributed valuable editorial feedback, in particular: John Moehrke, Manuel Metz, Marion Ball, and Susan Carver. *Content reused with permission from IHE and IBM.*

Chapter 7
Health Informatics Standards

Anne Casey

Abstract Health informatics standards help to ensure that health specific applications used by clinicians, patients and citizens are safe, usable, and fit for purpose. They support interoperability between systems so that information communicated electronically can be accurately interpreted and used for decision-making, continuity of care, and other purposes. This chapter covers HI practice standards, guiding the integration of ICT into clinical practice, and HI specialist standards including standards for semantic content, data structures, data interchange, security and safety. Examples of professional and technical HI standards are provided to demonstrate how each type of standard is dependent on the other to help nurses deliver safe, effective care and to communicate across boundaries.

Keywords eHealth • Nursing informatics • Informatics standards • Nursing systems

Key Concepts

eHealth
Nursing informatics
Informatics standards
Nursing systems

Introduction

Nursing informatics and health informatics are no longer the domain of specialists. As this book demonstrates, information management and the use of information and communication technology (ICT) are an integral part of the delivery of quality health care. In future, ICT will become even more essential for the delivery of affordable health and nursing care, as the number of people living with multiple chronic

The online version of this chapter (doi:10.1007/978-1-4471-2999-8_7) contains supplementary material, which is available to authorized users.

A. Casey, RN, MSc, FRCN
Knowledge and Information Service, Royal College of Nursing, London, UK
e-mail: tbacasey@hotmail.co.uk

© Springer-Verlag London 2015   97
K.J. Hannah et al. (eds.), *Introduction to Nursing Informatics*,
Health Informatics, DOI 10.1007/978-1-4471-2999-8_7

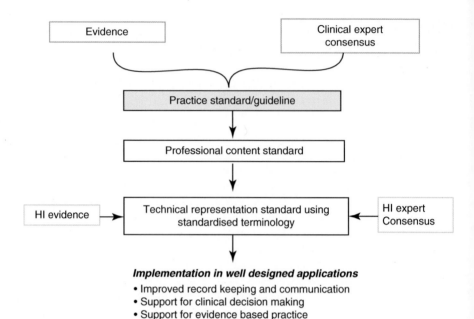

Fig. 7.1 Relationship between evidence based and consensus practice standards, HI practice standards and HI specialist standards

conditions increases and the number of qualified nurses continues to fall [1]. The integration of health informatics (HI) practice with nursing practice is a key theme of this chapter on HI standards. Standards for nursing practice and standards for the information and communication technologies (ICT) that support nursing practice are intertwined, each dependent on the other to help nurses deliver safe, effective care and to communicate across boundaries. Using the example of record content standards, Fig. 7.1 shows the relationship between evidence based and consensus practice standards, HI practice standards and HI specialist standards. This theme will be revisited throughout the chapter.

In this chapter, the nature of standards in health informatics is explained and key concepts such as conformance and consensus are explored. Table 7.1 provides definitions of relevant terms, some of which are also explained in the text. HI practice standards and HI specialist standards are described in the context of clinical nursing. Examples of standards from different countries are used to demonstrate how standards guide practice and support interoperability. Many of the examples are standards published by the International Organization for Standardization (ISO). These are referred to by number and not fully referenced – Table 7.2 explains how to obtain copies of all ISO standards. Examples of HI practice standards are mostly drawn from the UK partly because the author is more familiar with these but also to encourage readers to look beyond local policies and state or national standards to international sources. This is not only necessary, given that there are significant gaps in national standards' portfolios, but also relatively easy to do with the potential of internet searching to identify appropriate resources from across the globe.

Table 7.1 Terms and definitions

Standard	Document established by consensus and approved by a recognized body that provides for common and repeated use, rules, guidelines or characteristics for activities or their results, aimed at the achievement of the optimum degree of order in a given context (International Organisation for Standardisation) [94]
HI standard	Document, established from evidence and by consensus and approved by a recognized body, that provides rules, guidelines or characteristics for activities or their results, in the field of information for health, and health information and communications technology
Default standard	Way of doing things or artefact that is widely accepted as best practice/ gold standard even though it has not been officially recognised or documented by a recognized body
Regulation	Legal or professional rule or principle that directs activities or their results; also known as 'regulatory standard'
Clinical guideline	Systematically developed statements to assist practitioner and patient decisions about appropriate health care for specific clinical circumstances [15]
Mandation	Term that groups the categories of conformance requirement specified in standards: 'mandatory', 'conditional' and 'optional'

	Mandatory:	Always required
	Conditional:	Required under certain specified conditions. Anything specified as Conditional … shall be treated as Mandatory if the associated condition is satisfied, and shall otherwise be not present
	Optional:	Permitted but not required
		(ISO/IEC 11179–3 2003) [95]

Conformance	Degree to which the requirements in a standard specification are met
Compliance	Used interchangeably with 'conformance' but with a flavour of a mandatory regulation. Conformance implies some degree of choice whereas compliance suggests sanctions for not complying
Conformity assessment	Process used to show that a product, service or system meets specified requirements (International Organization for Standardization) [96]
Recognized body	Legal or administrative entity that has specific tasks and composition, with acknowledged authority for publishing standards (International Organization for Standardization) [96]
Interoperability	Ability of two or more systems or components to exchange information and to use the information that has been exchanged (Institute of Electrical and Electronics Engineers, 1990) [7]

	Functional interoperability – capability to reliably exchange information without error
	Semantic interoperability – ability to interpret, and, therefore, to make effective use of the information so exchanged. (Health Level Seven International HL7)

Information Governance	Framework of policies and procedures for handling personal health information in a confidential, secure and accurate manner to appropriate professional, ethical and quality standards; concerns keeping, obtaining, recording, using and sharing such information [97, p9]

(continued)

Table 7.1 (continued)

UMLS	Unified medical language system – a terminological resource from the National Library of Medicine – www.nlm.nih.gov/research/umls/about_umls.html
Clinical LOINC	A universal code system for identifying laboratory and clinical observations – www.loinc.org
SNOMED Clinical Terms	A terminological resource maintained by the International Health Terminology Standards Development Organization – www.ihtsdo.org

Table 7.2 Standards Development Organizations (SDOs)

ISO	International Organization for Standard (also known as the International Standards Organization) www.iso.org	ISO is an independent, non-governmental organization made up of members from the national standards bodies of 162 countries. It has published more than 19,500 International Standards and has around 3,400 technical groups developing standards.
		Technical Committee TC 215 is responsible for ISO Health Informatics standards.
		ISO standards can be purchased from the online ISO store or through the national standards body.
CEN	European Committee for Standardization www.cen.eu	CEN is an international non-profit association based in Brussels. It has 33 members (national standards bodies) who develop voluntary European Standards (ENs), which are then adopted as national standards in the member countries. It has formal arrangements for working with ISO to avoid duplication and promote harmonisation.
		Technical Committee TC 251 is responsible for CEN Health Informatics standards.
		CEN standards can be purchased from national member bodies.
JIC	JIC for Global Health Informatics Standardization www.jointinitiativecouncil.org	The Joint Initiative on SDO Global Health Informatics Standardization was formed to address gaps, overlaps, and counterproductive HI standardization efforts. Members include ISO TC215, CEN TC 215, HL7, CDISC, IHTSDO
HL7	Health Level Seven International www.hl7.org	Health Level Seven International is a not-for-profit, ANSI-accredited SDO providing a framework and standards for the exchange, integration, sharing, and retrieval of electronic health information that supports clinical practice and the management, delivery and evaluation of health services. HL7 has over 2,300 members. Membership is open to individuals and organizations for a fee – with a special low cost for health care professionals.
		HL7 standards are free to members and can be purchased from the HL7 online store.
openEHR	Open EHR Foundation www.openehr.org	The openEHR Foundation is a not-for-profit company providing 'an open domain-driven platform for developing flexible e-health systems'

Table 7.2 (continued)

CDISC	Clinical Data Interchange Standards Consortium www.cdisc.org	CDISC is a global, multidisciplinary, non-profit organization developing standards to support the acquisition, exchange, submission and archive of clinical research data and metadata.
		CDISC standards can be downloaded for free from the CDISC website.
ANSI	American National Standards Institute www.ansi.org	ANSI facilitates the development of National Standards (ANS) by accrediting the procedures of SDOs – groups working cooperatively to develop voluntary national consensus standards. It is the US national standards body member of ISO and encourages the adoption of international standards as national standards where they meet the needs of the user community.
		Membership is open to individuals and organizations. ANSI standards can be purchased from the online store.

NOTE: Hammond et al. [98] provide a helpful overview of standards development with a diagram showing how US and international SDOs relate to each other

In the final section of the chapter, the standards lifecycle is described and approaches to standards development and review are explained. After reading this chapter, the reader should be able to:

- Identify and access standards that are relevant to one's context (clinical practice, education, informatics specialist etc.)
- Use appropriate standards to assess conformance of HI practices, processes and applications
- Participate in standards development, conformance assessment and review.

Defining Standards and Related Concepts

What is a standard?

Standards are relevant to every aspect of our daily lives, from the way we drive to the food we eat. International standards are especially important. Consider the Automatic Teller Machine (ATM): people can use a personalized card to obtain money almost anywhere in the world because the banking systems have all adopted relevant international standards. In contrast, when travelling abroad, people have to carry an adaptor plug because different countries do not have the same standard for electricity power points. This chapter uses ISO 690, the international standard for bibliographic referencing, which is embedded in the word processing software.

Aside from personal convenience, international standards benefit us in numerous ways. They:

- Help to make the development, manufacturing and supply of goods more efficient, safer and cleaner.
- Make trade between countries easier and fairer.
- Support national technical regulations. For example, ISO 14971, *Application of Risk Management to Medical Devices*, has been adopted in the USA, Europe, and Japan [2].

ISO defines a standard as:

> A document established by consensus and approved by a recognized body that provides for common and repeated use, rules, guidelines or characteristics for activities or their results, aimed at the achievement of the optimum degree of order in a given context. [2]

Put more simply, a standard is '*an agreed way of doing something*' [3]

Both of these definitions conform to international standards for formulating good definitions [4] in that they state what the concept is without using the word that is being defined. The second definition conforms very well in that it is concise, unambiguous and states the essential meaning of the concept. The first definition includes a purpose ('*..aimed at the achievement of ...*') which goes against the recommendation that a good definition should '*be expressed without embedding rationale, functional usage, domain information, or procedural information*' [4; p7]. However, in order to understand HI standards we need to consider both their purpose and their 'functional usage', particularly conformance assessment.

Before discussing these topics however, there is one other aspect of the definition of a standard that needs to be considered, most easily understood as the difference between a noun and an adjective. ISO sees a standard as a **document** but people often refer to **things** as standards, for example: 'the Braden scale is the standard assessment tool for pressure ulcer risk in our organization'; 'we use a standard terminology in our electronic record system'; 'the X monitor is the standard device for measuring blood pressure in neonates'. In these examples, the Braden scale, the terminology and the device have been adopted by a clinical team, an organization or other body as their standard approach. In order to ensure quality and consistency, staff would be expected to use only these artefacts in the situations for which they have been adopted.

This meaning of the word 'standard' (i.e. as a descriptor that gives an artefact additional status) is not covered further in this chapter – here we focus on standards as documents that state 'rules, guidelines or characteristics'. Interestingly, many standards support the selection of artefacts for preferred use by describing the characteristics that make them safe, effective and useful. For example: ISO 9919 is a family of standards that specify the characteristics of medical electrical equipment such as pulse oximeters so that these can be assessed for safety and performance; ISO/TS 17117 sets out the essential features of controlled health terminologies to support evaluation as well as development. Supporting safety and evaluation are just two of the purposes of HI standards summarised below.

Purpose of HI Standards

At a general level, HI standards support clinical practice and the management, delivery, and evaluation of health services [5]. According to ISO, their specific purpose is '*to promote interoperability between independent systems, to enable compatibility and consistency for health information and data, as well as to reduce duplication of effort and redundancies*' [6].

Interoperability is '*the ability of two or more systems or components to exchange information and to use the information that has been exchanged*' [7]. Expanding on this definition, Health Level Seven International (HL7), a standards development organization (SDO), talks about functional and semantic interoperability:

- 'Functional interoperability is the capability to reliably exchange information without error.
- Semantic interoperability is the ability to interpret, and, therefore, to make effective use of the information so exchanged.' [8]

In all healthcare settings across the globe, we need to be able to exchange information reliably and then interpret and use it effectively: interoperability is essential. Reducing duplication of effort and redundancy are also important goals, as are making manufacture, supply and trade easier. However, there is something missing from this list of purposes for HI standards and that is the safe, effective integration of information management and ICT into clinical practice. This purpose fits well with definitions of nursing informatics which emphasise the integration of the science and art of nursing with information management and ICT [9]. This leads to the conclusion that HI standards have two main purposes: to support interoperability and to guide safe, effective HI practice. However, it is their 'functional usage' which is perhaps most important – we use standards to guide what we do and to measure conformance, discussed next.

Conformance

In the same way that we use practice standards to audit the quality of nursing care, we use HI standards to ensure that HI systems and the way we use them conform to agreed 'best practice'. The word 'conform' is key: a standard is something against which conformance or compliance can be measured – see Table 7.1 for definitions of conformance and compliance. In the two definitions above, I was able to evaluate the degree to which the definitions conform to the statements in the ISO standard for the formulation of data definitions [4].

A good test of the quality of a standard is whether it is specified in a way that makes assessment of conformance possible. Consider the two statements below related to on-screen display of medication:

1. *'Ensure that numbers and units of measure can be clearly distinguished'*
2. *'Leave a space between numbers and units of measure. Ensure that spacing is adequate by always leaving one blank, non-breaking space between a number and its unit of measure. In addition, use full English words instead of symbols and always use the standard abbreviation for units of measure.'* [10]

Imagine the process of evaluating a new medication administration system before it is introduced in the hospital. A subjective assessment is necessary against Statement 1 above, but Statement 2 allows for an objective and replicable measurement i.e. either there is 'one blank, non-breaking space' etc. or there is not.

Closely related to conformance is the idea of 'levels of mandation' – a term that groups the categories of 'mandatory', 'conditional' and 'optional'. Mandatory statements in a standard are those that must be complied with. Conditional ones must be complied with if certain specified conditions are met and optional ones are recommended but not required for conformance (ISO/IEC 11179–3). These terms are explained further in Table 7.1 but an example is given below from the *End of Life Care Co-ordination Information Standard* published by the English National Health Service (NHS) [11].

This standard specifies the required format for core content of the record to communicate a person's end of life care decisions and preferences. One of the requirements in the standard is that *Clinical governance and IT safety leads in each organization where the standard is implemented MUST ensure that the editing rights for specified clinical content elements are limited to the appropriate clinicians.* This mandatory (MUST) requirement aims to ensure that only the lead clinician records or amends critical information such as Do Not Attempt Resuscitation orders. Some content elements such as demographic details are mandatory in every record. Others should be recorded once the person has made a decision (conditional), for example, 'Preferred place of death'.

There are some similarities between these levels of mandation and the way we talk about professional standards. In health care, we terms like 'requirements', 'recommendations' and 'principles' which are found in Regulations, Clinical Guidelines and Practice Guidance. Regulations are legal or professional requirements for practising nurses mainly aimed at protecting the public. In the US, education and licensure requirements are set by the State Boards of Nursing [12] and a Code of Ethics for Nurses is published by the American Nurses Association [13]. In the UK, the Nursing and Midwifery Council is the regulatory body established in law that sets standards for education, conduct, performance and ethics [14].

In contrast, clinical guidelines are *'Systematically developed statements to assist practitioner and patient decisions about appropriate health care for specific clinical circumstances'* [15; p38]. 'Systematically developed' means that a systematic literature search and review of research evidence have been undertaken using agreed criteria and rigor. Practice guidance is generally evidence based but has not been systematically developed, depending rather on consensus among practice experts. The terms guideline, guidance, practice standard, practice parameter, quality standard and others are frequently used interchangeably. They are all standards in that they are 'agreed ways of doing something'. No matter what they are called, the important thing is to know how they were developed and who approved or endorsed them so that users can decide whether to comply with the recommendations made.

All nurses must comply with Regulations if they are to continue to practise. However, the degree to which a nurse is expected to comply with clinical guidelines or practice guidance will depend on national and local polices but often comes down to (a) the strength of the evidence that supports the recommendations and (b) the authority of the organization that has published or adopted the standard.

Continuing the example of End of Life Care, all clinicians would be expected to comply with the *End of Life Care Quality Standard* published by the English National Institute for Health and Clinical Excellence (NICE) [16]. NICE has the same kind of authority as the US Agency for Healthcare Research and Quality (AHRQ) [17] – clinicians would have to give a very good reason for not complying with guidelines from these organizations, for example, in a court of law or fitness-to-practise hearing.

Standards produced by less well known organizations can be equally authoritative provided the evidence cited is strong enough and the recommendations fit with nursing principles and best practice. The Registered Nurses' Association of Ontario's guideline on *End-of-life care during the last days and hours* [18] has good research evidence for many of its recommendations with the remainder being supported by consensus from leading experts in palliative care nursing. This balance of evidence and consensus is required in many areas of nursing where there is little empirical research to guide recommendations. However, as can be seen in the ISO definition of a standard in the introduction to this chapter, consensus rather than evidence seems to be the basis for the development of HI standards.

Consensus Or Evidence?

Consensus building by experts, technical committees and national standards bodies is used by most international HI standards organizations to prepare new standards. However, the initial drafting process also includes consideration of evidence such as what standards already exist in the area under consideration and how effective these are. Many standards are developed using the experience and lessons from applications that are well advanced in some settings. For example, the ISO standard for patient health card medication data (ISO 21549–7) was agreed among a number of countries that had implemented and evaluated health cards. The standard is therefore based on consensus underpinned by experience of what works but not necessarily from formal evaluation studies or other empirical evidence. For other applications and supporting processes there is less experience and consensus is more difficult to obtain. Personal Health Records (PHRs), for example, are not yet widespread in most countries so ISO's Health Informatics Technical Committee (TC215) published a Technical Report (TR) to summarise current knowledge on this topic and establish some definitions and principles (ISO/TR 14292). A standard may be developed for PHRs when more is known about any interoperability, safety or other requirements that would benefit from standardization.

If there is insufficient support for a full standard, ISO's experts may agree to publish a Technical Specification (TS) – this can be used as a standard but only has consensus within the Technical Committee, not across all the national standards organizations. For example, ISO/TS 21547 specifies principles for security requirements for archiving electronic health records – these have been adopted by a number of countries and the TS will most likely be updated and promoted to a full standard based on their feedback.

After a published standard has been in use for several years it will be reviewed. Evidence is collated on how it is being used, whether it is achieving its objectives and whether it needs to be revised or withdrawn. Until recently, fitness for purpose and implementation evaluations have not been sufficiently accounted for in the consensus approach to development and review of HI standards. More attention is being paid now to questions such as costs and outcomes of standards implementation, implications for staff, patients, application providers and others.

A combination of consensus and evidence should be used for the development and review of HI standards but there is still a question about how they are approved and adopted i.e. who are the HI standards 'authorities' equivalent to AHRQ and NICE?

'Recognized Body'

One of the greatest challenges in the standards world is that there are multiple sources for standards. Many different 'recognized bodies' and other organizations publish rules, guidelines and 'agreed ways of doing things', even in the specialised field of health informatics. Governments, Health Departments, Regulators and others adopt or develop their own HI standards for use in their countries and regions. Other organizations, such as the World Health Organization (WHO) and the International Council of Nurses (ICN), produce artefacts that are adopted as HI standards, for example, the WHO International Classification of Functioning Disability and Health (ICF) has been adopted in a number of countries as the standard to describe and measure health and disability [19].

A small but growing number of HI practice standards are developed by national and international professional bodies. Where no authoritative standard is available, the practice that is in common use may become known as the 'default standard' or 'de facto' i.e. it is widely accepted as best practice even though it has not been officially recognised or documented by a recognized body.

The most widely known HI SDOs are listed in Table 7.2 but perhaps more relevant to readers of this chapter are the national standards organizations in each country that contribute on their behalf to international developments and decide which standards should be adopted and promoted in their country. ANSI, the American National Standards Institute, is a good example of a national 'recognized body'. Founded in 1918, ANSI is 'the voice of the US standards and conformity assessment system' [20]. Many national organizations of this kind will also develop standards for their own country, which they can then contribute to the international arena when other countries identify a similar need.

The standards produced by these organizations may be entirely consistent, differing only in presentation such as when different versions are published for technical experts and for clinicians. Unfortunately, consistency across SDOs is not always the case. A very basic example is the spelling of the word 'organisation'. The European standards organisation (CEN) uses 's' whereas ISO uses 'z'. There are similar trivial examples specific to health informatics: the HI technical committee of ISO is called TC 215 – the equivalent committee in Europe is called TC 251.

At best, multiple HI standards lead to confusion; at worst they result in wasted resources and increase the risk of poor communication and unsafe practice and, concomitantly, risk to patient safety. To address existing inconsistencies and to prevent development of new competing standards, international HI standards organizations have established the Joint Initiative on SDO Global Health Informatics Standardization (see Table 7.2) [21]. Members of these SDOs consist mainly of HI experts and industry representatives. However, there is recognition that clinicians and health consumers should be part of standards development activity. In a presentation to the Joint Initiative Council meeting in October 2012, Professor Steven Kay emphasised the need for HI standards organizations to focus on 'usability' [22]. He cited the definition of usability from ISO 9241, a multi-part ISO standard covering ergonomics of human-computer interaction, i.e. usability is *the extent to which a product can be used by specified users to achieve specified goals with effectiveness, efficiency and satisfaction in a specified context of use*. According to Kay, 'users' are presently seen as representatives and experts from organizations with a vested interest in the standard under development, not the clinicians and patients who are often the ultimate 'consumer' of the standard [23].

ISO has recognised the importance of consumer participation: *a "good" standard means one that creates a good product – a product that you will want to use because it is safe, fit for purpose, and easy to operate* [24]. This sounds exactly what nurses, patients and public want from the systems and applications they use in health care. It is therefore essential that organizations representing, nurses, other clinicians and patients are an integral part of the 'recognised bodies' that develop, approve and adopt HI standards. Standards have a clear and defined development lifecycle or development process. In 2012, Canada Health Infoway [25] articulated a pan-Canadian Standards Product Life Cycle, which identified the four-stage development process for standards (Fig. 7.2). These include needs identification, options analysis, specification (standard) development, and maintenance [25; p.18].

This lifecycle is follows a traditional development process of identifying a health care challenge or 'business need' that requires a standards-based solution, exploring various options or potential standards solutions, proceeding to the adaptation of an existing standard or to developing a new standard, and finally reaching the stage of stability and on-going maintenance of that solution.

As standards progress through the development process, they may be awarded specific labels indicating their levels of maturity and readiness for use in health information applications [25]. These levels of maturity are intricately tied to the development process, as illustrated in Fig. 7.3. The *Canadian Strategy Selection* is the most introductory label of potential suitability for use as solution to a clinical challenge. The *Canadian Draft for Use* label is one that tells early adopters that this standard has undergone sufficient testing and validation to proceed with use but that future changes can still occur. The most important label is the *Canadian Approved Standards*, which designates the highest label of stability and that the standards is fully endorsed by the Infoway-sponsored inter-professional authorizing committees. When standards no longer meet business needs, they may become *Canadian Deprecated* or withdrawn from use.

Fig. 7.2 The pan-Canadian
Standards Product Life Cycle
[25]

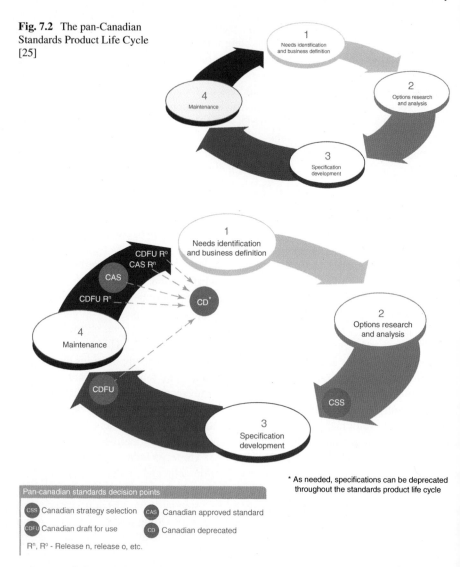

Fig. 7.3 The Pan-Canadian Standards Development Process and Decision Points [25]

Development, approval and adoption of standards follows a recognised standards lifecycle one example of which is given below with further detail in a later section.

Summary – Definition of An HI Standard

From the preceding discussion, we can adapt the ISO definition of a standard and extend it with notes about purpose and functional usage to conclude that an HI standard is:

A document, established from evidence and by consensus and approved by a recognized body, that provides rules, guidelines or characteristics for activities or their results, in the field of information for health, and Health Information and Communications Technology (ICT).

The purpose of HI standards is to:

- Support safe, effective HI practice;
- Promote interoperability between independent systems;
- Enable compatibility and consistency for health information and data;
- Reduce duplication of effort and redundancies.

HI standards should meet the needs of users, be practical to implement and be sufficiently well specified to enable assessment of conformance. Clinicians and consumers of health care should be involved in the development, implementation and review of HI standards.

HI Practice Standards

Scope of the Requirement for Standards

In this section, we consider the 'rules, guidelines and characteristics of activities or their results' that are needed to integrate information management and ICT into health care, particularly into nursing practice. For this purpose, the scope of health informatics can be considered as the scope of health care i.e. healthcare delivery; disease prevention and wellness promotion; public health and surveillance; clinical research [6].

HI also covers the use of information and ICT by patients, clinicians, managers, researchers and others. Many standards will be common to all, for example, anyone providing health care could be expected to have some level of competence in using technology, in accessing, understanding and using information to make decisions and in the secure management of information. Other chapters in this book go into more detail about specific topics such as education and competence, clinical and administrative applications, documentation systems, security, so the focus here will be on the standards that are available to support clinicians in their everyday practice including their support for healthcare consumers.

HI Standards for Clinicians

The term 'eHealth' is often used in place of 'health informatics' to convey a more general meaning i.e. *'healthcare practice which is supported by electronic processes and communication'* [26; p42] – see also Chap. 2. This definition places ICT in perspective – it is a support for practice rather than a separate subject, at last for the non-specialist. This is why, as mentioned in the introduction, HI standards must be so closely related to practice standards. Take the example of record content standards, which specify what must or should be recorded about the care of a patient in a particular context. It is impossible to talk about standardizing the content of a document used for handing over care between shifts, for example, without first defining best practice for shift handover. In the same way it is impossible to have a standard for recording falls risk assessment without reference to the evidence based guideline for assessing a person's risk for falls.

Examples of HI practice standards for all nurses and other clinical staff are given below, organised according to clinical eHealth themes identified by the NHS [26; p5]:

- Protection of individuals – confidentiality, privacy and security
- Data, information and knowledge
- Communication and information transfer
- Health and care records
- Terminology
- Clinical systems and applications
- Standards for Competence and Education

Protection of Individuals

Across the globe, nurse Practice Acts, Regulations and ethical codes require nurses to ensure confidentiality, privacy and security of information, irrespective of whether it is held and communicated on paper or electronically. The International Council of Nurses (ICN) requires National Nursing Associations to 'incorporate issues of confidentiality and privacy into a national code of ethics for nurses' [22]. Health departments and professional associations are the main sources of practice standards for Information Governance – see definition in Table 7.1. Such guidance documents range from statements of law and principles through to example templates and other tools to support implementation of these standards in practice. For example, the Royal College of Nursing provides a summary of the scope of the conversation that should be had with the patient regarding their health record, including:

- the kinds of information that is being recorded and retained.
- the purposes for which the information is being recorded and retained.
- the protections that are in place to ensure non-disclosure of their information.
- the kinds of information sharing that will usually occur.
- the choices available to them about how their information may be used and disclosed.
- their rights to access and where necessary to correct the information held about them on paper or electronic records [27; p3].

When and how to share patient information with others is a major issue for clinicians, including sharing with law enforcement and other non-health agencies. Legal requirements for obtaining consent to disclose patient information and for disclosing without consent differ between and even within countries, leading to confusion and communication failures. Failure to share information can result in significant harm as an Information Governance Review in England has found [28]. This report cites data from sentinel reviews in the US and a number of UK cases where professionals did not share confidential information about children who were at risk and were subsequently killed. Table 7.3 lists examples of standards for information sharing as well as for maintaining privacy and confidentiality.

Although there is plenty of guidance for seeking consent for information sharing, there do not seem to be any standards for recording consent or refusal, a necessary precursor for designing appropriate structure and content for electronic recording. However, ISO TC215 is currently collating international best practice to develop a Technical Specification (not yet a standard) for *Principles and data structures for consent in the collection, use, or disclosure of personal health information – Patient consent* (ISO 17915). Work is also progressing on *Data protection in transborder flows of personal health information* (ISO 16864). This kind of standard brings together practice and technical aspects but at a general level so that countries can extend the international provisions with content relevant to their different legal and professional jurisdictions (Table 7.3).

Table 7.3 Examples of practice standards – Confidentiality, privacy and information security

Organization	Title and year	URL
Centre for Disease Control (CDC) and the US Department of Health and Human Services	HIPAA Privacy Rule and Public Health (2013)	http://www.cdc.gov/mmwr/preview/mmwrhtml/m2e411a1.htm
College of Registered Nurses of British Columbia	Practice Standard – Privacy and Confidentiality (2010)	https://crnbc.ca/Standards/PracticeStandards/Lists/GeneralResources/400Confidentiality PracStd.pdf
Department for Education (England)	Information Sharing: How to judge a child or young person's capacity to give consent to sharing of personal information (2011)	http://media.education.gov.uk/assets/files/pdf/h/how%20to%20judge%20capacity%20to%20give%20consent.pdf
Nursing and Midwifery Council (UK)	Regulation in Practice: Confidentiality (2012)	http://www.nmc-uk.org/Nurses-and-midwives/Advice-by-topic/A/Advice/Confidentiality/
Palo Alto Medical Foundation	Privacy of Information (teens)	http://www.pamf.org/teen/sex/righttoknow.html
Royal College of Nursing (UK)	Consent to create, amend, access and share eHealth records (2012)	http://www.rcn.org.uk/__data/assets/pdf_file/0003/328926/003593.pdf

Data, Information and Knowledge

Nurses and other clinicians access and use data, information and knowledge in every aspect of their work, from checking the normal range of a laboratory result to performing an organizational audit or carrying out a nationwide research study. There is a vast array of standards to support these activities, most of them not specific to health informatics. However, health information literacy for clinicians is one area that has been extensively developed, recognizing firstly that they must be lifelong learners and secondly that they cannot retain all the information and knowledge required to practise health care in the modern age. Specifications of information literacy competencies by national organizations (including health library science organizations) provide default standards for healthcare staff in the various roles they may fulfil, including researchers and managers.

Standards for the data that are required to monitor healthcare quality and manage services are one of the most common HI standards available at local and national levels. These data set specifications are another example of how HI standards cannot be divorced from practice standards if they are to be an accurate reflection of care and outcomes and, most importantly, if the data are to be extracted from care records – the 'record once, use many times' principle. The UK Tissue Viability Society (TVS) publication *Achieving Consensus in Pressure Ulcer Reporting* [29] is a good example. Tissue viability specialist nurses had recognised that data about pressure ulcer incidence '*has little value if it is not collected in a rigorous and practical way, and that comparisons between organizations are pointless as there is no standardised data set used across the country*' [29; p6]. The TVS proposed a UK standard using the definitions agreed by the US and EU Pressure Ulcer Advisory Panels – the professional standard. Integrating the reporting of pressure ulcers with adverse event reporting and root cause analysis is a key part of the TVS standard, which specifies what should be reported, when and how. Being able to report then access, interpret and use data of this kind for quality improvement are core competencies for all qualified nurses.

Another core competency is supporting patients and health consumers to access, understand and use health related information. Nurses are frequently described as 'information brokers': Levy and Heyes [30] argue that, "the best way to ensure patients do not access poor quality or inaccurate information online is for healthcare professionals to act as 'information brokers' and guide users to high quality web resources" [30; p22]. This means that nurses must themselves have the skills needed to critique the accuracy, quality and authority of health-related websites.

There a number of standards and guidelines for ensuring the quality, readability and usability of health information. Specifications of the characteristics of good health information are used by accrediting organizations to indicate that the information itself or the organization producing the information meets specified quality standards. In 1999, the Agency for Healthcare Quality and Research (AHQR) in the U.S. identified seven quality criteria to guide evaluation of health information on the internet [31] which have been the basis for standards set by other organizations since then. These are:

- **Credibility**: includes the source, currency, relevance and editorial review process
- **Content**: accuracy and completeness
- **Disclosure**: informs the user of the purpose of the site, as well as any profiling or collection of information associated with using the site.
- **Links**: evaluated according to selection, architecture, content, and back linkages.
- **Design**: accessibility, logical organization (navigability) and internal search capability.
- **Interactivity**: feedback mechanisms and means for exchange of information among users.
- **Caveats**: whether site function is to market products and services or is a primary information content provider [31].

Table 7.4 lists examples of standards guiding practice related to information literacy (for clinicians and consumers) and to information quality. Note that information literacy of health consumers is one part of wider 'health literacy'. The National Network of Libraries of Medicine uses the Institute of Medicine definition of health literacy: '*the degree to which individuals have the capacity to obtain, process, and understand basic health information and services needed to make appropriate health decisions*' [32]. What this means for nurses is well illustrated by guidance on how to improve health literacy from the New Zealand Nurses' Organization [33].

Table 7.4 Examples of practice standards – Information Literacy and Information Quality

Organization	Title and year	URL
DISCERN (UK)	Quality criteria for consumer health information (includes a questionnaire to help users to assess information quality)	http://www.discern.org.uk/
National Library of Medicine. MedlinePLus	Evaluating Internet Health Information: A Tutorial from the National Library of Medicine	http://www.nlm.nih.gov/medlineplus/webeval/webeval.html
New Zealand Nurses Organization	Health Literacy Practice Position Statement (includes strategies for nurses to help improve consumer health literacy) (2012)	http://www.nzno.org.nz/LinkClick.aspx?fileticket=GPbcXpviZxM%3D
Royal College of Nursing (UK)	Finding, using and managing information – Nursing, midwifery, health and social care information literacy competences (2011)	http://www.rcn.org.uk/__data/assets/pdf_file/0007/357019/003847.pdf
US Dept of Health and Human Services. Office of Disease Prevention and Health Promotion	Quick Guide to Health Literacy (includes section on improving the usability of health information)	http://www.health.gov/communication/literacy/quickguide/

Communication and Information Transfer – Standards for What and How We Should Communicate

One of the most basic goals of nursing is that patients and those who care for them experience effective communication. The importance of good communication and information transfer is demonstrated when things go wrong, as almost every review of sentinel events/ critical incidents illustrates. Good quality information about care and treatment must be communicated to patients so they can make sense of what is happening and participate in decision-making and self care. Staff must communicate effectively with each other to ensure continuity, safety and quality of health care for all. These principles are enshrined in Practice Acts and Codes and in national and international standards and benchmarks [34].

Alongside face to face and telephone conversations, nurses are now using a greater range of communication tools such as SMS texting, social media and video links. Standards for use of these technologies to communicate with patients and with other clinicians are considered below in the section on applications and clinical systems.

In recent years there has been a major focus on hand-off/ handover communications involving the transfer of information between shifts, between agencies and between professionals when a patient is transferred from one setting to another, for example, from hospital to home or from the critical care unit to the operating room. In these circumstances, incomplete or delayed information can compromise safety, quality and the patient's experience of health care [35]. A number of principles have emerged that inform guidance for nurses and others on safe handover. These include:

- A standardized approach to handover communication.
- Use of a structured format for the information to be handed over [WHO recommends the SBAR (Situation, Background, Assessment, and Recommendation) technique] [36].
- Allocation of sufficient time for communicating and a location where staff won't be interrupted.
- Limiting the information to that which is necessary to provide safe care.
- Use of technologies and methods that can improve handover effectiveness, such as electronic records.
- Ensuring that processes which use electronic technology are interactive and allow for questions or updates [35–37].

A single standard format for the information to be transferred would not be appropriate in all care settings, but there are elements common to all handovers, including the patient's name, diagnosis and problems, plans and tasks to be done [35]. Guidelines developed for the NHS by the Centre for Health Care Informatics Design [38] identified a core data set for electronic handover communications that must be used in every electronic clinical handover, recognising that each healthcare

Table 7.5 Examples of practice standards – Communication and Information transfer

Organization	Title and year	URL
Agency for Healthcare Research and Quality (AHRQ) Patient safety Network	Transitions of Care (TOC) Portal (Joint Commission)	http://www.psnet.ahrq.gov/resource.aspx?resourceID=25778
Association of periOperative Registered Nurses (AORN) and the U.S. Department of Defense Patient Safety Program	Patient Hand Off Tool Kit (2012)	http://www.aorn.org/Clinical_Practice/ToolKits/Patient_Hand_Off_Tool_Kit/Patient_Hand_Off_Tool_Kit.aspx
British Geriatric Society	Transfer of Care for Frail Older People (2010)	http://www.bgs.org.uk/index.php/topresources/publicationfind/goodpractice
Royal Pharmaceutical Society	Keeping patients safe when they transfer between care providers – getting the medicines right. Good practice guidance for healthcare professions (2011)	http://www.rpharms.com/current-campaigns-pdfs/1303---rps---transfer-of-care-10pp-professional-guidance---final-final.pdf
World Health Organization	Communication During Patient Hand-Overs	http://www.who.int/patientsafety/solutions/patientsafety/PS-Solution3.pdf

setting will have its own, additional set of essential data. The content elements that are being considered for recognition as a national NHS handover standard are:

- Name, date of birth, unique identifying number (national identifier such as the NHS number).
- What is wrong with the patient e.g. active clinical problems.
- What has been done e.g. relevant investigations and treatments to date.
- What needs to be done e.g. action plan — including when and by whom.
- Anything else that is essential to inform the receiving clinician about e.g. risks, allergies, statuses, disability.
- Clinician making the handover.
- Clinician to whom the handover is being made.
- Current medications [39].

In 2012, the Cochrane Collaboration began a systematic review of the growing literature on handover, specifically focused on the *Effectiveness of different nursing handover styles for ensuring continuity of information in hospitalised patients* [40]. The rationale for this review was the absence of any evidence base for interventions to improve patient safety around handover. It is hoped that the review will provide the basis for more directive practice standards although it may be that further research is required to move from consensus to truly evidence based standards for information transfer.

There are too many examples of practice standards for good communication and information transfer to list in this chapter. A few examples are listed in Table 7.5.

Health and Care Records – Standards for Record Keeping and Record Content

Nurses are required to maintain up-to-date and accurate records of assessments, risks and problems, care, arrangements for ongoing care and any information provided to the patient [41, 42]. They must be able to record elements of the nursing process in a manner that reflects nursing practice including:

- the patient's views, expectations and preferences
- results of assessments
- judgments about the patient's needs and problems
- decisions made
- care planned and provided
- expected and actual outcomes
- communications with patients and carers and other professionals/ agencies [43].

Records should reflect core nursing values such as being patient focused, supporting patient decision making and self care. Their primary purpose is to support high quality care, effective decision-making and communication. Record keeping by nurses is supposed to be an integral part of practice, not 'an optional extra to be fitted in if circumstances allow' [41; p3]. However, many studies have identified that there is room for improvement in the quality of nursing documentation [43]. This will not happen unless records are valued and used rather than being viewed as a 'necessary evil' in case of litigation [34]. Although nurses are blamed for poor record keeping, it may be that the records themselves need to become more useful and usable as communication tools, a challenge for health informatics. A number of the studies cited in the review by Wang et al. [43] indicate that electronic applications and standardized documentation systems had the potential to improve documentation. However, a Cochrane Review of nursing record systems [44] concluded that there is a fundamental problem to be solved before both paper and electronic records can be improved: '*there needs to be more work with the nursing professions to understand exactly what needs to be recorded and how it will be used*' [44; p2]. Development of standards for the nursing content of patient records is a challenge that must be taken up by the profession, with support from informatics and terminology specialists.

Knowledge of standards for both record keeping practice and record content are essential for informatics specialists as these dictate the regulatory and professional requirements that must be incorporated into applications supporting record keeping and communication. Where national or regional standards exist (for example, as in Northern Ireland) [45], they provide a good basis for improving the quality of nurses' record keeping and for supporting the design of applications. It should be noted however, that uni-disciplinary standards are becoming less relevant as more provider organizations move to single patient records. Professional bodies and others who set practice standards need to collaborate more widely to ensure that there are clinical record standards common to all specialties and clinical disciplines. According to a UK joint professional working group, multi-professional standards:

'*will provide the foundation upon which to base the collection, storage, communication, aggregation and reuse of structured clinical information across organizational boundaries throughout health and social care*' [46].

Standards for recording, storing and retention/ destruction of records are not further addressed in this chapter. Instead we will now focus on the major gap in standards related to record keeping, that is: record content – the 'what' of record keeping, as distinct from the 'how, when and by whom'.

Nurses know in principle what they should be recording but may struggle with exactly what makes a good care record, either on paper or in electronic systems. In some countries, there are national requirements for what nurses should record but these are often at too high a level to direct practice. For example, Håkonsen et al. report that the Danish national guideline lists 12 areas about which nurses must document but it does not specify exactly what they have to document: '*It is an empty framework where nurses themselves must assess what is relevant to document … in the specific patient situations*' [47].

As well as supporting best practice, detailed record content standards are needed to inform the design of electronic records and communications. As the UK Joint Working Group noted, technical standards alone do not ensure the communication of interpretable health data; professionally agreed 'standard representations' for content are also needed [46]. Record content standards specify information elements that <u>must</u> and <u>should</u> be present for a specified record or communication context e.g. a discharge summary. Interestingly, these record content specifications can be found in some clinical practice guidelines. For example, a clinical guideline for managing head injury includes 'minimum acceptable documented neurological observations' such as: Glasgow coma score; limb movements; pupil size and reactivity; blood oxygen saturation; respiratory rate; heart rate; blood pressure; temperature [48]. Another example is the RCN's guidance on weighing infants and children in hospital which includes a section on standards and quality criteria for recording their weight [49]. If the recording practice standard were to be included routinely in practice guidelines there would be less need for separate content standards!

When content standards are separately specified, each information element in a record content set usually has a heading and a description with examples to ensure consistent use – Table 7.6 illustrates the structural (heading) and indicative content which may be a list of terms, numerical values or free text.

In summary, content standards:

- Are based on best/ evidence based clinical practice and Regulatory Standards.
- May (and should) be integrated with Clinical Practice Guidelines
- Define structural headings and may describe indicative content to populate the headings; they may define restricted content sets, for example, a list of terms and codes.
- May take account of what data is required for analysis (for example, to monitor and improve quality) but this is secondary to the primary purpose of supporting clinical care, communication and decision making.

Table 7.6 Examples of information elements that could be part of a content set for a discharge summary

Heading	Description
Information/ advice given to the patient	Detail of the verbal or written information or advice given to the patient and the patient's preferred form for such information. May be in the form a structured list of patient information leaflets or web links for a specific clinical context.
Advance decisions about treatment	List of and location of advance decisions i.e. written documents completed and signed when a person is legally competent, that explain a person's wishes in advance, allowing someone else to make treatment decisions on his or her behalf late in the disease process.

Table 7.7 Examples of professional record content standards

Organization	Title and year	URL
Patient Safety Organization Privacy Protection Center (US)	Hospital Common Formats (for adverse event reporting – including technical specifications)	https://www.psoppc.org/web/patientsafety/hospital-common-formats
Royal College of Physicians (UK)	Standards for the structure and content of medical records and communications when patients are admitted to hospital. (2008)	http://www.rcplondon.ac.uk/sites/default/files/documents/clinicians-guide-part-2-standards.pdf
NHS National End of Life Care Programme (England)	End of life care co-ordination record keeping guidance (2012) (includes practice principles and a technical specification – the 'national information standard')	http://www.endoflifecare.nhs.uk/search-resources/resources-search/publications/information-standard-record-keeping-guidance.aspx
Academy of Medical Royal Colleges, Royal College of Nursing, British Pharmaceutical Society (UK)	Standards for the design of hospital in-patient prescription charts (2011) – (includes content and format requirements)	http://www.aomrc.org.uk/projects/standards-in-patient-prescription-charts.html

- Are specified or endorsed by clinical professional organizations.
- Are the basis for related technical standards or specifications that support content design for clinical applications (refer back to Fig. 7.1 and see examples in Table 7.7).

Replicating paper record formats in electronic systems is not good user interface design therefore most content standards do not specify a layout of the content on a page, template or screen as these depend on the context of use and on good user interface design/ standards. Where necessary for safety or consistency, standards may specify a standard layout or include examples to demonstrate good practice. Wherever possible, content standards should also be independent of any specific technical or clinical implementation context. Again, a standard may reference good practice examples and implementation resources/ audit tools. To date, there are few professional standards for the structure and content of records – some examples are provided in Table 7.7.

A number of related standards are required as building blocks for content standards and their related technical specifications. These include terminologies, data dictionaries, data sets and detailed clinical models as well as interoperability resources such as terminology subsets and message specifications. These are discussed in the next section.

Terminology

Nursing has a relatively long history of terminology development and use. The American Nurses' Association (ANA) was the first to recognise the importance of standardised terminologies for supporting nursing practice, education, management and research [50]. Nurses in other countries have adopted terminologies developed in the US or have established their own to meet the specific needs of their populations. The International Council of Nurses has contributed to these efforts through the International Classification for Nursing Practice (ICNP) programme which 'serves as a unifying nursing language system for international nursing based on state-of-the-art terminology standards' (Fig. 7.4) [51].

A systematic review in 2006 suggested that use of standardised terminology improved documentation [52] but there has been no systematic review of the effect of standardized terminology on patient outcomes and experience of care. However, the International Journal of Nursing Terminology and Classification and other publi-

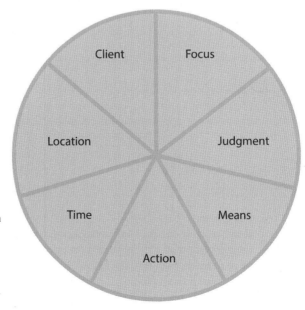

Fig. 7.4 ICNP® 7-Axis Model (With permission from the International Council of Nurses. ©2013 International Council of Nurses, 3, place Jean-Marteau, 1201 Geneva, Switzerland -All rights reserved)

cations do provide good examples of how standardised terminologies are used and the ways in which they could benefit nursing and patients. There are also examples of the positive effects of national initiatives to standardise the terminology used in practice instruments such as assessment scales. For example, evaluation of the Canadian Health Outcomes for Better Information and Care (C-HOBIC) project [53] indicated that use of the C-HOBIC approach to assessment using standardized terminology had a positive impact on professional practice, enabling nurses to share information and focus on patient outcomes. Benefits were more evident where C-HOBIC was integrated with existing systems, workflow and nursing processes [53; p5].

In recent years, the main challenge for terminology developers and application designers has been to incorporate adequate representations of nursing care into computer and digital applications. It is this aspect of terminology which concerns us here but it should be noted that any professionally endorsed terminology can add value to the ongoing work to develop and maintain the advanced terminological systems required in current and future healthcare applications. Many of the ANA recognised nursing terminologies have informed the integration of nursing content into major international multi-disciplinary terminological resources such as the Unified Medical Language System (UMLS), Clinical LOINC and SNOMED Clinical Terms. (See Table 7.1 for further description of these terminology resources.)

These latter resources are designed to support the entry and retrieval of clinical concepts in electronic record systems and their communication in messages. They are built using logical definitions, rather than definitions drawn from practice knowledge and evidence, and are intended only for use in computer applications. Several international standards developed by ISO TC215 focus on terminological resources for health informatics applications. These semantic content standards are introduced in the section below entitled Standards for Informatics Specialists.

Using Clinical Systems and Applications (see Also Chap. 8)

Guidance and training for nurses in the use of specific applications has traditionally been the responsibility of the supplier or the employing organization. However, the spread and variety of applications means that it is now possible to draw together practice principles that build on evidence and lessons learnt from evaluations of system implementations. There are many gaps in this relatively new area of standards development but where they exist, nurses and provider organizations can use agreed standards or adapt them (with caution) for their local context. This will help prevent duplication and ensure consistency and safety. Approaches to system safety and risk management are perhaps the most important standards for both informatics specialists and clinical nurses when considering clinical systems and applications.

Risk management and patient safety processes are core aspects of all clinical practice. Any new intervention, device or health technology will have undergone rigorous testing up to and including formal clinical trials. It is surprising then that HI technologies have not been subjected to the same evidence based/ risk management approaches – they should be no different. Serious harm can arise from the way systems are designed or the way they are used in practice, and any risk of harm must be identified and managed. These two example illustrate what can go wrong:

- Implementation of an administration system resulted in 20 % of patients having duplicate records. This increased the workload for staff, and created the potential for a patient being seen with wrong/ missing information.
- When prescribing data were migrated to a new system, a number of patients were issued prescriptions for discontinued repeat medications. During the data migration, these repeat prescriptions were incorrectly migrated as 'current' repeat prescriptions [54].

ISO has published a classification of safety risks from health software (TS 25238) citing concerns about the growing potential for harm to patients as the number, variety and sophistication of applications increases. Initial concerns focused on decision support systems with their obvious risks of errors but have now spread to all types of health software.

The NHS in England requires all healthcare organizations to comply with its standards for the application of clinical risk management to deployment and use of health IT systems [55]. There is a related standard for those who design and manufacture systems, including processes for handover of responsibility for clinical safety when a system is deployed or upgraded [56]. The principle behind these standards is that proactive safety risk management will help to reduce the likelihood of adverse events. According to these standards, healthcare organizations must have:

- A named lead for IT clinical risk who is independent from an implementation project manager or IT lead i.e. this is a clinical safety role.
- A clearly documented set of procedures covering clinical risk management of IT systems. This will include procedures for identifying and addressing hazards, and audit procedures to ensure the safety procedures are followed and are effective.
- Clear lines of escalation for safety concerns within the organization – linked to existing systems for raising concerns about clinical practice and existing routes for reporting adverse events/ near misses [57].

This last point is essential if nurses are to protect patients and fulfil the requirements of their ethical codes: if they have concerns about the safety of clinical systems and applications or the way these are being used they have a duty to act on their concerns. This responsibility extends to those who work for the companies that design and supply systems [57].

Safety standards apply to all systems and applications and are supplemented by specific standards and guidance for integrating mobile technology (mHealth), telehealth applications, social media, SMS text messaging, decision support and other clinical systems into practice. Examples of these types of standards, written for practitioners rather than informatics specialists, are given in Table 7.8. Over the coming years we should see more examples where telehealth and other applications are integrated into clinical practice guidelines as just another kind of intervention or mode of care delivery.

Table 7.8 Examples of professional standards and guidance for use of clinical systems and applications

Organization	Title and year	URL
College of Registered Nurses of Nova Scotia	Telenursing Practice Guidelines (2008)	http://www.crnns.ca/documents/ TelenursingPractice2008.pdf
National Council of State Boards of Nursing (NCSBN) (US)	White Paper: A Nurse's Guide to the Use of Social Media (2011)	https://www.ncsbn.org/2930.htm
Royal College of Nursing (UK)	Using text messaging services (2012).	http://www.rcn.org.uk/__data/assets/ pdf_file/0003/450246/004_230_ Using_text_messaging_V2.pdf
Royal College of Nursing (UK)	Using technology to complement nursing practice: an RCN guide for health care practitioners (2012).	http://www.rcn.org.uk/__data/assets/ pdf_ file/0019/450244/004_228_e-- Health_Using_technology_V3.pdf
Royal College of Nursing (UK)	Using telehealth to monitor patients remotely (2012).	http://www.rcn.org.uk/__data/assets/ pdf_file/0018/450252/004_232_ Using_telehealth_V3.pdf
Telecare Services Association (UK)	Telecare code of practice (2010).	http://www.telecare.org.uk/ standards/telecare-code-of-practice/ executive-summary

Standards for HI Competence and Education for Clinical Nurses (see Chaps. 20 and 21)

Chapters 20 and 21 cover HI educational needs so this brief mention is included for completeness. Given the widespread use of ICT in health care, a natural assumption is that all national and international standards of nursing proficiency or competence include the knowledge and skills necessary to manage information and to use ICT in daily clinical practice. Well known examples of such standards include the American Nurses' Association's *Nursing Informatics*: *Practice Scope and Standards of Practice* [58], the TIGER (Technology Informatics Guiding Educational Reform) Initiative competencies [59] and the Canadian Association of Schools of Nursing (CASN) Informatics Competencies, 2012. However, in this rapidly evolving area of practice where new terms like cloud computing and mHealth are almost immediately integrated into everyday use, it is doubtful that faculty everywhere will have the skills to successfully integrate new technologies and the latest standards into their programs. The National League for Nursing provides an Informatics Education Toolkit [60], as does CASN, to assist educators to achieve this integration and there is a similar resource from the NHS [26]. However, few such resources cite national or international HI standards with the exception of the TIGER Initiative report [59]. Raising awareness of HI practice standards is one way that informatics specialists could help to improve the education of non-specialists such as students and faculty.

Consumer Health Information Standards

The concept of consumer health informatics has been around for some time. It is defined as "the use of modern computers and telecommunications to support consumers in obtaining information, analyzing unique health care needs and helping them make decisions about their own health" [61]. In 2009, an invitational workshop entitled Personal Health Information Management: Tools and Strategies for Citizens' Engagement, was held in Finland in association with the 10th International Nursing Informatics Congress (NI2009). The report of this workshop included a discussion of the standards that are required to support people who wish to use technology as part of their approach to personal health management [62]. To support interoperability and safe, effective applications requires standards related to functionality, behaviour, work flow, information modelling, terminology, data, access control, identity, security and privacy. The authors concluded that there was much work to be done to identify which of the existing HI standards are relevant to consumer health applications and what gaps need to be filled.

A number of consumer-specific standards have been developed ranging from the international definition for personal health records (ISO/TR 14292) to guidance for nurses on how to support patients using technology [63] and guidance for patients on keeping their online records safe [64]. As more people engage with health information applications, they are becoming more involved with development of standards and dissemination to fellow consumers. We are already seeing a move away from health professionals and industry partners defining these standards to development in collaboration with patient organizations as well as consumer-led developments. However, there is still a need for national and international regulation and standardization. For example, rapid production of mobile apps for every conceivable health condition has led the U.S. Food and Drug Administration (FDA) to prepare guidelines for the regulation of medical apps, based on risk levels [65].

Interoperability among the many innovative applications that are improving personal health management, particularly in developing countries, also needs to be addressed. In 2012, a joint workshop hosted by the International Telecommunications Union and the World Health Organization considered what e-Health standards were needed in future to "leverage today's advanced communications capabilities to achieve more efficient, cost-effective and equitable health services worldwide" [66]. The roadmap discussed at that meeting informed a resolution by the World Health Organization in January 2013 on eHealth standardization and interoperability [67]. Standards development organizations such as HL7 are already actively working in this area, publishing regular updates from its Mobile Health Work Group.

HI Standards for Informatics Specialists

In 2011, the top three job responsibilities for nursing informatics specialists were:

- Systems implementation – preparing users, training and providing support;
- Systems development – customizing and/or updating a vendor system or an in-house system;
- Quality initiatives – including system evaluations/problem solving, quality improvement and patient safety [68].

Health informatics specialists support improvements in health outcomes, healthcare system performance and health knowledge discovery and management, through the application of technology [69]. In order to fulfil their responsibilities, HI specialists need to be clinical professionals and meet the standards of education and competence set by their professional organizations or government agencies. They also need to be very familiar with the practice and behavioural standards that support safe use of clinical systems and applications in order to educate and support their clinical colleagues.

One of the most important competencies for HI specialists is use of HI standards. In its 2009 report on Competencies for Public Health Informaticians, the US Department of Health and Human Services [70] listed four performance criteria to support this core competency:

- 'Communicates the origin and role of standards relevant to informatics projects and information systems within the enterprise
- Uses informatics standards in all projects and systems, where relevant standards exist
- Contributes to standards development efforts
- Supports orderly migration to a standards-based framework' ([70], Appendix p4-5).

To support better understanding of 'the origin and role of HI standards', this section considers the different kinds of specialist HI standards, i.e. those that are required to ensure safety and interoperability between systems: where two or more systems or components can exchange information (securely) and use the information that has been exchanged [7]. This requires standards for:

- Semantic content.
- Data structures.
- Data interchange.
- Security
- Safety.

A topic that seems to have received little attention outside the UK is user interface standards specific to healthcare so these are also introduced here. The scope of these areas and examples of standards are presented below; more detail can be found on the websites of the various standards organizations listed in Table 7.2.

Semantic Content

Semantics is the study of meaning – HI standards for semantic content aim to ensure that health information is meaningful and well-formed so that:

- Information in records is comprehensible and can be communicated between systems.
- Data can be re-used through consistent data aggregation and summary.
- Information in records can be linked to knowledge in decision support systems.

Working Group 3 of ISO TC215 and Working Group 2 of CEN TC251 address these goals by publishing standards and guidelines for the structure and format of HI terminologies (properly know as 'terminological systems'). They are not concerned with standardization of the content of terminologies, i.e. the individual terms within a terminology. In addition, these groups publish standards and guidance for the maintenance of terminologies, mapping between terminologies and classifications, and other related activities. ISO and CEN standards in the terminology space can be described as 'standards for terminology standardization'. They do not specify which terminology to use, nor do they include lists of terms. For example, the purposes of ISO 18104 *Categorial structures for representation of nursing diagnoses and nursing actions in terminological systems* are to promote interoperability by supporting:

- Analysis of the features of different terminologies and to establish the nature of the relationship between them.
- Development of terminologies for representing nursing diagnoses and nursing actions that are able to be related to each other.
- Identification of relationships between terminology models, information models and ontologies in the nursing domain.

The main target audience for ISO 18104 are developers of terminologies but it is also used by developers of models for health information systems such as electronic health records and decision support systems to describe the expected content of terminological value domains for particular attributes and data elements in the information models. Other semantic content standards of relevance to nursing include: EN/ISO 13940 *System of concepts to support continuity of care*; ISO/TS 22789 *Conceptual framework for patient findings and problems in terminologies*; ISO 13119 *Clinical knowledge resources — Metadata*; and standards in development for representing traditional medicine concepts in health records.

National standards are more likely to specify which specific terms to record in a given circumstance, for example, the NHS End of Life Care Coordination Standard includes terms and codes for content items where structured data rather than free text is required [11]. Iterative dialogue between clinical experts, terminology experts and system designers is required to develop and maintain these detailed terminology subset standards. This requires considerable resource and commitment which may be one reason why detailed content standards have been slow to emerge, the other reason being that the focus until recently has been on data sets for reporting rather than on clinical content of systems.

Data Structure Standards

According to ISO, the challenge for interoperability in health care is to be able to represent the structure of every kind of health information in a consistent way [71; p6]. At the most basic level, if we do not have common names for elements of electronic records and messages, we cannot expect them to be successfully communicated between systems. Standards for data types, record architecture, reference information models, detailed clinical models and other information components are developed by a number of organizations including ISO, CEN, HL7 and Open EHR (see Table 7.2).

ISO 18308 is a foundational structure standard that defines the requirements to be met by the architecture of systems and services that process, manage and communicate EHR information. It does not address the specific requirements of individual/localized applications but only the common set of requirements that all need to meet so that their EHR data can be safely communicated and combined. This is one standard that I would recommend all nursing informatics specialists to obtain and use as it defines core terms and covers essential system requirements (in plain English!) such as:

- Requirements for the representation of clinical information, including terms, quantities, numeric data and time.
- Representation and support of clinical processes and workflow including care planning.
- Communication and interoperability requirements.
- Ethical and legal requirements.

A complementary standard, ISO/HL7 10781, defines the requirements that must be met by individual EHR systems – a good example of international standards organizations working together to harmonise potentially conflicting standards and reduce duplication.

Multiple organizations are working together on standards to support detailed clinical models (DCMs), a way of structuring healthcare information that combines clinical knowledge, data specifications and terminology [72]. Once validated by clinical and technical experts, DCMs can be re-used multiple times in different applications – they are set to become content building blocks for clinical systems in the future. Experience with DCMs in nursing is just beginning: Park et al. [73] reported the development and validation of 429 DCMs for nursing assessments and 52 DCMs for nursing interventions as well as a test of an electronic nursing record system for perinatal care that is based on detailed clinical models and clinical practice guidelines [74].

The focus of international standards to support this kind of development is currently on how they should be represented and the quality criteria they must meet. ISO 13972 (in development) covers the following:

- Assuring clinician engagement and endorsement.
- Quality of the content that forms a proper DCM including metadata and appropriate terminology binding.

- Guidance on modeling of DCMs.
- Quality measures for repositories of DCMs – to be able to store, index, find, retrieve, update and maintain DCMs.
- Assuring patient safety in DCM specifications.

HL7's website [75] has a helpful summary of all aspects of detailed clinical models.

Data Interchange Standards (and Beyond)

In addition to consistency of representation using conformant terminologies and data structures, there needs to be consistency in the format of messages used to exchange health data electronically i.e. for communication transactions. This core aspect of interoperability has been a primary focus of HL7 standards and those of working group 2 of ISO TC215 although the latter's more recent role has been to enhance cooperation between the many different organizations involved in data interchange standards. Other examples of the vast array of standards in this space include:

- Basic standards that are used in exchanges of all information on the Internet e.g. HTTP (Hypertext Transfer Protocol).
- DICOM – Digital Imaging and Communication in Medicine.
- Interoperability profiles and specifications such as Health Information Technology Standard Panel (HITSP) Interoperability Specifications and Integrating the Healthcare Enterprise (IHE) Integration Profiles.

HL7 Version 2 messaging standards are widely used across the US and in many other countries. Version 3 standards, based on HL7's Reference Information Model (RIM), 'represent a new approach to clinical information exchange based on a model driven methodology that produces messages and electronic documents expressed in XML syntax' [76]. Version 3 standards are developed across a range of domains from Care Provision to Order Sets, Public Health and Clinical Genomics. By combining structure, content and syntax, they bring together all of the elements needed for achieving interoperability as illustrated in the description of the standard for order sets:

> This document proposes a multi-layered standard that supports the publication and mainte-
> nance of order set libraries, the sharing of order sets between collaborating institutions and
> entities, the structuring of order sets to support effective presentation and clinical use, and
> the importing and interoperation of order sets within advanced clinical guideline and care
> planning software [77].

Because these standards rely heavily on clinical expertise, HL7 encourages individuals and professional organizations to become members. There is a special membership category (with a much reduced cost) for clinical professionals such as physicians, nurses and pharmacists who are working for healthcare provider organizations and are directly engaged in providing care to patients – see Table 7.2.

Security Standards – Technical Safeguards

In the Security Rule adopted to implement provisions of the US Health Insurance Portability and Accountability Act of 1996 (HIPAA) technical safeguards are defined as *'the technology and the policy and procedures for its use that protect electronic protected health information and control access to it'* [78]. Related standards illustrate the scope of the controls required to ensure that electronic personal health data is not only protected but also made available when needed. This latter purpose is equally important so that privacy and confidentiality are not used as excuses to prevent data and information being communicated and used fairly and lawfully. These standards are:

- Access control standards covering unique user identification, emergency access procedure, automatic logoff and encryption.
- Audit controls.
- Integrity i.e. that the data or information have not been altered or destroyed in an unauthorized manner.
- Person or entity authentication.
- Transmission security. [78] – NOTE: this reference includes helpful checklists for people to check their organization's compliance to the standards.

In the UK, the Data Protection Act 1998 covers similar ground and requires that *'appropriate technical and organizational measures shall be taken against unauthorised or unlawful processing of personal data and against accidental loss or destruction of, or damage to, personal data'* [78]. This requirement covers any organization processing data and information, not just healthcare providers, as is the case with most ISO standards related to information security. ISO 27799 takes one of these overarching standards (ISO/IEC 27002) and specialises it for information security management in health, including practical actions for anyone seeking to implement 27002 in health care.

Safety

Health IT (HIT) is seen as a means for improving safety but it can also introduce new safety risks as illustrated in the preceding section on use of clinical systems and applications. The Institute of Medicine has produced a number of reports on HIT safety issues, identifying significant gaps in the HIT standards portfolio and infrastructure [79, 80]. In December 2012, the US government published a draft *Health IT Patient Safety Action & Surveillance Plan* which included two safety goals: 'use health IT to make care safer' and 'continuously improve the safety of health IT' [81]. Although the majority of actions related to the second goal were focused on standardised reporting and reduction of safety incidents, the proposals did include establishing safety standards and certification criteria for HIT applications.

The approach taken in the UK has been to focus on safety risk management throughout the application lifecycle – from design and manufacture to deployment and use, including decommissioning [82]. The UK standards draw heavily on a

Technical Specification from ISO *Application of clinical risk management to the manufacture of health software* (ISO/TS 29321). More standards and infrastructure will be established in the next few years as governments decide on what regulations are practical and necessary to ensure safe systems without stifling innovation or creating other barriers to development and implementation.

The importance of safety risk management and safety processes is at last being recognised in career frameworks for clinicians in health informatics roles. For example, one NHS health informatics career framework places the clinical risk management role at advanced practitioner level with the patient safety facilitator role at senior practitioner level [83]. Informatics specialists have a key role in raising awareness and educating non-clinical colleagues about safety risk assessment and mitigation as well as using and promoting existing safety standards and guidance throughout the system lifecycle.

Interface Design – Evidence-Based Safety Standards and Guidance

Good user or human interface design is based on usability principles/standards and makes application interfaces intuitive, easily learned, and consistent. A common 'look and feel' across multiple applications requires the same visual design and the same behaviour of elements such as buttons, icons and dialogue boxes. Anyone who switches between applications from major software vendors understands what 'intuitive use' means but most people never have to consider interface design – demonstrating its success.

General standards and guidelines for interface design range from legal requirements for accessibility such as large font size for the visually impaired to parts of NASA's 'human-systems integration design considerations' for the development of manned space stations [84]. Many of these general considerations are applicable to health care however there are some user interface issues that are specific to health care. In 2007, the NHS in England teamed up with Microsoft Health to develop a set of evidence-based guidance documents aimed at ensuring safe input and display of clinical information [85]. In the Medication Line guidance, for example, detailed guidance points are provided for: formatting drug names, displaying dose, strength, volume, rate and duration, wrapping, truncation, use of abbreviations and symbols [86].

A number of these guidance documents have been adopted as NHS Information Standards, including several apparently simple guides such as those for displaying dates [87]. The purpose of this guide is to achieve the important safety features of certainty (or removal of ambiguity), clarity and readability by:

- Eliminating confusion between the month and day values.
- Minimising the space required to display dates on a screen.
- Maintaining a reading pattern that is natural to users.
- Eliminating opportunities for misinterpreting the date as representing some other data.
- Promoting consistency across clinical applications by defining a set of two permissible date formats [88].

Another safety critical feature of interface design has been considered by ISO TC215: display of alert symbols as part of decision support. This is an area where consensus is difficult i.e. there may never be a global symbol for screen display of alerts and warnings in electronic health records. However, it is possible to draw up principles for the design and use of alert symbols and warning information, a task that TC215 is currently undertaking. Rather than producing an International Standard (IS) on this topic, ISO will publish either a Technical Report (TR) summarising the current state of knowledge or a Technical Specification (TS) with agreed principles and a limited set of universal rules. Sometimes the decision to develop a TR or TS rather than an IS cannot be made until well into the standards development lifecycle (described in the next section) when it becomes clear that the subject area is less mature than initially thought or that consensus will not be possible.

Standards Development and Review

Structured development processes always begin with statement of need or requirements, i.e. what is the problem, who is affected by it and what is needed to solve it. Standards development is no different and begins with industry or other stakeholders identifying a gap in the standards portfolio that needs to be filled at a national or international level. In this section, the steps in the ISO standards lifecycle are summarised, including the essential steps of dissemination and review. A useful summary of the process is provided on the ISO site: www.iso.org/iso/home/standards_development.htm. Other standards developers follow similar pathways involving multiple stakeholders in a consensus process based on expert opinion.

Challenges for HI standards development are discussed before moving on to the final section which considers how nurses can participate in the many activities required to promote safe, effective HI practice, the development of safe usable systems and to support interoperability.

The ISO Standards Lifecycle

Proposal

This stage begins with identification of stakeholders who can contribute to clarifying the requirement and the scope and purpose of a standard. Then a global scan is undertaken to identify what standards already exist and where there is recognised expertise in the area under discussion. At the end of this stage a decision is made whether to:

(a) **Adopt** or **adapt** an existing international or national standard OR
(b) **Develop** a new standard, drawing on what is already known to work.

The adopt/ adapt/ develop decision is an important ISO principle: standards should not duplicate each other and should build on what is already known. ISO may adopt a standard produced by CEN, HL7 or another standards body through a fast track process; joint working across standards development organizations is common. For example, work on ISO 18104 began in CEN as ENV 14032 *System of concepts to support nursing*. It was moved to ISO under an arrangement called the Vienna Agreement, a formal route for cooperation between ISO and CEN [89]. Ensuring harmonisation across all HI standards is the goal of the Joint Initiative Council for Global Health Informatics Standardization which now coordinates standards strategies and plans with the aim of making all future standards available through ISO [21].

If a decision is made to adapt or develop standard, an expert group then begins a preliminary draft document and puts a proposal forward to the governance structures of the standards organization. At ISO, a new work item proposal is submitted to the relevant Technical Committee (TC 215 for health informatics) where a vote by TC members determines whether this should become an ISO programme of work. The TC is looking for a clear international justification that reflects the benefits of implementing the proposed standard and/or the loss or disadvantage if a standard is not made available. At least five 'P-members' must commit to provide active support for the work in order for it to be approved. (P or Participating members are national member bodies rather than organizations with ISO Observer status – 'O-members').

Countries that put forward experts usually have a domestic standards infrastructure that mirrors ISO working groups. For example, ANSI's HI Technical Advisory Groups (TAGs) manage US contributions, including ballot responses [90]. They also promote the use of US standards internationally, advocating US policy and technical positions so that international and regional standards are more likely to align with domestic requirements.

Similar structures exist in all member countries so that, for example, health informatics experts in Japan can actively engage with relevant work items and send delegations to TC 215 working group meetings to represent consensus views from that country. In the US and UK, these experts are normally volunteers from industry, government, academia or healthcare provider organizations. The success of standards efforts is therefore dependent on the willingness of these bodies to commit the resources required for experts to participate – another challenge discussed below.

Preparatory Stage

The nominated experts from the five (or more) supporting countries form the core of a working group/ task force to prepare a working draft of the standard with a volunteer leader/ convenor to plan and coordinate the work. Development is open so the working group will often involve other experts. For ISO 18104, stakeholders that were involved from the beginning included the International Council of Nurses

(ICN), the Nursing Specialist Group of the International Medical Informatics Association (IMIA-NI) and ACENDIO, the Association for Common European Nursing Diagnoses, Interventions and Outcomes. Once the experts are satisfied with the draft, it goes as a Committee Draft (CD) to the parent working group and then to the TC for the consensus-building phase.

At this stage the document must be structured according to ISO rules with sections for Definitions, Normative References and Normative Content and Conformance requirements. Explanatory information, discussion, implementation examples, additional references etc. are contained in Informative Annexes i.e. they are not included in the Normative (mandatory) provisions of the standard. Extracts from 18104 below illustrate the differences in content and the formality of the language used.

Definition example

4.1 concept

Unit of knowledge created by a unique combination of **characteristics**

NOTE: a **concept** can have one or more names. It can be represented using one or more terms, pictures, icons or sounds.

Normative content example

A nursing action expression (in a terminology) shall have a descriptor for **action** and at least one descriptor for **target**, except where the **target** is the **subject of record** and implied in the expression.

Informative discussion content example

'Nesting' refers to relationships between concepts where one or more concepts can be parts of another concept. For example, *eye care* may be made up of a number of sub-actions such as *assessment of eye*, *cleansing of eye* and *instillation of eye drops.*

Committee Stage

The Committee Draft is registered by the ISO Central Secretariat and distributed for comment and voting by the P-members of the TC. Successive Committee Drafts may be considered until consensus is reached on the technical content. Once consensus has been attained, the text is finalized for submission as a Draft International Standard (DIS). One of the issues with this voting process is that it is based on ISO's national member body structure and other stakeholders such as the three international nursing groups mentioned above have no say in the formal comment and voting rounds. During the revision of 18104 in 2011/12, we got round this challenge by requesting comments from international stakeholders and including them in the formal feedback.

ISO and many other SDOs use a structured and very helpful approach to feedback comments. This requires the country making the comments to categorise them to indicate whether they are editorial (such as spelling and format) or technical (e.g. errors in definitions or unclear/ unsupported Normative content) and to include a suggested amendment to the relevant part of the document. The expert group is required to respond to every comment made and must provide a rationale for any comments and suggested amendments that are not accepted. Any contentious issues are taken back to the wider TC so that other experts can provide input and reach consensus before the DIS enquiry stage.

Enquiry Stage

Next the Draft International Standard (DIS) is circulated to all ISO member bodies by the ISO Central Secretariat for voting and comment. It is approved for submission as a final draft International Standard (FDIS) if a two-thirds majority of the votes are in favour and not more than one-quarter of the total number of votes cast are negative. If the approval criteria are not met, the text is returned to the originating TC for further work following which a revised document will be sent out voting and comment as a Draft International Standard.

Approval and Publication

In the last development stage, the FDIS is circulated to all ISO member bodies requesting a final Yes/No vote within a period of 2 months. If further technical comments are received during this period, they are not considered but are registered for consideration during a future revision. The document is approved as an International Standard if a two-thirds majority of the members is in favour and not more than one-quarter of the total number of votes cast are negative. Again, if these approval criteria are not met, the standard is referred back to the originating TC for reconsideration in light of the technical reasons submitted in support of the negative votes. Once the FDIS has been approved, only minor editorial changes are permitted before the final text is sent to the ISO Central Secretariat for translation into the three official languages of ISO (English, French and Russian) and publication.

Figure 7.5 identifies the various stages of balloting or review and feedback cycles employed by the International Organization for Standardization (ISO) in the standards development lifecycle.

Implementation

Regions and countries have different approaches to the adoption and implementation of international standards. For example, every country uses ISO 3166 – country codes – exactly as it is published. Some countries take a particular international standard and build it into their national standards, for example ISO ISO/IEC 5218 – Codes for the representation of human sexes – is the basis for a more extensive entry

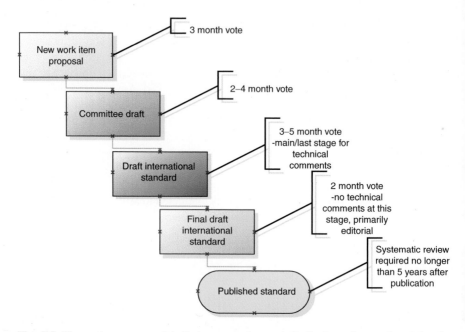

Fig. 7.5 The various stages of balloting or review and feedback cycles employed by the International Organization for Standardization (ISO) in the standards development lifecycle. *NOTE: Certain stages may be omitted depending on development needs (e.g. Committee Draft or Final Draft International Standard stages). Further information: ISO/IEC Directives, Part 1 Consolidated ISO Supplement — Procedures specific to ISO Fourth edition, 2013*

in the NHS data dictionary that defines 'person sex' for use in all health data reporting data sets.

In some European countries, CEN standards automatically become national standards whereas in the UK as decision will be made whether or not to adopt a standard as a mandatory/ contractual requirement for those supplying HI solutions to the NHS. The specification of relevant standards in national laws/regulations (e.g. medical devices regulations) and vendor contracts are the major implementation drivers. For other standards, a number of approaches may be required including: endorsement by organizations such as professional associations; awareness raising; education; supported change management; and incentives.

A few organizations support a coherent, user driven approach to implementing proven standards. One example is IHE which brings together users and developers of healthcare applications in a four-step process:

1. Clinical and technical experts define critical use cases for information sharing.
2. Technical experts create detailed specifications for communication among systems to address these use cases, selecting and optimizing established standards.
3. Industry implements these specifications called IHE Profiles in their systems.
4. IHE tests vendors' systems [91].

Review of International Standards (Confirmation, Revision, Withdrawal)

International Standards are reviewed at least every 5 years and a decision made by a majority vote of the P-members on whether the standard should be confirmed, revised or withdrawn. Countries are asked to indicate whether they use the standard and if they have any issues with it that would require revision or withdrawal. Revised standards follow a similar pathway with an expert group steering the work through ballot/ voting stages, seeking international consensus, approval and publication.

When the revision of ISO 18104 was due, the initial request for comment identified that it had been used in at least 11 member countries and by several international terminology development organizations. Inputs from those countries and from the original professional stakeholder organizations identified several areas that needed to be addressed in a revision including:

1. Updating normative references and definitions and considering more recent international terminology developments.
2. Consideration of a model for outcomes (in addition to models for diagnoses and actions)
3. Adding an informative annex to clarify the relationship between the model for diagnoses and the model for actions as well as points of intersection between terminology models and information models.
4. Adding implementation guidance/ examples, and simplifying the language used in the document so that it is better understood by target groups.

Some reviews will elicit more concrete technical requirements, based on live use of a standard in multiple systems or settings. For example EN/ISO 13940 – *System of concepts to support continuity of care* – was used to restructure the NHS Data Dictionary in England. This work validated the provisions of the standard and confirmed its value but also identified a number of issues with relationships between data elements as they were specified in the standard. These have been taken forward to the next version.

Standards Development Challenges

The core principles for national and international standards development are that this activity is voluntary, open to all, consensus based and stakeholder driven. However, there are a number of challenges with achieving these goals, particularly at the international level. The 'open standards' process must balance the interests of those who will implement the standard with the interests and voluntary cooperation of experts who may own intellectual property rights (IPR) associated with it. The word 'open' does not imply free – there may be a need for some form of licensing to protect IPR and often there is a fee to obtain a copy of the standard which offsets the costs of the development and maintenance process.

Volunteer effort sometimes limits the level and type of expertise available and means that a standard can take longer to develop than is required in a rapidly developing field like health informatics. Organizations such as HL7 have made significant advances in the way it engages stakeholders and develops standards in an effort to be more responsive to the urgent demands of the industry. However, end users of health informatics standards such as health professionals and health care consumers are still not actively engaging to the extent that ISO would expect. In 2008, a multi-disciplinary task group led by nursing members of TC 215 made a number of recommendations for improving clinical stakeholder engagement in international HI standards development and review (ISO/TR 11487). Progress has been slow on these recommendations which included:

- Establish communications with international health professional organizations, particularly those that have a health informatics profile/component. This could include regular information exchanges and invitation for liaisons to attend TC 215 meetings.
- Explore mechanisms by which input of such international stakeholder organizations can be recognized within formal TC215 processes, including lessons from other ISO domains (engineering, chemical, etc.).
- Require that proposers of new work items identify relevant clinical and other stakeholder groups, their input to the proposal and how they may be involved in the work item.
- Request national member bodies to report on the measures being taken to engage and facilitate the participation of clinical stakeholders at the domestic level as a basis for further action and to identify models of good practice that other members could adopt.

Participation of developing countries and non-English speaking members has also been limited although this is changing slowly. In 2004, a survey of participation in ISO's standards development processes reported that Western Europe represented *'almost half the voting base in ISO's standards development work, despite representing approximately 6% of the world's population'* [92]; p2]. It has been good to see the active engagement of Korea, Japan and China in TC215 meetings in recent years.

Given these challenges, it is no surprise that there are significant gaps in the HI standards portfolio. Global policy making organizations such as the European Union (EU), the Joint Initiative Council, WHO and HITSP have all identified the need for improved and coherent action to address the healthcare interoperability requirements of the future. The European eHealth Interoperability Roadmap was published in December 2010 with a number of standards related key actions for EU member states:

- Equip Europeans with secure online access to their health data and achieve widespread deployment of telemedicine services
- Define a minimum common set of patient data for interoperability of patient records to be accessed or exchanged electronically across Member States
- Foster EU-wide standards, interoperability testing and certification of eHealth systems.

Similar objectives are being addressed in the US by HITSP whose members *'work together to define the necessary functional components and standards – as well as gaps in standards – which must be resolved to enable the interoperability of healthcare data'* [93]. The high profile of HI standards and the huge amount of national and international standards-related activity presents a particular challenge for nursing as we will see in the final section below.

Participation in Standards Development and Review

There are a number of routes and opportunities for nurses to engage in the development of HI practice standards. Researchers, practising nurses, policy leaders and others can collaborate to influence what standards get developed, creating and collating evidence to support standard/guideline development and promoting their use through education, practice audit and change management. Individual nurses can engage by contacting their professional organizations some of which may need to be made aware of the need for HI practice standards but may welcome interested volunteers.

Participating in the development and review of national and international HI specialist standards is less straightforward. There are very few clinicians involved in general and too few nurses in particular. Those who are involved come in several guises:

- The practising clinician who has an interest in a specific aspect of health information and participates on a part time basis. Many of these people do this work in their own time although some employers recognise the value of this activity and provide varying levels of support to attend events and undertake development/ review work.
- The health informatics specialist i.e. someone who has developed a career in health informatics. This person can have a significant role in helping technical people understand the clinical world and vice versa. However, unless he/she maintains clinical networks, this person may become distanced from the world of practice.
- The practising clinician who becomes involved for a short time on a particular project. Facilitation of this input can result in new skills for this person who could be encouraged to participate further.

A major area of interest for nurses is HI terminology and content standards but only a few are involved in this kind of international standards activity, mainly at HL7, ISO and CEN. It is a complex world for new members to enter at any level; time and support are needed to develop sufficient understanding to participate effectively. Efforts to recruit and develop new participants have had little success for a number of reasons including:

- Lack of time and financial support to participate – some countries provide funding but this is limited to national delegates.
- Perceived lack of relevance to nursing practice and therefore to managers.

- Perceived complexity of the domain: jargon, technical knowledge requirements etc.
- Lack of awareness of the need or of how to get involved.

There is plenty of entry-level material on the websites of the major SDOs to inform anyone of the need, relevance and development processes. Each country that has a participating organization will include on its website information about how to participate and many provide online training opportunities. Willing volunteers are usually welcomed with open arms but there is a fee to join some organizations including ANSI and HL7. Before signing up, consider some of the factors that support those who are involved:

- Employer's support: time to undertake reviews and attend meetings.
- Payment of expenses and employer's support for time.
- Learning opportunities provided at meetings.
- Dialogue/ interaction with other nurses engaged in the work.
- Direct mentorship by more experienced nurse or other clinician.

Conclusion

A 2013 Kings Fund report on the future of UK health and social care [1] estimated that by 2016 the majority of the population will access the web through mobile devices. Routine use of electronic records will be achieved by 2017; by 2021 there will be a shortfall of between 40,000 and 100,000 nurses – teleconsultations and remote monitoring will become routine to manage the growing number of elderly people with multiple chronic conditions and the million or more people with dementia. Information and communications technology, including robots in health care settings and homes, are central to the future of health and social care.

To support the rapid advances needed for future solutions, health information standards are being developed and implemented across the globe. These will have a profound impact on nursing, patient care and outcomes. HI practice standards are needed to support integration of information management and ICT into clinical practice. They will provide guidance for clinicians, patients and public on how to make best use of information and technology and are closely linked to standards for practice, including record keeping. Specialist HI standards are also lacking and are required to ensure that applications are safe, usable and fit for purpose. They must support interoperability between systems so that information that is communicated electronically can be accurately interpreted and used for decision-making, continuity of care and other purposes.

Although the number of nurses working in health informatics roles is increasing, the number participating in standards development and review is, if anything, decreasing. Health informatics specialists need to work with their clinical colleagues, professional organizations and developers of clinical guidelines to produce, maintain and measure conformance to HI practice standards. They should also engage with national and international HI standards organizations, helping to fill gaps in the standards' portfolio and promoting the use of standards in their own organizations. New approaches to participation that do not involve expensive and time consuming travel must be found so that nursing can continue to have an active, leadership role in this important activity.

Downloads

Available from extras.springer.com:

Educational Template (PDF 103 kb)
Educational Template (PPTX 116 kb)

References

1. King's Fund. The Future of ehealth and social care timeline 2013–2033. [Online] [Cited 4 Mar 2013] http://www.kingsfund.org.uk/time-to-think-differently/timeline.
2. International Organisation for Standardisation. What are standards and how do they help? [Online] [Cited: 13 Feb 2013] http://www.iso.org/sites/ConsumersStandards/en/1-1-what-standards-context.htm.
3. British Standards Institute. Information about standards. [Online] [Cited: 14 Feb 2013] http://www.bsigroup.co.uk/en-GB/standards/Information-about-standards/.
4. ISO/IEC. Information technology — Metadata registries (MDR) — Part 4 Formulation of data definitions. Geneva: ISO; 2004. ISO/IEC 11179–4:2004.
5. Health Level Seven International. Introduction to HL7 standards. [Online] [Cited: 20 Feb 2013] http://www.hl7.org/implement/standards/index.cfm.
6. International Organisation for Standardisation. TC 215 Health Informatics. [Online] [Cited: 20 Feb 2013] http://www.iso.org/iso/iso_technical_committee?commid=54960.
7. Institute of Electrical and Electronics Engineers. IEEE Standard Computer Dictionary: a compilation of IEEE standard computer glossaries. New York: Institute of Electrical and Electronics Engineers; 1990.
8. Health Level Seven International HL7. HL7 FAQs. [Online] [Cited: 20 Feb 2013] http://www.hl7.org/about/FAQs/index.cfm.
9. IMIA Special Interest Group on Nursing Informatics. cited in Working Group Nursing Informatics. AMIA. [Online] 2009. [Cited: 20 Feb 2013] http://www.amia.org/programs/working-groups/nursing-informatics.
10. National Patient Safety Agency. Design for patient safety: guidelines for the safe on-screen display of medication information. [Online] 2010. [Cited: 20 Feb 2013] http://www.nrls.npsa.nhs.uk/resources/collections/design-for-patient-safety/?entryid45=66713.
11. NHS Information Standards Board. End of life care co-ordination: core content standard specification. [Online] Oct 2012. [Cited: 20 Feb 2013] http://www.isb.nhs.uk/documents/isb-1580/amd-29-2012/1580292012spec.pdf.
12. National Council of State Boards of Nursing. About NCSBN. [Online] [Cited: 20 Feb 2013] https://www.ncsbn.org/about.htm.
13. American Nurses Association. Code of ethics for nurses. [Online] [Cited: 20 Feb 2013] http://www.nursingworld.org/codeofethics.

14. Nursing and Midwifery Council. The code: standards of conduct, performance and ethics for nurses and midwives. [Online] [Cited: 20 Feb 2013] http://www.nmc-uk.org/Publications/Standards/The-code/Introduction/.

15. Feild MJ, Lohr KN, editors. Clinical practice guidelines: directions for a new program. Washington, DC: National Academy Press; 1990.

16. National Institue for Health and Clinical Excellence. QS13 Quality standard for end of life care for adults. [Online] Aug 2011. [Cited 20 February 2013.] http://publications.nice.org.uk/quality-standard-for-end-of-life-care-for-adults-qs13.

17. Agency for Health Research and Quality. Agency for Health Research and Quality (AHQR). [Online] [Cited: 20 Feb 2013] http://www.ahrq.gov/.

18. Registered Nurses' Association of Ontario. Guideline summary end-of-life care during the last days and hours. Agency for Healthcare Research and Quality. [Online] Oct 2011. [Cited: 20 Feb 2013] http://www.guideline.gov/content.aspx?id=34759&search=palliative+and+end+of+life.

19. World Health Organisation. International Classification of Functioning, Disability and Health (ICF). [Online] http://www.who.int/classifications/icf/en/.

20. American National Standards Institute. About ANSI. ANSI. [Online] [Cited: 20 Feb 2013] http://www.ansi.org/about_ansi/overview/overview.aspx?menuid=1.

21. Joint Initiative Council. Joint initiative on SDO global health informatics standardization. [Online] [Cited: 20 Feb 2013] http://www.jointinitiativecouncil.org/.

22. International Council of Nurses. Code of ethics for nurses. International Council of Nurses. [Online] 2012. [Cited: 20 Feb 2013] http://www.icn.ch/about-icn/code-of-ethics-for-nurses/.

23. Kay S. Presentation and discussion by Steven Kay on usability of health informatics standards. Joint Initiative Council. [Online] October 2012. [Cited: 20 Feb 2013] http://www.jointinitiativecouncil.org/.

24. International Organisation for Standardisation. Why consumer participation in standards improves products and services improves products and services. ISO. [Online] [Cited: 20 Feb 2013] http://www.iso.org/sites/ConsumersStandards/en/2-4-consumer-participation.htm.

25. Canada Health Infoway. pan-Canadian Standards Decision Making Process Version 2.2. 2012. https://www.infoway-inforoute.ca/index.php/programs-services/standards-collaborative/pan-canadian-standards.

26. National Health Service (NHS). Learning to manage health information: a theme for clinical education 2012. Embedding information in clinical education . [Online] April 2012. [Cited: 20 Feb 2013] http://www.cln.nhs.uk/eice/images/learningtomanage_12.pdf.

27. Royal College of Nursing. Consent to create, amend, access and share eHealth records. [Online] 2012. [Cited: 20 Feb 2013] http://www.rcn.org.uk/__data/assets/pdf_file/0003/328926/003593.pdf.

28. Severs M. Failure to share – meeting of Information Governance Review. [Online] 28 Feb 2012. [Cited: 20 Feb 2013] https://www.wp.dh.gov.uk/caldicott2/files/2012/06/Failure-to-share.pdf.

29. Tissue Viability Society. Achieving Consensus in Pressure Ulcer Reporting. [Online] 2012. [Cited: 8 Mar 2013] http://www.tvs.org.uk/sitedocument/TVSConsensusPUReporting.pdf.

30. Levy S, Heyes B. Information systems that support effective clinical decision making. Nurs Manage. 2012;19(7):20–2.

31. Agency for Healthcare Research and Quality. Assessing the quality of internet health information . [Online] 1999. [Cited: 20 Feb 2013] http://www.ahrq.gov/data/infoqual.htm.

32. National Network of Libraries of Medicine. Health literacy. [Online] [Cited: 20 Feb 2013] http://nnlm.gov/outreach/consumer/hlthlit.html.

33. New Zealand Nurses' Organisation (NZNO). Health literacy practice position statement. NZNO. [Online] 2012. [Cited: 20 Feb 2013] http://www.nzno.org.nz/LinkClick.aspx?fileticket=GPbcXpviZxM%3D.

34. Casey A, Wallis A. Effective communication: principle of nursing practice E. Nurs Stand. 2011;25(32):35–7.

35. British Medical Association. Safe handover: safe patients. Guidance on clinical handover for clinicians and managers. London: BMA; 2004.

36. World Health Organization. Communication during patient hand-overs. [Online] 2007. [Cited: 20 Feb 2013] http://www.who.int/patientsafety/solutions/patientsafety/PS-Solution3.pdf.
37. Joint Commission Center for Transforming Healthcare. Hand-off communications. [Online] [Cited: 20 Feb 2013] http://www.centerfortransforminghealthcare.org/projects/detail.aspx?Project=1.
38. Centre for Health Care Informatics Design, City University. NHS Connecting for Health Safer Handover Project: ER-08-0300. Final Report on Safer Handover. London: Centre for Health Care Informatics Design, City University; 2009.
39. Galliers J, Wilson S, Randell R, Woodward P. NHS Connecting for Health Safer Handover Project: ER-08-0300. Final Report on Safer Handover. London: Centre for Health Care Informatics Design, City University; 2009.
40. Smeulers M, van Tellingen IC, Lucas C, Vermeulen H. Effectiveness of different nursing handover styles for ensuring continuity of information in hospitalised patients (Protocol). Cochrane Database of Systematic Reviews. 2012;(7):CD009979. doi:10.1002/14651858.CD009979.
41. Nursing and Midwifery Council. Record keeping: guidance for nurses and midwives. [Online] 2009. [Cited: 1 Mar 2013] http://www.nmc-uk.org/Documents/NMC-Publications/NMC-Record-Keeping-Guidance.pdf.
42. Royal College of Nursing. Nursing content of eHealth records . [Online] 2012. [Cited: 1 Mar 2013] http://www.rcn.org.uk/__data/assets/pdf_file/0005/328928/003596.pdf.
43. Wang N, Hailey D, Yu P. Quality of nursing documentation and approaches to its evaluation. J Adv Nurs. 2011;67(9):1858–75.
44. Urquhart C, Currell R, Grant MJ, Hardiker NR. Nursing record systems: effects on nursing practice and healthcare outcomes (Review). [Online] 2010. [Cited: 8 Mar 2013] http://onlinelibrary.wiley.com/doi/10.1002/14651858.CD002099.pub2/pdf/standard.
45. Northern Ireland Practice and Education Committee. NIPEC improving record keeping. [Online] [Cited: 1 Mar 2013] http://www.nipec.hscni.net/recordkeeping/.
46. Royal College of Physicians. Developing standards for health and social care: report of the Joint Working Group. [Online] 2012. [Cited: 1 Mar 2013] http://www.rcplondon.ac.uk/sites/default/files/devoloping-standards-for-social-care-records-report-of-joint-working-group.pdf.
47. Hakonsen S, Madsen I, Bjerrum M, Pedersen P. Danish national framework for collecting information about patients' nutritional status. Nursing Minimum Dataset (N-MDS). Online J Nurs Inform. [Online] 03 Nov 2012. [Cited: 1 Mar 2013] http://ojni.org/issues/?p=2044.
48. (NICE), National Institute for health and Clinical Excellence. Head injury: triage, assessment, investigation and early management of head injury in infants, children and adults. [Online] 2007. [Cited: 1 Mar 2013] http://publications.nice.org.uk/head-injury-cg56.
49. Royal College of Nursing. Standards for the weighing of infants, children and young people in the acute health care setting. [Online] 2010. [Cited: 1 Mar 2013] http://www.rcn.org.uk/__data/assets/pdf_file/0009/351972/003828.pdf.
50. Rutherford M. Standardized nursing language: what does it mean for nursing practice? Online J Issues Nurs. [Online] 31 January 2008. [Cited: 1 Mar 2013] http://www.nursingworld.org/MainMenuCategories/ANAMarketplace/ANAPeriodicals/OJIN/TableofContents/vol132008/No1Jan08/ArticlePreviousTopic/StandardizedNursingLanguage.html.
51. International Council of Nurses. Vision, goals & benefits of ICNP. [Online] [Cited: 1 Mar 2013] http://www.icn.ch/pillarsprograms/vision-goals-a-benefits-of-icnpr/.
52. Muller-Staub M, Lavin M. Nursing diagnoses, interventions and outcomes – application and impact on nursing practice: systematic review. J Adv Nurs. 2006;56(5):514–31.
53. Praxia Health Informatics Research. C-HOBIC Initiative Benefits Evaluation Final Report. [Online] 20 October 2009. [Cited: 1 Mar 2013] http://www2.cna-aiic.ca/c-hobic/documents/pdf/Evaluation_Final_Report_2009_e.pdf.
54. NHS Connecting for Health. Nine steps for safer implementation. [Online] 2009. [Cited: 1 Mar 2013] http://www.isb.nhs.uk/documents/isb-0160/dscn-18-2009/0160182009guidance.pdf.
55. Information Standards Board for Health and Social Care. Clinical risk management: its application in the deployment and use of health IT systems version 2 – specification. [Online] 2013. [Cited: 1 Mar 2013] http://www.isb.nhs.uk/documents/isb-0160/amd-38-2012/0160382012spec.pdf.

56. Clinical risk management: its application in the manufacture of health IT systems version 2 – specification. [Online] 2013. [Cited: 1 Mar 2013] http://www.isb.nhs.uk/documents/isb-0129/amd-39-2012/0129392012spec.pdf.

57. Royal College of Nursing. Making IT SAFER. [Online] 2011. [Cited: 1 Mar 2013] http://www.rcn.org.uk/__data/assets/pdf_file/0004/328927/003594.pdf.

58. American Nurses' Association. Nursing Informatics: Practice Scope and Standards of Practice. Silver Spring, MD: Nursesbooks.org; 2008.

59. TIGER Collaborative. Informatics competencies for every practicing nurse: recommendations from the TIGER Collaborative. [Online] nd. [Cited: 1 Mar 2013] http://tigersummit.com/uploads/3.Tiger.Report_Competencies_final.pdf.

60. Nursing, National League for. NLN competencies for nursing education: informatics. [Online] [Cited: 1 Mar 2013] http://www.nln.org/facultyprograms/facultyresources/informatics.htm.

61. International Medical Informatics Association. Consumer health informatics. [Online] [Cited: 1 Mar 2013] http://www.imia-medinfo.org/new2/node/137.

62. Goossen W, Casey A, Juntilla K, Newbold S, Park H-A. Technical and infrastructure requirements for personal health information management systems. [book auth.] Brennan PF, Casey A, Saranto K, editors. Personal health information management, tools and strategies for citizens' engagement. Kuopio: University of Kuopio; 2009.

63. Royal College of Nursing. Personal health records and information management: helping patients, clients and parents/carers to make the most of information. [Online] 2012. [Cited: 1 Mar 2013] http://www.rcn.org.uk/__data/assets/pdf_file/0005/465458/16.12_Personal_Health_Records_Briefing_-_18_July_2012.pdf.

64. British Computer Society and Department of Health. Keeping your online health and social care records safe and secure. [Online] 2013. [Cited: 1 Mar 2013] http://www.bcs.org/category/17485.

65. Strickland E. The FDA takes on Mobile Health Apps. IEEE Spectrum. [Online] 2012. [Cited: 1 Mar 2013] http://spectrum.ieee.org/biomedical/devices/the-fda-takes-on-mobile-health-apps.

66. International Telecommunications Union. ITU-WHO Workshop produces roadmap to guide the development of global e-health standards. [Online] 2012. [Cited: 1 Mar 2013] http://www.itu.int/ITU-T/newslog/ITUWHO+Workshop+Produces+Roadmap+To+Guide+The+Development+Of+Global+Ehealth+Standards.aspx.

67. World Health Organisation. eHealth standardization and interoperability. [Online] 28 January 2013. [Cited: 8 Mar 2013] http://apps.who.int/gb/ebwha/pdf_files/EB132/B132_R8-en.pdf.

68. HIMSS. 2011 HIMSS nursing informatics workforce survey. [Online] 2011. http://himss.files.cms-plus.com/HIMSSorg/content/files/2011HIMSSNursingInformaticsWorkforceSurvey.pdf.

69. Australian Health Informatics Education Council. Health informatics: scope, careers and competencies. [Online] November 2011. [Cited: 1 Mar 2013] http://www.ahiec.org.au/docs/AHIEC_HI_Scope_Careers_and_Competencies_V1-9.pdf.

70. US Department of Health and Human Services. Competencies for Public Health Informaticians. [Online] 2009. [Cited: 1 Mar 2013] http://www.cdc.gov/informaticscompetencies/downloads/PHI_Competencies.pdf.

71. European Committee for Standardization (CEN). EN 13606–1 health informatics – electronic health record communication – part 1: reference model. Brussels: CEN; 2007.

72. Goossens W, Goossen-Baremans A, van der Zel M. Detailed clinical models: a review. Healthc Inform Res. 2010;16(4):201–14.

73. Park H-A, Min Y, Kim Y, Lee M, Lee Y. Development of detailed clinical models for nursing assessments and nursing interventions. Healthc Inform Res. 2011;17(4):244–52.

74. Park HA, Min YH, Jeon E, Chung E. Integration of evidence into a detailed clinical model-based electronic nursing record system. Healthc Inform Res. 2012;18(2):136–44.

75. Health Level 7 (HL7). Detailed clinical models. [Online] [Cited: 4 Mar 2013] http://wiki.hl7.org/index.php?title=Detailed_Clinical_Models.

76. HL7. HL7 Version 3 product suite. [Online] [Cited: 1 Mar 2013] http://www.hl7.org/implement/standards/product_brief.cfm?product_id=186.

77. HL7 Version 3 Standard: Order Set Publication, Release 1. [Online] [Cited: 4 Mar 2013] http://www.hl7.org/implement/standards/product_brief.cfm?product_id=287.
78. Department of Health and Human Services. HIPPA security series – security standards: technical safeguards. [Online] 2007. [Cited: 4 Mar 2013] http://www.hhs.gov/ocr/privacy/hipaa/administrative/securityrule/techsafeguards.pdf.
79. Information Commissioner's Office. Data protection principles. [Online] [Cited: 4 Mar 2013.] http://www.ico.gov.uk/for_organisations/data_protection/the_guide/the_principles.aspx.
80. Institute of Medicine. Health IT and patient safety: building safer systems for better care. [Online] 2011. [Cited: 8 Mar 2013] http://www.iom.edu/~/media/Files/Report%20Files/2011/Health-IT/HealthITandPatientSafetyreportbrieffinal_new.pdf.
81. Office of the National Coordinator of Health Information Technology. Health IT patient safety action & surveillance plan for public comment. [Online] 2012. [Cited: 8 Mar 2013] http://www.healthit.gov/sites/default/files/safetyplanhhspubliccomment.pdf.
82. NHS Information Standards Board for Health and Social Care. Patient safety. [Online] [Cited: 8 Mar 2013] http://www.isb.nhs.uk/use/baselines/safety.
83. NHS Wales Informatics Service. Health informatics career framework. [Online] [Cited: 8 Mar 2013] https://www.hicf.org.uk/.
84. (NASA), National Aeronautics and Space Administration. Man-systems integration standards. [Online] [Cited: 4 Mar 2013] http://msis.jsc.nasa.gov/Volume1.htm.
85. Microsoft Health. Common user interface. [Online] [Cited: 4 Mar 2013] http://www.mscui.net/.
86. Microsoft Health. Design guidance: medication line. [Online] 2009. [Cited: 4 Mar 2013] http://www.mscui.net/DesignGuide/Pdfs/Design%20Guidance%20--%20Medication%20Line.pdf.
87. National Health Service (NHS). NHS common user interface. [Online] [Cited: 4 Mar 2013] http://www.cui.nhs.uk/Pages/NHSCommonUserInterface.aspx.
88. Microsoft Health. Design guidance: date display. [Online] [Cited: 4 Mar 2013] http://www.mscui.net/DesignGuide/Pdfs/Design%20Guidance%20--%20Date%20Display.pdf.
89. International Organisation for Standardization (ISO). Cooperation with CEN (Vienna Agreement). [Online] [Cited: 4 Mar 2013] www.iso.org/iso/standards_development/processes_and_procedures/cooperation_with_cen.htm.
90. American National Standards Institute (ANSI). Introduction to ANSI. [Online] [Cited: 4 Mar 2013] www.ansi.org/about_ansi/introduction/introduction.aspx.
91. Integrating the Healthcare Enterprise (IHE). About IHE. [Online] [Cited: 4 Mar 2013] http://www.ihe.net/About/.
92. Morikawa M, Morrison J. Who develops ISO standards? A survey of participation in ISO's international standards development processes. [Online] October 2004. [Cited: 4 Mar 2013] http://www.pacinst.org/reports/iso_participation/iso_participation_study.pdf.
93. Healthcare Information Technology Standards Panel (HITSP. Welcome to www.HITSP.org. [Online] [Cited: 4 Mar 2013] http://www.hitsp.org/.
94. International Organization for Standardisation ISO. Standards catalogue TC215 health informatics. ISO. [Online] [Cited: 20 Feb 2013] http://www.iso.org/iso/home/store/catalogue_tc/home/store/catalogue_tc/home/store/catalogue_tc/catalogue_tc_browse.htm?commid=54960&published=on.
95. ISO. What are standards and how do they help? [Online] [Cited: 13 Feb 2013] http://www.iso.org/sites/ConsumersStandards/en/1-1-what-standards-context.htm.
96. International Organization for Standardization. What is conformity assessment? [Online] [Cited: 8 Mar 2013] http://www.iso.org/iso/home/about/conformity-assessment.htm.
97. European Commission. EU eHealth Interoperability Roadmap. [Online] 2010. [Cited: 4 Mar 2013] http://www.ehgi.eu/Download/European%20eHealth%20Interoperability%20Roadmap%20%5bCALLIOPE%20-%20published%20by%20DG%20INFSO%5d.pdf.
98. Hammond WE, Jaffe C, Kush RD. Healthcare standards development: the value of nurturing collaboration. J AHIMA. 2009;80(7):44–50. Available at http://library.ahima.org/xpedio/groups/public/documents/ahima/bok1_043995.hcsp?dDocName=bok1_043995.

Additional Reading

International Organization for Standardization. Glossary of terms and abbreviations. [Online] [Cited: 8 Mar 2013] http://www.iso.org/sites/ConsumersStandards/en/5-glossary-terms.htm.

National Guideline Clearinghouse. Inclusion criteria. [Online] [Cited: 20 Feb 2013] http://www.guideline.gov/about/inclusion-criteria.aspx.

Nursing, National Council of State Boards of. About NCSBN. [Online] [Cited: 20 Feb 2013] https://www.ncsbn.org/about.htm.

Agency for Health Research and Quality (AHQR). [Online] [Cited: 20 Feb 2013] http://www.ahrq.gov/.

Feild MJ, Lohr KN, editors. Clinical practice guidelines: directions for a new program. Washington, DC: National Academy Press; 1990.

ISO. TC 215 Health Informatics . [Online] [Cited: 20 Feb 2013] http://www.iso.org/iso/iso_technical_committee?commid=54960.

Kay S. Presentation and discussion by Steven Kay on usability of health informatics standards. Joint Initiative Council. [Online] October 2012. [Cited: 20 Feb 2013] http://www.jointinitiativecouncil.org/.

International Organisation for Standardisation. ISO/TS 17117:2002 health informatics – controlled health terminology – structure and high-level indicators. Geneva: ISO; 2002.

Kind A, Smith M. Documentation of mandated discharge summary components in transitions from acute to subacute care. [Online] nd. [Cited: 1 Mar 2013] http://www.ahrq.gov/downloads/pub/advances2/vol2/advances-kind_31.pdf.

Royal College of Nursing. Delegating record keeping and countersigning records. [Online] October 2012. [Cited: 1 Mar 2013] http://www.rcn.org.uk/__data/assets/pdf_file/0005/486662/004337.pdf.

College of Nurses of Ontario. Practice standard: documentation. [Online] 2008. [Cited: 1 Mar 2013] http://www.cno.org/Global/docs/prac/41001_documentation.pdf.

Hardiker NR, Casey A, Coenan A, Konicek D. Mutual enhancement of diverse terminologies. AMIA annual symposium proceedings, 2006. pp. 319–23.

Nursing and Midwifery Council. Standards of proficiency for nurse and midewife prescribers. [Online] 2006. [Cited: 1 Mar 2013] http://www.nmc-uk.org/Documents/NMC-Publications/NMC-Standards-proficiency-nurse-and-midwife-prescribers.pdf.

Eysenbach G. Consumer health informatics. Br Med J. 2000;320:1713.

European Committee for Standardization (CEN). European Standards (EN). [Online] [Cited: 4 Mar 2013] http://www.cen.eu/cen/products/en/pages/default.aspx.

Health Level 7 International (HL7). About HL7. [Online] [Cited: 4 Mar 2013] http://www.hl7.org/about/index.cfm?ref=nav.

Union, World Health Organisation and International Telecommunications. [Online]

Goossen W. Personal health records: infrastructure and standards. [book auth.] Brennan PF, Casey A, Saranto K, editors. Personal health information management, tools and strategies for citizens' engagement. Kuopio: University of Kuopio; 2009.

Chapter 8
Nursing Documentation in Digital Solutions

Sally Remus, Margaret Ann Kennedy, Breane Manson Lucas, and Tracy Forbes

Abstract The imperative of accurate and timely nursing documentation has never been higher than in contemporary professional practice. Increasingly, electronic clinical information systems (CIS) are available in practice settings across the continuum of care to record care. Electronic documentation is not simply the reproduction of paper-based records in a digital format. The design and functionality of solutions in a technology-enabled environment are critical elements to ensure ease of use, alignment to clinical processes, and the achievement of the full range of potential benefits.

Keywords Clinical Information System (CIS) • Clinical documentation • Interprofessional care teams • Point of Care (POC) • Point of Service (POS) • Workaround • Functionality • Text notes

Key Concepts

Clinical Information System (CIS)
Clinical documentation
Interprofessional care teams
Point of Care (POC)
Point of Service (POS)
Workaround
Functionality
Text notes

The online version of this chapter (doi:10.1007/978-1-4471-2999-8_8) contains supplementary material, which is available to authorized users.

S. Remus, RN, BScN, MScN (✉)
Doctoral Student, Arthur Labatt Family School of Nursing, Western University,
London, ON, Canada
e-mail: sallyremus1@gmail.com, sremus@uwo.ca.

M.A. Kennedy, RN, BScN, MN, PhD, CPHIMS-CA, PMP, PRINCE2 Practitioner
Atlantic Branch, Gevity Consulting Inc, Halifax, NS, Canada
e-mail: mkennedy@gevityinc.com

B.M. Lucas
Cerner Corporation, Kansas City, MO, USA
e-mail: Breane.Lucas@Cerner.com

T. Forbes, BComm
Gevity Consulting Inc, Vancouver, BC, Canada
e-mail: tforbes@gevityinc.com

© Springer-Verlag London 2015   145
K.J. Hannah et al. (eds.), *Introduction to Nursing Informatics*,
Health Informatics, DOI 10.1007/978-1-4471-2999-8_8

Introduction

The value, issues, and challenges with respect to nursing documentation and its quality, whether paper-based or electronic-based, have been well cited in a number of publications by nursing professionals. This chapter will address nursing documentation and the electronic solutions that support accurate and effective clinical documentation. The initial sections will examine nursing documentation as a key component of professional practice and how it contributes to patient/client care (includes individuals, families and communities), other clinical team providers, health service organizations, the nursing profession, and health system at large. The role nursing documentation plays, whether paper, electronic, or both, will also be related to the dimensions of patient safety, quality of care and health system use. Industry lessons that influence the quality of electronic nursing documentation will be highlighted within the context of health systems that continue to evolve to paperless practice settings as a result of electronic medical/patient/health record implementations. Finally, specific electronic documentation solutions will be presented as examples of clinical documentation solutions that readers may encounter in practice.

The Role and Value of Nursing Documentation

Publication findings and practice experiences yield one major theme, the central role played by nursing documentation. Specifically, it is a multi-dimensional communication tool which supports patient/client centred care, patient safety, and quality of care/service provided by the nurse and the nursing profession. From the perspective of patient safety and quality of care/service, the role of nursing documentation is intended to share relevant clinical information on behalf of the patient/client and care provided by the nurse during a shift in a typical health institution (e.g., hospital, long term care, etc.) or community based service encounter (e.g., home care, public health, primary care office, etc.). Documentation elements that address patient/client preferences position the nursing profession to achieve its accountability as patient advocates in clearly expressing the patient story. From a different perspective, the extent of the nursing process components (i.e., assessments, plans, interventions and outcomes) documented reflects the nursing care provided, and extends the utility of nursing documentation as a communication vehicle that monitors the patient/client progress and communicates with all relevant providers in the circle of care [1]. If nursing documentation clearly and concisely articulates the observations, actions and outcomes of care in a timely and accurate manner, it will accurately report the quality of service/care provided. If the quality of documentation is poor and has gaps or limited detail, it can place patients/clients, clinical providers, and health service organizations at considerable risk of physical and/or legal harm [2, 3]. If documentation fails to share essential patient/client information between nurses during a shift or service encounter hand-off to other health team members, continuity of care will be disrupted, resulting in potential harm and/or unnecessary treatment delays.

Nursing documentation's role as a multidimensional communication tool also influences the 'health' of the interprofessional care team at the departmental level, which may extend throughout the organization. Effective communications across the clinical care team can influence the 'health' of the work environment where team work and collaboration is essential in providing safe, quality patient care/services, and also if patient satisfaction will be achieved according to the IOM study, 'Keeping patient's safe: Transforming the work environment of nurses' ([4], p2008) Emphasis is placed on 'healthy work environments' (HWE) by provider organizations today, ensuring that quality, healing work environments are created to support staff retention and recruitment trends. Further, positive work environments with 'happy', motivated staff are strongly associated with positive patient satisfaction results, safe patient care and quality outcomes, and professional work satisfaction [5, 6]. The latter demonstrates a different lens of the multidimensional role played by nursing documentation. Further impacts may be realized across organizational teams as well as vertically through the administrative structures of an organization through the role of nursing documentation as expressed by the effects (positive or negative) of nurse-patient relationships, and safe, quality care provided as a result of effective inter-professional team communications and collaborations.

At a systems level, nursing accountability is another responsibility enabled though nursing documentation whether it be paper-based, electronic or both. Nursing documentation standards are established by regulatory bodies that are responsible for nursing licensure and/or registration where nurses work. In Ontario Canada, two key regulatory roles of nursing documentation include professional accountability and demonstration of nursing competencies as outlined by professional practice standards [College of Nurses of Ontario (CNO)] [1]. Professional accountability is demonstrated through the nurse's practice commitment to providing safe, effective and ethical care and the successful knowledge transfer of the care through nursing documentation in a patient/client history ([1], p3). Further, nursing documentation must demonstrate that the nurse has applied nursing knowledge, skill and judgement within a therapeutic nurse-client relationship, as required by the professional practice standards (i.e., regulatory and legislative practice requirements) ([1], p3). Although the professional practice standards in Ontario represent only one jurisdiction where nurses are registered to work, similar requirements of nursing documentation applies to most regulatory bodies' expectations across jurisdictions where nurses work.

Also, at the system level, data from nursing documentation can play a significant role and serves a number of purposes. Nursing documentation data at the system level can be and is used for four main purposes: (1) to evaluate professional practice as part of quality improvement activities, (2) to determine types of patient care/services required and/or provided, (3) to inform and advance evidence based nursing practice research and (4) to assist nurses' learning via documentation (chart) reviews (see Table 8.1) ([1], p4)

Table 8.1 Nursing documentation data purposes

Purpose	Examples
Evaluate professional practice as part of quality improvement processes	Informs/maintains: – Regulatory practice standards & guidelines – Organizational professional practice policy & procedures – Decision support tools required at POS
Determine types of care/ services required or provided	Informs jurisdictional health human resource strategies
	Facilitates the visibility of nursing contributions through nursing documentation data
	Informs the visibility of patient outcomes through nursing documentation data
	Informs and innovates healthcare delivery models
Inform and advance evidence based practice research	Mining and analysis of nursing documentation content (data, information) informs nursing care research requirements
	Informs nursing decision support needs at POS
Facilitate/assist nurses' learning via chart reviews	Facilitates nursing professional development plans
	Facilitates nursing reflective practice, a regulatory accountability in ON Canada

Adapted from: Canada. College of Nurses of Ontario (CNO) [1]

The latter purposes of nursing documentation are more difficult to realize with paper-based documentation processes, where searching through volumes of unstructured, isolated health record information (facts) can yield minimal results in a timely manner, resulting in nurses not being significant users of information or even know how to use the information when available [7]. Working in an information free zone and relying on memory-based practices is a residual effect from the industrial revolution era that lingers in nursing practice but can no longer support contemporary, complex healthcare environments [7, 8]. A consequence of 'volumes of unstructured information' found in paper-based documentation practices render nursing practice contributions very difficult to detect or even invisible. Visibility of nursing's contributions through the role nursing documentation at the health system level is essential for the sustainability of the profession.

Documenting Nursing in Technology Enabled Environments

As healthcare systems forge ahead with the implementation of electronic records (includes electronic patient/medical/health records), electronic clinical documentation is replacing paper-based documentation practices. Numerous benefits have been anticipated with 'point of care' or 'point of service' (POC/POS) systems, where clinical documentation systems are the most commonly used application in health care settings [9, 10]. Electronic nursing documentation at the POS has been recognized to improve both patient care and nurse experience by facilitating nursing productivity with documentation, eliminating redundancies and inaccuracies of charted

Table 8.2 Intended roles of nursing documentation as a multidimensional communication tool

Dimension/level	Practice or process	Outcome
Health system level	Nursing accountability & Nursing competencies	Informs & maintains currency of regulatory practice standards across jurisdictions
	Nursing documentation standards	Facilitates a common communication standard or clinical language
		Informs nursing health human resource strategy across jurisdictions
		Informs care coordination across the continuum of care (i.e., health systems)
Organizational-departmental level	Nursing documentation standards	Facilitates a common communication standard or language across the inter-professional team
	Care coordination and communications across the intra & inter disciplinary teams	Facilitates 'seamless' shift or service encounter hand-offs
		Facilitates healthy work environments – staff retention/recruitment & professional work satisfaction
Patient-client level	Nursing documentation standards	Clearly conveys care/service provided & patient/client story
	Nursing accountability	Advocates preferences on behalf of the patient/client
		– Facilitates patient satisfaction when nurses are better informed

information, improving timely access to data/information, and expediting interprofessional team communications [9, 11]. In addition, the 'quality' of completeness in electronic nursing notes has been demonstrated to improve the effectiveness and quality of the nursing visit from both a patient and nursing perspective [12].

Many assume that transitioning to electronic documentation practices automatically equates with success in achieving the intended roles of nursing documentation at the patient-client, organizational-departmental, and/or health system levels. Specifically, assumptions relate to documentation being able to: convey the quality of service/care provided, advocate patient-client preferences, facilitate 'seamless' care coordination by the interprofessional team, meet professional accountability requirements, and so forth. Table 8.2 highlights the aforementioned intended roles of effective electronic nursing documentation systems as a multidimensional communication tool at each dimension (i.e., patient-client, organizational-departmental and health system levels) with select practices/processes and aligned outcomes.

However, the success of achieving the intended roles with electronic clinical documentation systems involves a number of other considerations that will influence its success. Factors such as system design, system functionality, nursing computer proficiencies and nursing competencies (skills/knowledge) can result in both strengths and weaknesses in executing the process of nursing documentation. Effective design of electronic nursing documentation systems is a key consideration. The design of electronic nursing documentation system templates are critical if a 'user friendly interface' between the nurse and electronic documentation system will support clinician 'usability' as intended and successful adoption. Does the design of the electronic templates align with clinical assessment cognitive workflows? Specifically, does the data captured on the template align/resonate with the way clinicians think and document when performing patient/client clinical assessments, interventions, etc.? When electronic documentation applications fail to reflect or facilitate clinical practice (i.e. process) workflows or the priorities of clinicians for documentation, clinicians can develop some creative approaches (i.e. "workarounds") to documenting the care provided despite the limitations of the application. Such "workarounds" will be created when electronic documentation applications do not reflect professional values or workflow [13]. Adler, Manager of Practice Standards describes Varpio's system "workaround" phenomena as a "conflict" between the nurse and the electronic documentation system. Such conflicts arise when nurses cannot perform (document) adequately what is necessary to meet professional regulatory practice mandates ([14], p18).

System "workarounds" may be revealed when clinicians do not leverage the electronic tools as designed, which has consequences in achieving the intended benefits (e.g. improve patient safety, outcomes, team communications) when converting from paper to electronic nursing documentation. Workarounds may include not using the standard electronic template features (e.g. drop down menus, radio buttons) to select standard data elements in electronically documented nursing entries. Instead, nurses opt to document electronic assessments via text box entries or as text notes which mimics traditional paper based documentation processes and generates clinical data that is considered "unstructured" and not codified. The text note workarounds that model traditional paper-based documentation practices result in nursing data that is not readily available to be electronically 'mined' for analysis, losing one of the key advantages of electronic documentation tools. Here, relevant patient information at the point of care will not be easily accessible to the interdisciplinary team for timely, clinical decision-making. An additional consequence of text based workarounds impacts nursing productivity with timely nursing documentation and impacts the ability to clearly communicate the patient's story and/or condition potentially affecting effective communications, patient safety and outcomes. To avoid these workaround pitfalls, Adler ([14], p18) indicates that contemporary regulatory standards of practice need to direct new nursing responsibilities/accountabilities with electronic documentation systems. Specifically, nurses must assume expanded advocacy roles in practice settings where involvement in choosing, implementing, and evaluating new electronic documentation systems is essential. Thus, documentation system design would more likely conform to practice policies and support quality nursing care ([14], p18). Further, active nursing participation in system selection, implementation and evaluation will facilitate successful adoption where the system features are leveraged as intended.

Documentation design surrounding content or data elements embedded in the electronic templates is a controversial topic. Numerous authors [13, 15] point out that the anticipated benefits of electronic clinical documentation may never be realized for those documentation applications developed without gaining an in-depth understanding of the use of paper-based documentation or the importance of oral and paper-based communications. Specifically, tensions can be created during electronic documentation design sessions between traditional professional practice leaders and nurse informaticians and/or clinical informaticians when data elements and content design decisions are being made. Such tensions can be even more pronounced when such design teams lack an informatics resource and the professional practice leaders are left to design system applications with only technical resources that lack any clinical knowledge or experience. Also, the tendency of many design teams is to duplicate existing paper documentation forms in the design/build of electronic documentation applications, which once implemented, are minimally used with limited documentation value. If efficiencies and successes of documentation benefits are to be realized, then conversion from paper-based documentation tools to electronic documentation (eDoc) must be recognized as more than mere replication of paper forms into an electronic format [16, 17]. To avoid the latter content design pitfalls and ensure that key episodic or unresolved patient issue data is "surfaced" for quick identification and follow up, it would benefit organizations to understand, value, and embrace the role of skilled nurse informatician (NI) resources to lead, partner, and guide documentation system design decisions with professional practice and technical resources. Healthcare trends leveraging NI resources are demonstrating successful system designs and implementations [8, 18].

Electronic documentation design that incorporates recognized/approved standardized nursing languages (e.g. ICNP – International Classification of Nursing Practice, C- HOBIC – Canadian Health Outcomes for Better Information and Care) enables nurses to more easily access, search, and view relevant interpretable patient information to make informed care decisions across the inter professional team. See Chap, 7 for a more in depth discussion of standards and standardized nursing languages. Enabling clear, succinct, and legible electronic documentation reduces the risk of misunderstanding, and improves patient outcomes as a result of effective communications [2].

Extending the use of standardized nursing languages in electronic nursing documentation tools across jurisdictions (i.e., in electronic health records) has the potential to generate health system level benefits from three perspectives. First, it facilitates patient centred care, as relevant health information follows the patient/client and is accessible across the continuum of care wherever care is provided. Patients/clients are no longer required to rely on memory for sharing important information (e.g. allergies, medications, etc.), and this enables consistent, accurate information that is captured once and used many times. Second, use of standardized languages demonstrates nursing professional practice's accountability in the delivery of care and third, it enhances the 'visibility' of nursing's contributions through electronic documentation. With nursing standardized languages embedded in electronic documentation tools, nurses can be freed up to focus on their work, and data can be captured demonstrating nursing's effectiveness, contributions and accountability. This also supports accurately attributing nursing actions and outcomes to nursing rather than to other professions, and enables accurate cost analysis of nursing [3, 19]. Without standardized languages embedded in electronic documentation tools, nursing will never realize the advantages of the EHR at the system level, namely having relevant patient information at the point of care, real-time decision support, and or computer generated nursing data that is evidenced-based [20].

Functionality in Nursing Documentation

System design features or available functionality (e.g. copy/paste, structured drop down menus, data carry forward features) available in nursing documentation applications/tools, which are not found in paper documents, can have both positive and negative impacts in electronic documentation. The investigation by Pare et al. [12] reveals numerous positive impacts at the nurse-patient level with the introduction of an electronic documentation tool across various community health centres. Results included nursing satisfaction related to ease of adapting to a new system, perceived value of electronic documentation as a useful "clinical tool" (with features/functionalities), not a "computer tool", and perceived value in how this clinical tool improved the care provided through its clinical content. Specifically, the electronic documentation application fostered a structured approach to nurses' reasoning, resulting in nursing documentation that was more complete and consistent. In fact, nurses no longer viewed their patient interventions as prescribed tasks (e.g., vital signs, dressing changes, etc.) but reported a focused view on their patient holistically. This supported both quality and care continuity across multiple provider visits and was identified as a benefit by the patients themselves ([12], p15–16).

On the contrary, author experiences suggest that the new electronic system features coupled with the experience and/or proficiency of the nurse user (i.e. skills/ knowledge – novice versus expert, computer skills, etc.) can affect the quality of the electronic documentation. Current healthcare is staffed with multiple generations of nurses, ranging from the new 'millennials' (20-somethings) who have grown up with technology and are considered to be 'tech savvy' to more experienced nurses (baby boomers) who have extensive clinical expertise but may lack computer proficiencies and/or confidence required to effectively leverage the electronic documentation tools as designed or intended. According to Nemeth et al. (2006) as cited in Kelley et al. ([15], p155), these system features may alter how nurses document, make decisions and/or communicate with other caregivers, potentially impacting the quality of care. Quality of care measured by nursing outcomes, and ensuring patient safety is a cornerstone of good electronic documentation and an essential nursing accountability as a professional regulatory requirement. However, insufficient evidence is available today with how system features/functionality, system content design of electronic clinical documentation tools, and/or user characteristics' influence the intended roles of electronic clinical documentation [9, 15].

Clinical Documentation Interfaces

This next section presents some of the common clinical or nursing documentation applications. Nurses, depending on their practice setting will encounter a variety of solutions in acute care, community health and public health. It is important to note that clinical applications are distinct in terms of their functionality and interfaces and are designed to support the specific clinical needs (or business needs) of the domain in which they are used. Although there are many vendors and applications available, it is beyond the scope of this text to include all possible options.

The following examples are presented as known credible documentation applications and no endorsement over other applications is intended by their inclusion.

Cerner Solutions – An Integrated Clinical Environment

Cerner has completely automated the acute care nursing workflow with the solutions described below. From the time the nurse receives a patient assignment for their shift, he or she can review the patient's medical record, document a head-to-toe assessment, leverage medical device integration, begin a nursing care plan, and safely administer medications to efficiently discharge patients – all while improving the outcomes of the patient population.

Cerner's Power Chart: Advanced Care Documentation

Advanced Care Documentation (Fig. 8.1) provides the patient chart for clinicians in a centralized location to access activities, view patient data, update orders, and receive important notifications, such as new orders or new results. The clinician's care process works as a seamless flow of information with an integrated system [21].

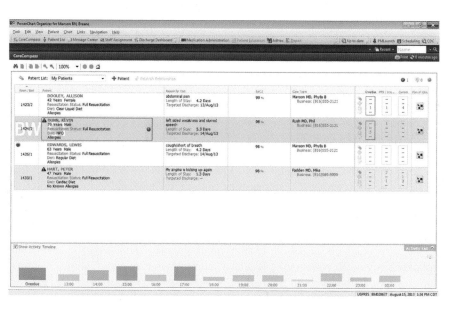

Fig. 8.1 Advanced Care Documentation

Key benefits include:

- Increases efficiency by automatically populating orders and results [21]
- "Improve outcomes by making decisions based on patient information from a single source of truth" [21]
- Medical device integration with the electronic medical record to review clinical data in the patient record [21]

CareCompass, is the home base that provides 80 % of the information clinicians need with the rest of the information only a single click away. It is the clinician's patient assignment for the day. *CareCompass* guides the clinicians and nurse managers in the organization, planning and prioritization of patient care [22] and:

- Provides Single and Multi Patient summary views
- Provides Summary Driven Workflows
- Presents clinicians with relative information through Push technology rather than memory-based information
- Captures patient information once and leverages it elsewhere
- Tells the comprehensive patient story allowing for better communication and safer patient handoffs

Start on the left of the screen to begin navigation. The nurse can easily determine where the patient is and any information needed, such as isolation status, before going into the room. *CareCompass* also displays who the patient is and "up front" information that the nurse needs to know all the time – Resuscitation status, diet, and allergies [22]. The middle of the screen displays why the patient is hospitalized, the expected date of discharge, their level of acuity, and who is caring for them. On the right side of the screen is where the nurse needs to go next. Along the bottom of the screen is an indication of what a rolling 12 h of the nurse's day looks like or how busy the nurse will be. Hovering over this section will display details across the assigned patients regarding the activities that are coming up.

It is a "cheat sheet" or summary, updated in real time that enables clinicians to obtain complete, accurate and up-to-date alerts (see Fig. 8.2), orders, abnormal lab values, and other information on their assigned patients. It is the 'who, what, when, where and why' of the nurse's assigned patients – utilizing both multi-patient and single patient views (see Fig. 8.3).

There are many places to go within the chart. In reality, clinicians only go to 4–5 places in the record on a regular basis. Quick access is provided to the places that clinicians go most frequently so that they can quickly navigate from a 10,000-foot view to a 1,000 foot view of a patient. With one click in the *CareCompass,* the nurse can see the Inpatient Summary.

The view in Fig. 8.4 brings all clinical information (labs, vital signs, orders, quality measures) face up for the clinician to quickly access and obtain a status update (tells the story of the patient) [3]. It is also actionable, so the nurse can place orders, document vital signs, and update patient problems directly from this view [23].

Flowsheet documentation improves outcomes by supporting clinical reasoning and critical thinking. This is based on accessible patient information and the ability to view information across time so the nurse can see trends developing, how the

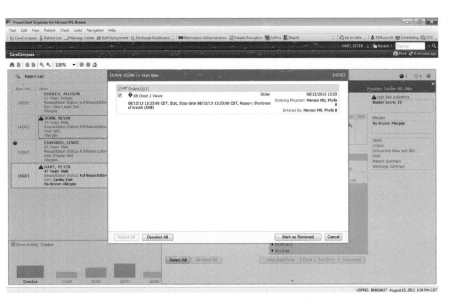

Fig. 8.2 CareCompass "cheat sheet" or summary, updated in real time that enables clinicians to obtain complete, accurate and up-to-date alerts, orders, abnormal lab values, and other information on their assigned patients

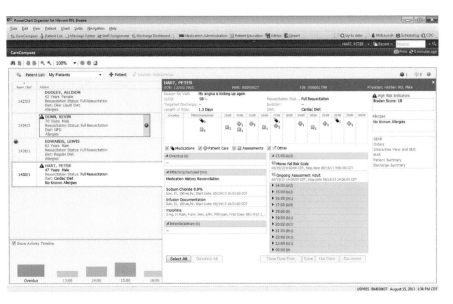

Fig. 8.3 CareCompass 'who, what, when, where and why' of the nurse's assigned patients – utilizing both multi-patient and single patient views

patient is progressing or not progressing, which will further enable proactive patient care. It provides the capability for clinicians to review clinical data from medical devices directly into the patient record, for example, vital signs (Fig. 8.5), ventilators,

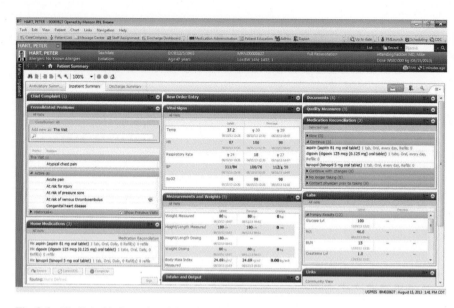

Fig. 8.4 All clinical information (labs, vital signs, orders, quality measures) face up for the clinician to quickly access and obtain a status update (tells the story of the patient)

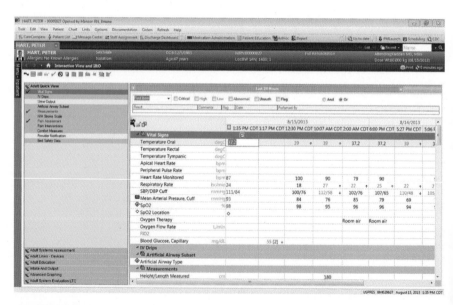

Fig. 8.5 Flowsheet documentation provides the capability for clinicians to review clinical data from medical devices directly into the patient record, for example, vital signs ventilators, beds, and infusion pumps

beds, and infusion pumps. The clinician documents head-to-toe assessments (Figs. 8.6, 8.7, and 8.8), lines, wounds, tubes and drains, patient education, input and output, and also has the ability to see patient data in a graphical view. Clinical

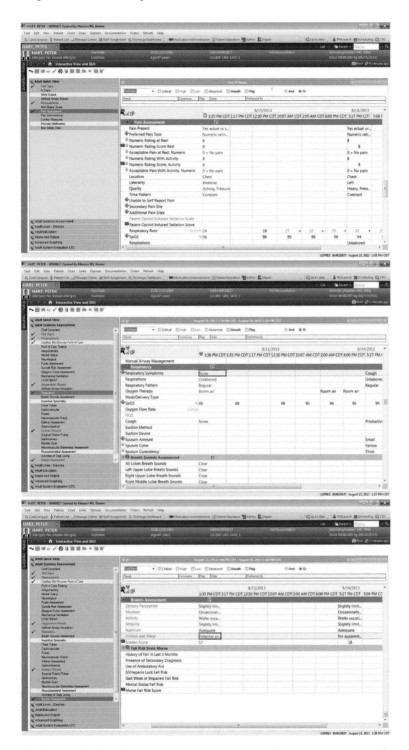

Figs. 8.6, 8.7, and 8.8 The clinician documents head-to-toe assessments, lines, wounds, tubes and drains, patient education, input and output, and also has the ability to see patient data in a graphical view

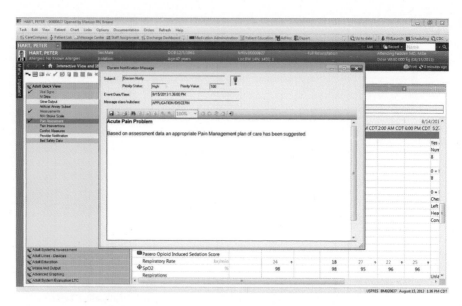

Fig. 8.9 Clinical Decision Support and Evidence Based Practice Nursing Care Plans help health care facilities deliver the highest quality of care by preventing and managing conditions such as pain, pressure ulcers and falls

Decision Support and Evidence Based Practice Nursing Care Plans (Fig. 8.9) help health care facilities deliver the highest quality of care by preventing and managing conditions such as pain, pressure ulcers and falls (Figs. 8.10 and 8.11) [24].

The benefits of Clinical Decision Support and care plans include the following [24]:

- "Leverage technology and data to improve outcomes"
- "Improve patient safety and care quality"
- Increase return on investment and reduce costs
- "Access the latest evidence at the point of care via order sets, plans of care, alerts and notifications, and documentation"
- "Identify patients at risk and provide consistent, cost-effective treatment"
- "Achieve and sustain performance improvement"

The nurse uses the eMAR (Medication Administration Record) to view and document all active medications and "as necessary" (PRN) response activities for a specific patient (Figs. 8.12 and 8.13). To safely and accurately administer medications by verifying the "five rights" (right patient, right drug, right dose, right route, right time), clinicians can use barcode scanning for positive patient identity at the bedside.

The discharge process can be daunting and time consuming; the primary objective of the *Discharge Summary* and *Discharge Readiness Dashboard* is to streamline the discharge workflow for clinicians (Fig. 8.14) [25]. The *Discharge Summary* is an interdisciplinary "checklist" of everything that has been done and remains

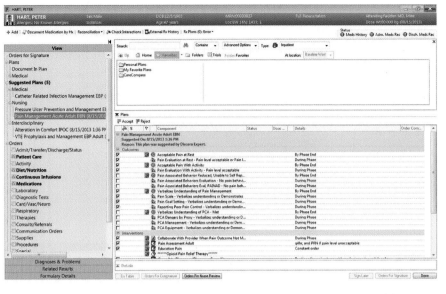

Fig. 8.10 Clinical Decision Support and Evidence Based Practice Nursing Care Plans help health care facilities deliver the highest quality of care by preventing and managing conditions such as pain, pressure ulcers and falls

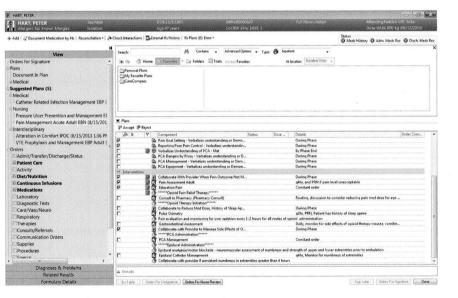

Fig. 8.11 Clinical Decision Support and Evidence Based Practice Nursing Care Plans help health care facilities deliver the highest quality of care by preventing and managing conditions such as pain, pressure ulcers and falls

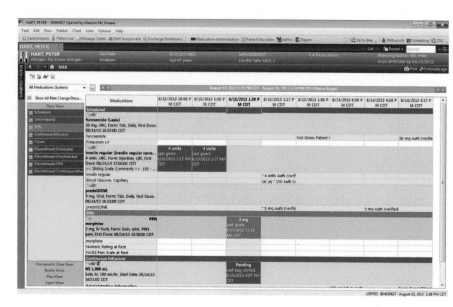

Fig. 8.12 The nurse uses the eMAR (Medication Administration Record) to view and document all active medications and "as necessary" (PRN) response activities for a specific patient

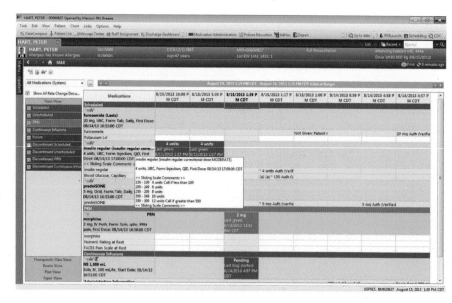

Fig. 8.13 The nurse uses the eMAR (Medication Administration Record) to view and document all active medications and "as necessary" (PRN) response activities for a specific patient

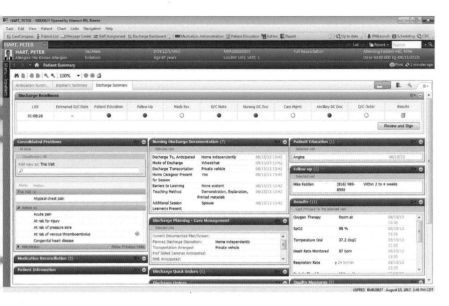

Fig. 8.14 The discharge process can be daunting and time consuming; the primary objective of the *Discharge Summary* and *Discharge Readiness Dashboard* is to streamline the discharge work flow for clinicians

pending on the date the nurse received the discharge order from the provider. It presents a patient-specific view of detailed information regarding the components pertinent to discharge. "Clinicians can add documentation, add a discharge order, and link to the "add" modules within the chart" [25].

The unit view of the *Discharge Readiness Dashboard* provides clinicians with a view of patients' progress toward discharge – including whether or not a discharge order (or pending discharge order) has been placed, as well as other key steps including Medication Reconciliation, Patient Education, and Follow-up appointments for all patients (Fig. 8.15). This is a highly effective interactive dashboard for nurse managers and case managers that are focused on having timely discharges.

The following video shares user experiences by nursing staff at the Truman Medical Centre: http://www.youtube.com/watch?v=O7Z8BCdN9_A&feature=youtu.be

Siemen's Soarian Clinicals

Figures 8.16, 8.17, and 8.18 provide an alternate approach to nursing documentation in acute care using the C-HOBIC Tool, embedded in the Siemen's Soarian interface.

Discharge Dashboard
Discharge Readiness
Patient List: My Patients
Patient Name
Length of stay (DD:HH:MM)
Estimated Discharge Date
D/C Order
Dx
Patient Education
Follow-Up
Meds Rec
D/C Note
Nursing DC Doc
Care Mgmt
QM
Ancillary DC Doc
Results
HART, PETER
Male 47 Years
1433/1
01:08:27
EDWARDS, LEWIS
Male 63 Years
1426/1
04:05:41
08/14/2013
DUNN, KEVIN
Male 70 Years
1424/2
05:06:46
08/14/2013
DOOLEY, ALLISON
Female 42 Years
1423/2
04:05:45
08/13/2013

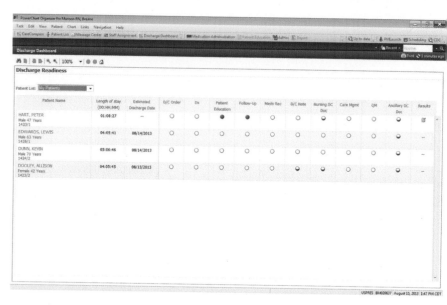

Fig. 8.15 The unit view of the *Discharge Readiness Dashboard* provides clinicians with a view of patients' progress toward discharge – including whether or not a discharge order (or pending discharge order) has been placed, as well as other key steps including Medication Reconciliation, Patient Education, and Follow-up appointments for all patients

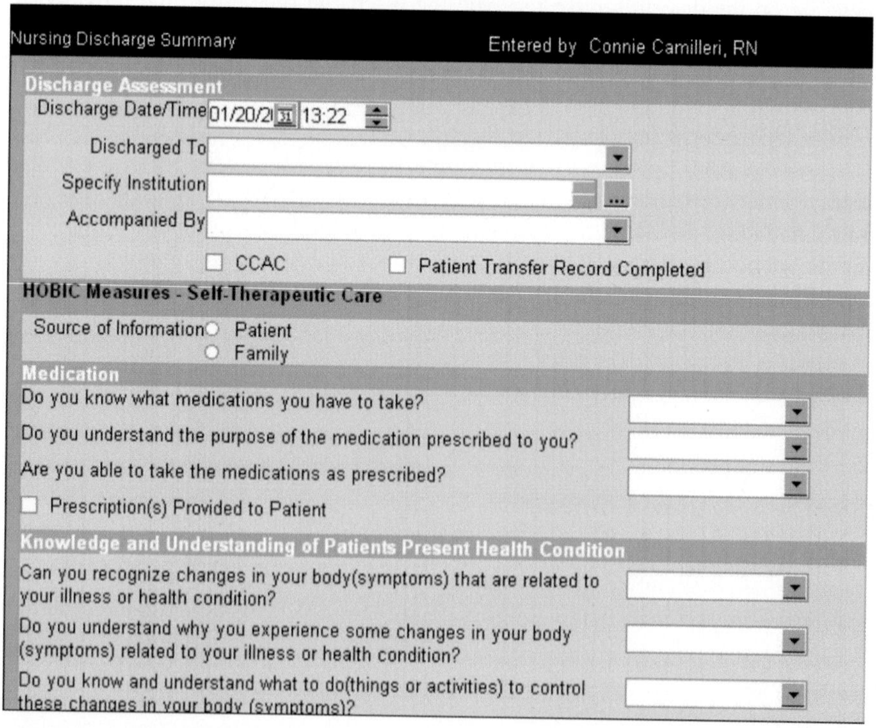

Nursing Discharge Summary
Entered by Connie Camilleri, RN
Discharge Assessment
Discharge Date/Time 01/20/2 13:22
Discharged To
Specify Institution
Accompanied By
CCAC
Patient Transfer Record Completed
HOBIC Measures - Self-Therapeutic Care
Source of Information
Patient
Family
Medication
Do you know what medications you have to take?
Do you understand the purpose of the medication prescribed to you?
Are you able to take the medications as prescribed?
Prescription(s) Provided to Patient
Knowledge and Understanding of Patients Present Health Condition
Can you recognize changes in your body(symptoms) that are related to your illness or health condition?
Do you understand why you experience some changes in your body (symptoms) related to your illness or health condition?
Do you know and understand what to do(things or activities) to control these changes in your body (symptoms)?

Fig. 8.16 Nursing admission assessment: HOBIC measure – therapeutic self-care (Courtesy of St Michael's Hospital, Toronto, ON Canada: cited in White and Remus [26])

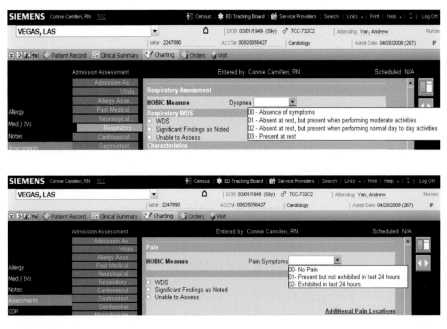

Fig. 8.17 Nursing admission assessment: HOBIC measures – dyspnea & pain (Courtesy of St Michael's Hospital, Toronto, ON Canada: cited in White and Remus [25])

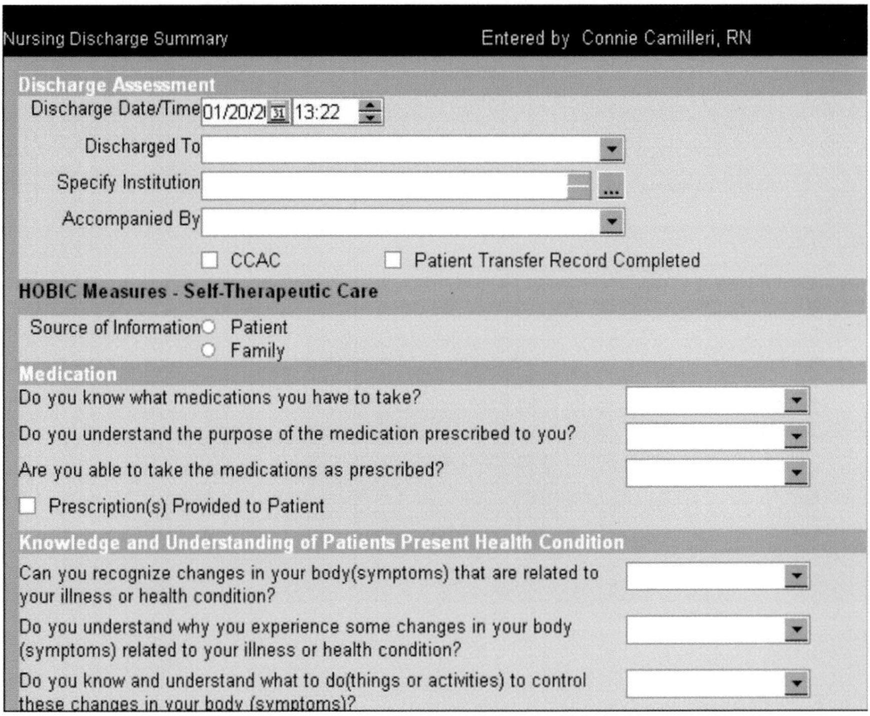

Fig. 8.18 Nursing discharge summary: HOBIC measures (Courtesy of St Michael's Hospital, Toronto, ON Canada: cited in White and Remus [25])

Panorama – a Public Heath Surveillance Application

An example of a clinical information system or clinical application outside of acute care is a public health surveillance solution. Public health professionals need an operational support system to help manage day-to-day public health responsibilities and effectively detect and manage health problems such as SARS, tuberculosis, influenza, and other communicable diseases that may pose an outbreak threat.

The IBM Public Health Solution for Disease Surveillance and Management, or Public Health SDSM application was designed by IBM Canada in partnership with Canada's public health professionals to meet these specific needs. In Canada, the official name of this solution is Panorama.

Panorama supports public health's unique requirement to accommodate both population and single clients for managed care. Public health also needs to monitor and collect data from many health care systems, in order to fulfill their program mandates. Panorama supports the exchange and interface with feeder systems such as physician offices and laboratories, and also acts as a provincial repository or data storage mechanism for specific areas where public health is the source of truth – such as Immunization Registries.

Initially designed and developed for implementation and use by provincial and territorial jurisdictions across Canada, Panorama is available globally. It provides public health professionals with integrated tools that assist in monitoring, managing, and reporting on public health (see Fig. 8.19). Both front-line service providers and public health decision makers have access to critical information through a centralized data repository. This improves client and population health outcomes, resulting in cost savings.

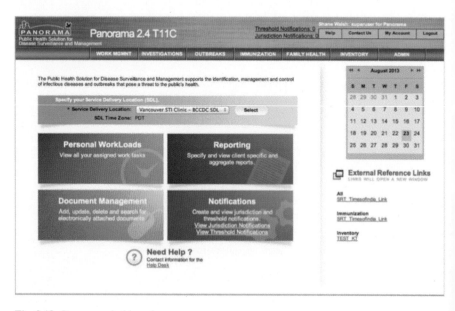

Fig. 8.19 Panorama dashboard

Panorama is a comprehensive, integrated public health information system that will help public health professionals work together to efficiently manage individual cases, outbreaks, immunizations, and vaccine inventories. Unique characteristics of Panorama include:

- Protects public health through the prevention, detection and management of communicable disease occurrences
- Enables collaboration (interoperability)
- Follows industry communication tools and terminology standards (Web services, HL7, SNOMED CT)
- Modules can be implemented separately or together
- Enables role-based access to personal health information and client records, according to the specific responsibilities of the clinician's official employment role

The Panorama Solution is organized into seven major components or "modules", which reflect the clinical priorities in public health.

1. Communicable disease Investigations management
2. Outbreak management
3. Immunization management
4. Family Health
5. Materials/ vaccine inventory management
6. Notifications Management (eReferral)
7. Work Management (Task Management)

Shared Services are those services that are available to all modules or underlying services to all modules. They are divided into four main categories: Technical Services, Domain Services, User Services and Domain UI (user interface) Services.
Some examples of Panorama's shared services are:

1. Domain UI Services

   (a) Recent Work
   (b) UI Context
   (c) Left Navigation

2. Domain Services

   (a) Issue Management
   (b) Audit
   (c) Logging

3. Technical Services

   (a) Batch Scheduler

4. User Services

   (a) Geocoding
   (b) Mapping
   (c) TypeAhead

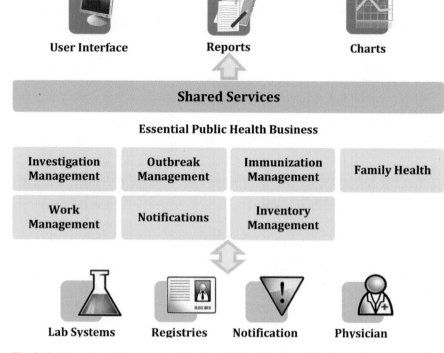

Fig. 8.20 Overview of Panorama application showing 7 key modules, integration opportunities, and shared services

This can also include items such as Clinical Notes, Document Management, and Reports. Once a client is registered in Panorama, the clinician can update and add to the record without having to enter data in each module, ensuring consistent, accurate, and timely health information (Fig. 8.20).

Panorama's Seven Key Modules

Panorama delivers the tools to manage individual outcomes while monitoring and assessing the population's health. The complexity of this architecture is balanced across seven distinct but integrated modules that work seamlessly to provide public health clinicians with the full scope of their information needs. Using a single integrated dashboard, the clinician is able to select the appropriate module and engage with the data as necessary.

As noted, Panorama uses role–based access to provide authorized clinicians with the appropriate access to personal health information, aggregate information, and functionality supporting their specific role. This also means that some clinicians, dependent on their specific role, will not have access to all seven modules – but only to those relevant to the work within their formal role and job description. For example, a community health nurse (CHN) in a family health clinic would not require access to the investigations or outbreak management modules. Access to these modules would be limited to the clinician who is formally responsible for following up on communicable disease contacts and outbreak management.

Investigations

Investigation Management provides tools for public health professionals to identify, investigate, and manage cases and contacts of communicable diseases. It provides a longitudinal view of the public health record of a client or non-human subject and is designed to act like an "index file" by providing summary information with the ability to "drill down" for additional detail. These tools help contain a disease event and reduce risk to the public (Fig. 8.21).

Outbreak Management

Outbreak Management supports the needs of investigation, monitoring, management, analysis, and reporting of communicable disease outbreaks at both the client support and surveillance levels. Outbreaks can include a combination of clinical investigations and aggregate counts of unidentified people infected with the disease (Figs. 8.22 and 8.23).

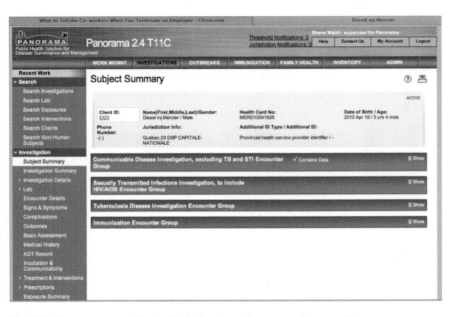

Fig. 8.21 Summary screen: longitudinal view for a client or non-human subject

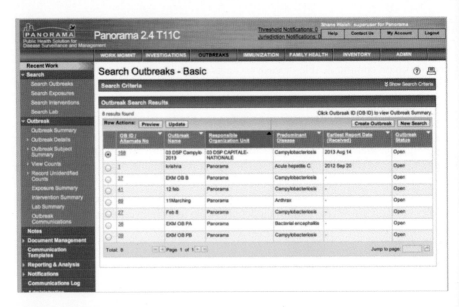

Fig. 8.22 Outbreak management

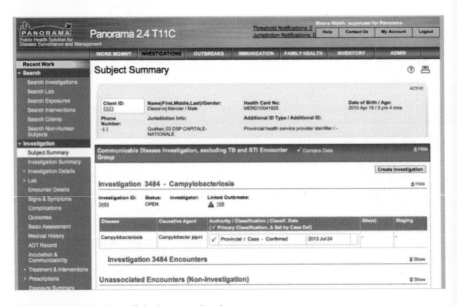

Fig. 8.23 Individual case linked to an outbreak

Immunization Management

Immunization Management provides tools required to create and manage immunization schedules and determine eligibility to produce a forecast. This component assists users in planning, delivering, and keeping track of individual and mass

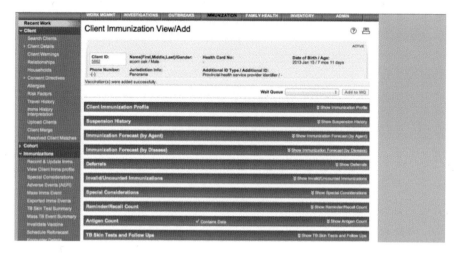

Fig. 8.24 Immunization management

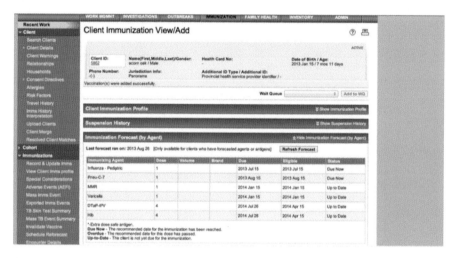

Fig. 8.25 Immunization forecast by vaccine agent

immunization events. It also includes the ability to capture adverse reactions, precautions, contraindications, and exemptions, and evaluate immunization coverage for a population (Figs. 8.24 and 8.25).

Inventory Management

Inventory Management helps to maintain appropriate levels of vaccine and other materials at locations where they are needed. By improving distribution and the process of identifying aging product, vaccine wastage is reduced. This component

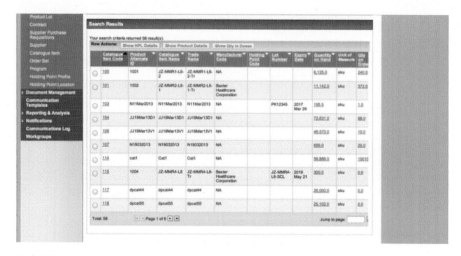

Fig. 8.26 Inventory-view vaccine

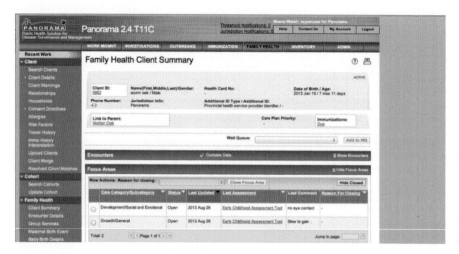

Fig. 8.27 Family health screening results

manages vaccine and supply inventories, supports vaccine cold chain maintenance, and supports sharing and transfer of vaccine in the case of an outbreak (Fig. 8.26).

Family Health

Family Health supports a single record for multidisciplinary holistic care of mother and baby. It is a comprehensive primary care record with customized screening, assessment and long-term care planning tools (Fig. 8.27).

Notification Management

Notifications Management provides three types of notifications to support the communication needs of public health professionals:

- Jurisdictional notifications are unstructured messages that can be created and posted to a specified group.
- Threshold notifications are system-generated messages to specific users or groups when a particular set of rules is met (for example, inventory level, number of TB cases). Users can create and edit threshold notifications within a jurisdiction to monitor any change or addition of data over a defined period.
- Client warnings serve for the protection of the client. For example, noting drug allergies, or for the public health worker, potential client site visit risks such as aggressive dogs.

Work Management

Work Management helps to ensure the quality and effectiveness of the business processes for the analysis and management of investigations, outbreaks, and immunization. Users can electronically manage the allocation of work, and monitor the status of tasks.

Key Features and Benefits

A variety of benefits may be achieved through the use of a health information system in public health, particularly since many public health systems lack a comprehensive, integrated health information management system. Panorama offers a number of specific benefits that enhance the clinician's ability to delivery services, and include:

- Powerful case management capabilities to communicate with laboratory systems
- Sophisticated filtering and analytical tools
- Outbreak management tools to detect, manage, and analyze incidence of a particular disease beyond what is expected for a particular time and place
- Strong immunization management capabilities for immunization recording, scheduling, reporting of adverse events and reminder recalls
- Extensive supply chain management capabilities for vaccines and related materials
- Family health management component summarizes all non-disease related health activity including primary care and planning management
- Solution can be deployed as a suite or by individual module
- Multi-language support
- Predefined ad hoc reporting capabilities to enable extraction and analysis of data

- Designed to be highly interoperable and to integrate with other health systems (such as client and provider registries, lab systems, EMR etc.).
- Follows latest industry standards such as HL7 messaging and SNOMED
- Multi-platform support

High-Level Application Benefits

As a by-product of public health staff using Panorama to manage their day to day work, aggregated, non-nominal information is available real time, to inform future planning of the public health business continuum in order to provide:

- Improved population immunization coverage that prevents occurrence of communicable diseases
- Improved adverse events reporting and follow up
- Earlier detection of communicable disease outbreaks
- Improved management of cases and contacts
- Improved capacity to respond to communicable diseases through more efficient use of public health resources
- Reduced vaccine spoilage costs
- Improved productivity of front line public health workers
- Improved management and reporting reduces the risk of potential trade and travel advisories that can have dramatic economic impacts
- Improved productivity and effectiveness though central work management and client records

Additional Benefits

Panorama has solved other complex public health policy problems such as medical terminology management, user-defined assessment tools, and complex privacy and consent management requirements that have either been missing from the public health users application toolkit prior to Panorama, or else so manual and labour intensive, often involving significant duplication of effort and data, with it's corresponding impact on timeliness and quality, that is becomes very costly to support and manage.

Panorama's fundamental goal was to improve public health around communicable diseases. The pan-Canadian stakeholders identified seven major outcomes expected of the solution. Panorama is able to deliver on all seven:

1. Appropriate immunization puts up firewalls to the spread of disease. Factors that have to be taken into account include concentration of population, groups at risk such as aboriginal populations and likely vectors of transmission.
2. Many people are allergic to vaccines or the preservatives used within them. Identifying those allergies before vaccination to avoid negative impacts, and managing the impacts when they inevitably occur reduces resistance to immunization. This substantially increases the benefits of immunization programs.

3. Communicable diseases are detected through direct observation of symptoms, analysis of exposures and through lab results. Ensuring that this information is available as soon as possible and as completely as possible to primary care providers and outbreak management teams can enable outbreaks to be significantly reduced in intensity and duration through aggressive interventions such as boil water advisories, quarantine and isolation and appropriate treatment.
4. An infected person can travel broadly and quickly in today's global economy. Witness the lawyer who traveled from the United States to Paris while infected with multi-drug resistant tuberculosis. Tracking down his contacts required the plane crew and passenger manifest, hotel service staff and family members be identified and contacted quickly. Efficiency in contact management and in managing the investigations that result can be invaluable in large-scale epidemics. During SARS, stacks of paper reached ever higher in Toronto.
5. Rapid dissemination of lab results and appropriate interventions can mean that newly exposed people and populations can be diagnosed and treated quickly. Rapid action can substantially reduce the death toll from a major outbreak. Note – morbidity refers to the relative incidence of a particular disease
6. Major outbreaks will more than consume the average country's limited public health specific staff, and rapidly encroach on private health care staff. Making the most efficient use of the constrained human resources available maximizes both the ability to respond to the outbreak, and the ability to continue to provide primary care around other health concerns.
7. Robust tracking and management can substantially reduce the death toll from a major outbreak. Note – morbidity refers to the relative incidence of a particular disease.

Improving Practice Systems

The application provides the following functional improvements and advantages over today's public health practice systems (both computer-based and human practices):

- Built-in functionality to assist health care professionals in forecasting Immunizations, determining vaccination needs, and validating immunization records
- Case classifications through use of automated case definitions
- Inventory tracking to the local level with automatic decrement by immunization for real-time tracking
- Integrated communications and work management
- Business intelligence: in-application reports for typical public health information needs including Immunization Coverage Reports and Immunization Reminders and aggregated notifiable disease exposures, counts and age and sex distribution
- Ad hoc reporting and data extract tools
- Designed to meet the needs of a region, province, state or country using a single shared database instance – one client, one record.

Flexibility

Panorama consolidates the needs of public health professionals into a single Web-based application with a flexible design that can evolve with public health practice, policy, and research. The system also offers a high degree of configuration options and multilingual support.

A key application component is the availability of user-defined forms (UDFs). This feature provides a way for users to enter unique information into the system using data collection forms to meet jurisdictional, program (for example, early childhood, newborn and post partum, and audiology) and situational (for example, outbreak) needs. There is no need to wait for a version release of the application, in order to managed reporting and Business Intelligence requirements. Authorized users may refine or update existing in-application reports, case questionnaires or screening tools, in real time so that users of the application are always using the most up to date versions that reflect the business needs. In addition, Panorama has a Universe for those with appropriate permissions, to allow the creation of ad hoc reports and extract data using SAP Business Object Universes within the application.

These universes provide the capability to address any unforeseen epidemiological or legislative reporting need. The SAP Business Objects tool is an enterprise-strength query and reporting application integrated seamlessly into Panorama, that helps users ask questions about client or other data and create clear reports in an easy to use "drag and drop" manner. The results can be exported to CSV or Excel format for import into SAS, EPIINFO, or other statistical analysis tools.

Privacy

The privacy of a client's medical information can be protected in accordance with local privacy legislation. Panorama's security features enable each instance to be implemented with security settings that comply with a particular region's specific legislation.

Summary on Nursing Documentation

This chapter elaborated on the role of nursing documentation as a multidimensional communication tool, how its role serves nurses at the patient-client level, organizational level, and health system level, and how this distinct role will influence the sustainability of the nursing profession. Further, it was illustrated that the multidimensional role that nursing documentation plays will only be fully achieved through electronic nursing documentation. A variety of nursing documentation applications were provided as examples of the solutions nurses will encounter in practice. The authors note that functionality of any specific application may vary significantly based on the practice needs in the domain and nurses are necessary contributors to teams mandated to make design and build decisions or purchase decisions.

In the electronic environment, meaningful data/information will be available and actionable at the point of care to nurses and interprofessional team members across the continuum of care. Achieving this latter vision, where nurses finally having credible information to inform their care will enable the profession to be true coordinators of care and collaborators on behalf of their patients [18].

Downloads

Available from extras.springer.com:

Educational Template (PDF 89 kb)
Educational Template (PPTX 125 kb)

References

1. Canada. College of Nurses of Ontario (CNO). Practice standard: documentation, revised 2008. Toronto: The Standard of Care; 2008. pp. 1–12.
2. Blair B, Smith B. Nursing documentation: frameworks and barriers. Contemp Nurse. 2012;41(2):160–8.
3. Tornvall E, Wilhelmsson S. Nursing documentation for communicating and evaluating care. J Clin Nurs. 2008;17:2116–24.
4. Page A. Practice implications of keeping patients safe. In: Hughes R, editor. Patient safety and quality: an evidenced-based handbook for nurses. Rockville: Agency for Healthcare Research and Quality; 2008. pp. 609–20. Retrieved: www.ahrq.gov/qual/nurseshdbk/nurseshdbk.pdf.
5. Kramer M, Maguire P, Brewer B. Clinical nurses in Magnet hospitals confirm productive, healthy unit work environments. J Nurs Manag. 2011;19:5–17.
6. Maiden J. Is your work environment healthy? Nurs Manage. 2010;41(11):36–9.
7. Pringle D, Nagle L. Leadership for the information age: the time for action is now. Nurs Leadersh (Tor Ont). 2009;22(1):1–6.
8. Kennedy M, Remus S. Chief nursing information officers: key roles and competencies in effective health informatics leadership. eHealth Vancouver; 2012.
9. Waneka R, Spetz J. Hospital information technology systems' impact on nurses and nursing care. J Nurs Adm. 2010;40(12):509–14.
10. Tyler D. Administrative and clinical health information systems. In: McGonigle D, Mastrian K, editors. Nursing informatics and the foundation of knowledge. Sudbury: Jones and Bartlett; 2009. p. 205–18.
11. Hughes S. Point-of-care information systems: state of the art. In: Ball M, Hannah K, Newbold S, Douglas J, editors. Nursing informatics: where caring and technology meet. New York: Springer; 2000. p. 242–51.
12. Pare G, Moreault M, Poba-Nzaou P, Nahas G, Templier M. Mobile computing and the quality of home care nursing practice. J Telemed Telecare. 2011;17:313–7.
13. Varpio L. Electronic patient records and professional practices: a rhetorical analysis of the impact of changing media and interface design. Paper presented at London Health Sciences Centre – Nursing Professional Practice Council, London, 2005.
14. Canada. College of Nurses of Ontario (CNO). Struggling with electronic documentation. The Standard. 2012;37(1):18–9.

15. Kelley T, Brandon D, Docherty S. Electronic nursing documentation as a strategy to improve quality patient care. J Nurs Scholarsh. 2011;43(2):154–62.
16. Ball M, Hannah K, Newbold S, Douglas J, editors. Nursing informatics: where caring and technology meet. 3rd ed. New York: Springer; 2000.
17. Monegain, B. "EHR usability: A love/hate relationship." *HIMSS and Healthcare IT News* 2012;9(10): 4–6,8. Retrieved November 12, http://www.HealthcareITNews.com.
18. Remus S, Kennedy M. Innovation in transformative nursing leadership: nursing informatics competencies and roles. Nurs Leadersh (Tor Ont). 2012;25(4):14–26.
19. Remus S. RNs participating at the policy table. Canadian Nursing Informatics Association Conference – Nurses & Informatics: Transforming Healthcare, Toronto, 10 Sept 2005.
20. Lunney M, Delaney C, Duffey M. Advocating for standardized nursing languages in EHRs. J Nurs Adm. 2005;35(1):1–3.
21. Advanced Care Documentation. Kansas City, Missouri, U.S.A: Cerner Corporation; 2009 (copyright 2009–2011). Available: https://store.cerner.com/items/200.
22. CareCompass. Kansas City, Missouri, U.S.A: Cerner Corporation; 2009 (copyright 2009–2011). Available: https://store.cerner.com/items/1482.
23. Inpatient Summary. Kansas City, Missouri, U.S.A: Cerner Corporation; 2009 (copyright 2009–2011). Available: https://store.cerner.com/items/284.
24. Lighthouse Performance Improvement. Kansas City, Missouri, U.S.A: Cerner Corporation; 2009 (copyright 2009–2011). Available: https://store.cerner.com/items/242.
25. Discharge Readiness. Kansas City, Missouri, U.S.A: Cerner Corporation; 2009 (copyright 2009–2011). Available: https://store.cerner.com/items/173.
26. White P, Remus S. Health outcomes for better information and care: making nursing visible. HIMSS'09 – Nursing Informatics Symposium: Leaders Optimizing Healthcare Outcomes through Informatics, Chicago, 4 April 2009.

Chapter 9
Independent Living Applications

Julie Doyle and Lorcan Walsh

Abstract Countries globally have been experiencing an unprecedented increase in the number of older adults. As a result there has been an elevated interest in understanding the factors that may support the maintenance of independent living and quality of life of older adults. There is a large role for innovative technology to support monitoring, early detection and management of health and wellbeing in the home. Most diagnostic and treatment approaches to health are centered in clinical settings, and very few have focused on improving the self-management of wellbeing using novel in-home, ICT (information communication technology) based intervention systems. Utilizing combinations of ambient sensor data acquisition, telehealth and ICT it is possible to predict changes in wellbeing, and to deliver feedback and interventions to support personal wellness management.

Keywords User needs • Self-management of health and well-being • Reactive to proactive method of healthcare • ICT services • Telehealth • Smart homes • Independent living

Key Concepts

Focusing on patient or user needs and supporting them in self-management of their health and wellbeing

Moving from a reactive to a more proactive method of healthcare

ICT services to support physical, social and cognitive wellbeing and promote independent living

Telehealth

Smart homes, including ambient sensor monitoring, to support independent living

The online version of this chapter (doi:10.1007/978-1-4471-2999-8_9) contains supplementary material, which is available to authorized users.

J. Doyle, BSc, PhD (✉) • L. Walsh, B.Eng, PWD
CASALA and the Netwell Centre, Dundalk Institute of Technology,
Dundalk, County Louth, Ireland
e-mail: julie.doyle@casala.ie; lorcan.walsh@casala.ie

Introduction

Globally, populations are ageing [1, 2]. From 2006 to 2026, within the 65 and over age group, the dependency ratio[1] is expected to increase from 16.4 to 25.1 % for Ireland, and increase from 25.2 to 36.6 % for the EU [3]. In the US, the dependency ratio was 22 % in 2010 and is estimated to climb to 35 % in 2030 [4]. According to the British Government's Actuary Department, there are currently around 10 million adults over 65 in the UK, with this figure expected to rise to almost double to 19 million by 2050 (Parliament UK Statistics). The health statistics released by the Irish Department of Health (2005) mirror this trend and indicate that average life expectancy of the Irish population has grown by 10 years over the past 50 years. In the US, average life expectancy has grown from 69.9 years for those born in 1959–1961 to 77.9 years for those born in 2007 [5]. Older adults are a diverse group and many enjoy long term, good health. However to varying degrees, national health and social care systems are preparing for potentially higher incidences of chronic disease and dependency problems [6]. There is a cost element. Across developed countries approximately half of healthcare spending is attributed to older adults. In the UK, hospital readmission has risen by over 30 % due to lack of appropriate support at home [7]. In 2003, 13.2 million hospital readmissions among 35.4 million US adults were for those aged 65+ [8]; amongst 11.9 million Medicare beneficiaries in the US, 19.6 % of those who are discharged are re-admitted within 30 days and the estimated cost to Medicare of unplanned re-hospitalizations in 2004 was $17.4 billion [9]. Thus, a critical challenge exists in supporting older adults to live healthy lives in the place of their choice.

Relatedly, there has been a growing interest in preventative or restorative health care, including assisted living technologies, designed for and with older adults [10–12]. These include a broad spectrum: from video-monitoring, remote health monitoring, electronic sensors and equipment such as fall detectors, door monitors, smoke and heat alarms and bed alerts. There are also smart and telecare technologies, including electronic assistive technologies (EAT), information and communication technologies (ICT) and environment control systems (ECS).

From a nursing informatics perspective Prof Patricia Flatley Brennan at University of Wisconsin has engaged in pioneering research on independent living for many years. Her current research is as Leader of the Living Environments Laboratory at the Wisconsin Institutes for Discovery[2] demonstrates innovations in advanced visualizations and architectures, which support and facilitate specific behaviors promoting independence in the home. Her early research work included Computer Link: An electronic resource for the home caregiver supporting clients with dementia [13] and Heart Care, an Internet-based information

---

[1] The dependency ratio is an age population ratio of those typically not in the labor force (the dependent part) and those typically in the labor force. It is calculated as (number of people aged 65 and over/number of people aged 15–64) × 100.

[2] http://wid.wisc.edu/research/lel/

and support service for patients recovering at home from coronary artery bypass graft (CABG) surgery [14].

Technology aims to improve a person's functioning by preserving dexterity and mobility, helping with some household chores, reinforcing some kinds of memory, providing information, monitoring and detecting critical health situations and facilitating and strengthening communication with family, friends, caregivers and professionals [15] and publications by Flately demonstrate the nursing contribution to research in this domain has been in existence for over 30 years or more. Turner et al. [7] assert that much of this technology depends on computer based systems, with advanced sensor networks and interaction interfaces for the provision of services aimed at supporting daily living, possibly based on the monitoring of environmental conditions and of inhabitants' behavior.

As will be discussed throughout this chapter, such technologies have had varying levels of success in terms of effectiveness of supporting independent living. Telehealth has been shown to be very effective, particularly in the UK where the large scale Whole Systems Demonstrator project (discussed further in Section on "Telehealth") has reported results including a 45 % reduction in mortality rates, a 20 % reduction in emergency admissions and a 15 % reduction in emergency room visits [16]. Trials of ICT to support independent living have been on a smaller scale, usually pilots, and thus more longitudinal research is required to fully evaluate their effectiveness and cost benefits. While the goal of such technologies is to support independent living, many operate at less than full capacity and with little scope at present to assess everyday aspects of wellbeing. They focus on detecting sudden critical physiological and behavioral changes and offer few mechanisms to support preventative actions or wellness maintenance.

As an example, interventional therapies exist to act on particular signals of ill health. Raised blood pressure recordings prompt the ensuing prescription of blood pressure lowering drugs. Blood pressure monitoring then follows within a looped process of target setting and evaluation of variance above or below the set standard. Interventional treatment, when operating in this way, translates easily to the tele-medicine context: at one end, discrete data is gathered or sensed by readily available devices, processed via a simple decision tree computer program, and output to an action stream linked to clinician or pharmacist opinion. Such systems, whether they apply to blood pressure management, falls detection, or blood sugar assessment, have intrinsic value, yet they do not provide a holistic overview of the person's general wellbeing, including emotional state, fatigue, somnolence, and cognitive performance. Such determinants represent key predictors of quality of life and related mental health in older person cohorts, having a similar magnitude of effect to disease-related disability – yet it is the latter component which has dominated interventional telemedicine systems of care as they easily permit the distinct delivery of a specific intervention in response to a significant, macro-event.

By way of example, an alarm-activated fall occurrence precipitates a nurse visit, which in turn precipitates an emergency admission. Thus a "red flag" (emergency) process is detected and enacted. An acutely stressful, potentially life-threatening event, with a financial consequence for the healthcare system has occurred. However, the personal fear and anxieties that may have preceded, and indeed follow, the red flag incident are ignored. Such fears and anxieties constitute examples of so-called "orange flag" healthcare data.

There is obvious purpose in *detecting* such emotional responses: for the individual concerned living in fear of a health event such as a fall, it may create a sufficiently strong motivation so as to force the person to give up their home, and seek a supervised environment, possibly within an institutional care setting. A series of life changing events has thus occurred. Furthermore, there is also obvious purpose in *intervening* based on an orange flag alert in so far as medical morbidity, social disruption, and healthcare system expenditure is avoided, and crucially for the individual, an improved state of wellbeing is offered. This paradigm allows an ambient assisted living (AAL) home environment to remain focused on key metrics of ill health and disease status (so called *pathological mode*) on one level, but to additionally operate within a novel tier in which psychological, behavioral and other aspects of daily functioning (the *psychosocial mode*) are recorded, analyzed and managed.

Thus independent living technologies should support 'orange flag' healthcare – promoting wellness and prevention rather than solely 'red flag' or critical care. However, predicting changes and prompting positive preventative intervention measures, aiding the avoidance of severe physical or mental harm, still remains a challenge. The case study presented in Section "Case study – independent living in great northern haven" of this chapter describes an initiative addressing this challenge.

Research at Casala and the Netwell Centre

The authors of this chapter are researchers within the Netwell Centre and the Centre for Affective Solutions for Ambient Living Awareness (CASALA) located in Dundalk, Ireland. Together, these cross-sectoral, multi-disciplinary research centers are developing new ideas that support ageing-in-place and enhance the quality of life and well-being of older people through technology, community and environment-based interventions. Specifically, the Netwell Centre focuses on integrated community-oriented services, more sustainable home and neighborhood design, and age-friendly initiatives. CASALA is focused on technology development, industrial engagement, commercialization and market stimulation for innovative systems and services for older people. A large part of the ongoing research at Netwell and CASALA involves **Great Northern Haven (GNH)** a demonstration housing project consisting of 16 purpose-built homes, each equipped with a combination of sensor and interactive technology to support independent living for older adults. Each of the apartments at GNH is occupied by an older adult, all of whom have been living there since June 2010. As will be described in the GNH case study in the section on Great Northern Haven, such longitudinal monitoring of residents living in these smart homes provides very powerful information on how older adults live their lives and supports the monitoring of wellness and the promotion of timely interventions to prevent or slow down health decline.

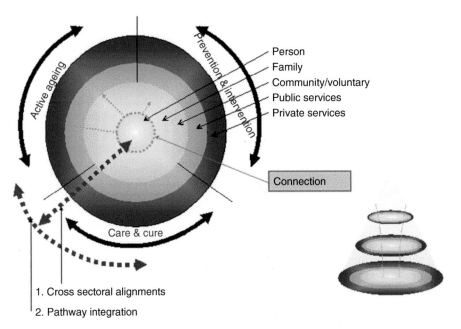

Fig. 9.1 The person at the heart of the eco-system

The remainder of this chapter is organized as follows. The section on "User needs" discusses user needs in relation to independent living technologies, highlighting that the person should be at the centre of any initiative that promotes independent living. Varying ICT-based services to support independent living are outlined in the section on "ICT-based services supporting independent living" whilst telehealth applications are discussed in the section on "Telehealth". A discussion on how Ambient Assisted Living and smart homes can support ageing-in-place is presented in the section on "Ambient assisted living and smart homes". A case study is outlined in the section on "Case study – independent living in great northern haven" that demonstrates the use of ICT, telehealth and AAL technologies in practice in an assisted living facility for older adults. Finally, the "Summary/discussion" section summarizes the chapter.

User Needs

While this chapter is focused on technologies to support independent living, it is important to note that technology should act as an enabler to healthy ageing rather than a replacement for current practice and services. Any initiative to promote independent living should place the person at the centre of its thinking. Looking at Fig. 9.1, we can see the person supported by family, community services, public and private services. Furthermore, in addition to supporting care and cure of the person, promoting active ageing, wellness and prevention through interventions is an important part of independent living. The remainder of this chapter will discuss various types of technologies that help achieve this. However, first we discuss the needs of end users of these technologies – older adults – with respect to their use of technology.

Technology can often represent a barrier for older adults, acting as an inhibitor to usage rather than a facilitator. There are many reasons for this including unfamiliarity, computer anxiety and inaccessible technology [17]. Furthermore, cognitive disabilities resulting from age degenerative processes can significantly increase the learning curve of older adults, making it more difficult and time consuming for this group to learn new skills, compared to younger adults. Physical impairments related to sensory loss are another obvious effect of ageing [18]. Such impairments affect visual, auditory and tactile capabilities, further distancing older adults from technology. Sainz Salces et al. [19] provide a detailed discussion on the physical and cognitive effects of ageing. The above-mentioned factors are not only important in designing a usable system for older adults. They also affect whether or not an older adult might want to use such technology. While it is generally agreed that older people are capable of learning new skills [20], as noted in [21] the effort required to learn something new may be perceived as not worth the trouble for the expected gain. Therefore, it is important to understand what might motivate older people to want to use such technology. Designers of applications that target older adults as a user group must understand this cohort's attitudes towards technology and communication and ensure applications are designed with their unique needs in mind.

Predicting the usage of a system has been a topic of research for many years. One of the earliest attempts was the proposal of the Technology Acceptance Model (TAM) by Davis [22]. It stated that system use is a response that can be explained or predicted by user motivation, which in turn is directly influenced by an external stimulus consisting of the actual system's features and capabilities. Davis [22] stated that perceived usefulness and perceived ease of use were sufficient to predict the attitude of a person towards using a technology system, and this attitude had a direct influence on actual system use. There have been many additions and refinements to TAM over the years. While it is a highly cited model in the field of technology acceptance, many researchers have raised questions regarding its effectiveness. Furthermore, it is typically used to assess motivation to use technology within the workplace, with little empirical research focusing on the older adult cohort. Oppenauer [23] suggests extending TAM for use with older adults, by including the psychological variables of motivation (to maintain social contacts) and user needs (both health and psychological). Indeed, there are presumably a number of additional factors affecting technology acceptance amongst the older adult cohort that must be examined to gain a better understanding of what might motivate this cohort to use technology.

A number of factors influence the acceptance, adoption and use of technology by older adults, including age, computer anxiety, fluid intelligence, crystallized intelligence, cognitive abilities and computer self-efficacy [17]. Many studies have highlighted the negative association between age and computer use, computer knowledge and computer interest, showing that acceptance is mainly influenced by the individual's learning history with technology [24] as well as comfort with and interest in using computers [25] describes generational differences, education, socioeconomic status, attitudes towards technology and cost as primary factors. Other important factors to consider include perceived benefits gauged by felt-need or actual physical, cognitive or social need, a desire to live independently, desirability, cost and access to technology, the potential stigmatism associated with certain healthcare technologies, vulnerability, security and privacy.

It is therefore crucial to involve older adults in the design of technologies that will support them in living independently in their homes. At CASALA and the Netwell Centre, this involves user requirements gathering through interviews and focus groups, involving older adults as co-designers in technologies at each stage of the design and development process and evaluating usability, effectiveness, satisfaction and impact of such technologies with older adults.

ICT-Based Services Supporting Independent Living

Advances in technology have enabled healthcare information and communication technologies (ICT) to become increasingly pervasive, moving from controlled clinical environments to real homes. As a result, many academic and industrial initiatives have been launched to promote the design and development of ICT, which monitors health, increases mobility, facilitates social connection and enhances cognitive function [26–28]. These independent living technologies may enable older adults to live independently in the place of their choice as they age, and ultimately increase their quality of life and wellbeing, in addition to reducing the cost of healthcare. Much progress has been made in recent years in developing technology interventions to support ageing in place [29]. These include ambient assisted living technologies [19], technologies to monitor activities of daily living [30], health management systems [31], and more interactive 'wellness' technologies such as applications delivered through interactive TV [27] or standalone devices [28, 32] to name but a few. Further examples are given below.

Physical Wellbeing

While a majority of older adults can live independently and enjoy a reasonable quality of life, there is a high prevalence of falls and frailty amongst this cohort. The proportion of community dwelling adults who sustain at least one fall over a 1-year period, ranges from 28 to 35 % in the ≥65 year age group to 32–42 % in the ≥75 year age group, with 15 % of older people falling at least twice [33, 34]. Within Ireland, falls are the leading cause of injury related visits to emergency departments. It has been estimated that while 80 % of falls in older persons are non-injurious, the remaining 20 % can have serious consequences [35]. These may include disability, mobility impairment, dependency, psychological problems, including fear of falling and social isolation [36]. The cost of falls each year among older adults in the US alone has been estimated to be in the region of US $20 billion [37].

Frailty is an issue that is central to ageing, transcending specific diseases and compromising quality of life [38]. By the age of 80, approximately 40 % of older adults have some degree of functional decline and 6–11 % of older people are considered frail [39]. The prevalence of frailty in community-dwelling older Europeans (>65) varies between 5.8 and 27.3 % and is reported at 22 % in the US; in addition, between 34.6 and 50.9 % are classified as 'pre-frail' in Europe and 28 % in the US [40, 41]. Research is beginning to emerge suggesting that frailty and emotional wellbeing are closely linked. The 'frailty identity crisis' is a psychological syndrome that may accompany the transition from robustness to the "next to last" stage of life [42]. The emotional and psychological challenges resulting from the development of frailty include sadness, regrets and depression, and can complicate frailty itself.

There is a large role for innovative technology to support monitoring, early detection and management of physical wellness in the home. Most diagnostic and treatment approaches are centered in clinical settings, and very few have focused on improving the self-management of physical wellbeing using novel in-home, ICT based systems.

As a result, there has been a surge in exercise and rehabilitation technology development for older adults, with the aim of making exercise fun and interactive. These include SilverFit a system that uses virtual reality video games to make exercising fun for this cohort [43], Motivating Mobility, a home-based technology solution for stroke rehabilitation, specifically helping people to reach and grasp with the shoulder, arm and fingers [44] and 'Wii-habilitation' which has become popular in retirement homes and day care centers, whereby groups of older adults come together to play Nintendo's Wii, which both encourages physical exercise and social communication.

BASE (balance and strength exercises) is a technology solution to deliver the Otago strength and balance re-training program in the homes of a number of older adults [32]. The aim is to focus specifically on improving older adults' lower limb strength and balance. Otago has been shown to reduce falls in older adults by over a third [45], but is typically not delivered through technology. BASE uses sensing technology to track older adults as they are performing their exercises and provides real-time feedback on correctness of exercises using animations, repetition counters and audio prompts, delivered on the person's television (Fig. 9.2). It therefore overcomes some of the traditional problems associated with the delivery of Otago, and indeed physiotherapy in general, including lack of motivation to perform exercises or incorrect execution, which in some cases may lead to further problems.

Social Connectedness

Loneliness is prevalent among older adults for a number of reasons. As people age, social connections can be lost as a result of widowhood, dispersed family members or a shrinking peer network. Further factors affecting reduced social interaction include illness, a lack of mobility or a fear of falling, each of which can confine a person to their home, reducing their engagement in social activities and potentially

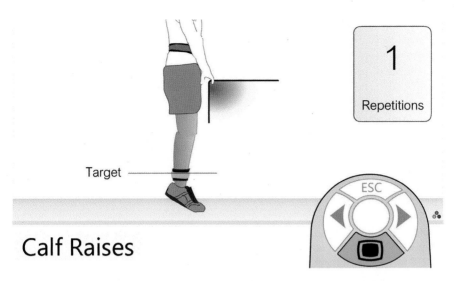

Fig. 9.2 BASE Calf exercises feedback. Feedback in BASE for a calf raises exercise showing number of repetitions remaining and the exercise target to be met, along with information on how to control movement through the program by remote control

resulting in a loss of independence. Given the associations amongst loneliness and significant health problems, including hypertension [46, 47], cognitive decline [48] and increased mortality [49], warrants alleviating interventions.

Technology can facilitate communication between older adults and their peers and family members, stimulating new relationships and maintaining existing ones [50]. A number of ICT-based approaches have developed to facilitate social connectedness; some use direct contact means (such as video conferencing software), while others use more ambient means of communication (also known as ambient awareness). Building Bridges is a project that uses communication technology to foster social connectedness amongst older adults, their peers and family and friends [28]. It does so through the shared experience of a video or radio broadcast, following which, listeners have the opportunity to take part in a group chat to discuss the broadcast. Other systems include photo sharing amongst family members [51] and social TV [52]. Examples of non-direct communication include MarkerClock [53], which is a communications appliance that allows users to improve their awareness of each other's rhythms and routines. The interface is built inside a standard analog clock; the levels of activity per hour are highlighted over the preceding 6 h.

Supporting People with Dementia and Their Caregivers

Dementia can affect people of any age, but it is most common in older people. Ferri et al. [54] provided dementia prevalence estimates for every World Health Organisation (WHO) region, for men and women, in 5-year age bands from 60 to 84 years, and for 85 years and older. It was estimated that worldwide (in 2005) approximately 24.3 million people had been diagnosed with dementia, with 4.6 million new cases every year (one new case every 7 s). Assuming that there were no changes in mortality and no effective prevention strategies or curative treatments; the number of people affected was estimated to double every 20 years to 42.3 million by 2020, and 81.1 million by 2040.

Technologies to support dementia can ease the burden on caregivers, providing peace of mind concerning the dementia patient's security in addition to improving the quality of life for both caregiver and patient. When considering the design of technologies to support dementia patients and their caregivers, there are additional challenges and thus additional guidelines that should be adhered to beyond what has been discussed previously in this chapter. It is often difficult to involve dementia patients in the design process given their memory impairments and cognitive and social difficulties; many caregivers are themselves older adults who might not be familiar with technology and paid care staff are often not aware of the benefits of technology and how it can be integrated into care practice [55].

ICT has significant potential to address the unmet needs of dementia sufferers and their caregivers. Research in this space examines how technologies can support:

- Activities of daily living – such as dressing, food/drink preparation, medication adherence.
- Domestic tasks – locking up, washing up.
- Leisure activities – addressing loss of interests.
- Interpersonal interaction – communication, person recognition, appointments.
- Risks – Cooking safety, wandering.

Typical ways in which such activities are supported by caregivers include the use of verbal cues such as prompts and notes, visual cues such as making items visible and increasing lighting, and familiarity of surroundings, appliances and routines. Technologies for dementia patients should integrate these supports. Furthermore, there are additional usability issues that must be considered keeping in mind the unique needs of dementia sufferers. When designing technologies for dementia patients, it is important to present affordances for action – for example 'do what this message says' or 'touch this picture' – that do not require the learning of multi-step procedures.

Monitoring technologies are widely used to support dementia patients, primarily for purposes of safety and security. Infrared sensors are commonly used with nursing homes and specialized dementia units to detect wandering or to alert care staff when a patient gets out of bed at night. But people in the early stages of dementia who are still living at home typically do not have such technology. Furthermore, such sensors can be used for many additional purposes, such as monitoring activities of daily living, ensuring someone is getting up out of bed, has turned the stove off etc.

ICT has been used to support communication between people with dementia and their caregivers. The CIRCA system is a multimedia interactive reminiscence and conversational aid to support satisfying, meaningful communication between people with dementia and their caregivers [55]. Other work has examined the use of cognitive 'prostheses' to support diminished cognitive capabilities [56, 57]. Cooking safety and kitchen tasks have also been examined [58]. Wherton and Monk [59] provide a detailed description of the opportunities for technology to support people with dementia to live at home.

There are many therapies for people with dementia that are suitable to be applied using multiple technologies. Reminiscence therapy for dementia patients discusses past events, experiences and activities between people with dementia and their care-givers and has been associated with improvements in cognition, mood and behavioral function as well as decreased caregiver strain [60]. Traditionally, this has been performed directly with the person often recording stories in a reminiscence diary for the person with dementia to review afterwards.

However ongoing research is examining technology-based approaches, such as creating personalized, computerized interventions [61] or using video-based thera-pies such as life-logging [62, 63]. The personalized computer interventions may take the form of displaying comforting messages or videos from close friends or family, pictures from their childhood, and/or a computerized reminiscence diary. The video-based therapies may include capturing images from throughout a per-son's day and allowing them to review it at the end of each day. The images may be recorded using a body-worn camera or cameras embedded in their environment.

Caregivers themselves commonly experience depression, sleep disturbances, anxiety and loss of companionship as a result of providing continuous care. Technological support provided to these caregivers may serve to alleviate stress, reduce the feeling of being over-burdened, or provide helpful advice. Two examples of this include an online teleconferencing schedule [64] and a caregiver support tool [65] which included videos and support content provided by caregiver 'champions' and experienced health care experts. The EU project Discover for Carers [66] also aims to support caregivers of people with dementia.

Medication Prompting

Medication adherence is a challenging problem, particularly when multiple medica-tions need to be taken or for those with a reduced cognitive capacity. Pill boxes labelled for each day have been traditionally used to alleviate some issues, however problems still arise when individuals forget to take their medication, or when differ-ent medications are required to be taken at various times of the day. Many technolo-gies have been developed to prompt the user to take particular medications at certain times of the day; some of which have been based on using reminder messages on mobile phones and/or customized pill boxes. However, context-sensitive prompting (e.g. reminding the user to take their medication while they are in their bathroom) can be more effective as individuals may not adhere to the reminder using standard reminder-based prompting (e.g. their medication prompts occur while they are not in the house, on the telephone, or with a visitor) [67]. Furthermore an instrumented pillbox can also report if/when a person does take their medication and this can be used to highlight and quantify forgetfulness.

Self Report Applications

Recent times have seen the advent of the quantified-self movement, whereby individuals have begun to use computers, mobile phones, tablets etc. to 'self-track'. Self-tracking typically involves recording some aspect of your life, including your work, sleep, exercise, diet or mood and supports self-management of such through the provision of informative and educational feedback. This feedback is typically *persuasive* and aims to help the person to change their behavior to live the lifestyle they wish to lead.

UbiFit is an application that uses on-body sensing and activity inference to encourage and promote physical activity [68]. It uses the screen of a mobile phone to display a wallpaper that consists of a garden that blooms as the person performs physical activities throughout the week. The user can set goals (outlining the amount of activity they would like to achieve) and if they meet their goals, a butterfly appears in the garden. However, UbiFit only supports tracking of one single parameter of wellbeing. BeWell is a smartphone application to monitor, model and promote wellbeing across three parameters – quantity of sleep, physical activity and social interactions [69]. All sensing happens through the smartphone, for example levels of social interaction are determined by microphone measurement of ambient conversations and duration of sleep is inferred by examining phone usage patterns. Similar to UbiFit, BeWell uses the wallpaper of a mobile phone to display a metaphor of an aquarium, For example, a turtle depicts the user's sleep habits. If the person has had enough sleep, the turtle 'wakes up' and comes out of its shell. If the turtle remains in its shell, it means the user should try to get more sleep. Both BeWell and UbiFit are targeted at the general population rather than older adults. They are stand-alone applications rather than subsets of a larger integrated home self-management system. Furthermore, evaluations carried out at CASALA have indicated that older adults find it difficult to interpret such metaphors, i.e. they would find it difficult to remember what the butterfly or turtle represent [70].

Other more commercial applications include MindBloom[3] – an application that supports people in improving their quality of life by helping them focus on what aspects of their life are important to them and motivating them to improve these areas. While there are a number of smartphone and tablet applications that support monitoring and tracking of mood, for example MoodJam[4] and MoodPanda,[5] they fall short in providing an effective, clinical tool for monitoring and supporting emotional wellbeing of older adults. However, a number of research efforts have begun to appear in this space. Monarca is a persuasive monitoring and feedback system for mental illness and is an excellent example of a closed feedback loop to patients [71]. With Monarca, mental health patients self-report on their mood, sleep, activity and medication adherence on a daily basis, using a mobile phone.

---

[3] https://www.mindbloom.com/

[4] http://moodjam.com/

[5] http://moodpanda.com/

The patient has access to an overview of their data on their phone and their clinician also has access to this data through a Web interface. Together, they can explore historical data. Triggers can also alert both the patient and the clinician as to potential warning signals, for example if the person has not taken their medication or if their mood is particularly low.

Telehealth

Telehealth is emerging as a solution to deal with the increasing prevalence of chronic disease amongst ageing populations. The NHS reports spending 70 % of its budget on the 15 million people who have one or more chronic conditions, with patient numbers expected to grow by 23 % over the next 20 years, given the ageing population [72]. In the US, the Center for Disease Control (CDC) reports that nearly half of US adults are living with at least one chronic illness.[6] These diseases are the top killers in the US and represent a significant portion of healthcare spending.[7] The NHS recognizes that the current approach to healthcare of people with long term conditions is unsustainable in terms of both quality of care and cost and their goal is to move towards a more proactive intervention model.

Telehealth involves the remote exchange of data between a patient and healthcare professionals as part of the patient's diagnosis and healthcare management [73]. For example, telehealth applications exist to monitor blood pressure, COPD, diabetes and heart failure. They aim to support the person in monitoring and managing their own health and provide encouragement to adhere to healthy lifestyle practices. They are typically monitored by healthcare professionals, who are alerted if an abnormal reading is recorded. Numerous studies have evaluated the effectiveness and benefits of telehealth in terms of improved health outcomes for patients, reduced mortality and cost benefits for healthcare systems [74–76]. While some research suggest telehealth has positive effects on patients with chronic conditions, such as improved quality of life and patient satisfaction, others have found no effect or even negative effects.

A number of telehealth pilots have been carried out worldwide. However, the majority does not make it past pilot stage, given the complexity involved in implementing telehealth projects, and are thus not implemented on a large scale. However, it is generally agreed that larger scale trials, rather than small pilots, are necessary to determine the true effectiveness of telehealth. The UK had been leading the way in large-scale telehealth deployment with the Whole Systems Demonstrator (WSD) and three million lives (3ML) projects [77].

---

[6] Centers for Disease Control: Chronic Disease at a Glance 2009. See: http://www.cdc.gov/nccdphp/publications/AAG/chronic.htm

[7] Gerard Anderson, "Chronic Conditions: Making the Case for Ongoing Care" (Partnership to Fight Chronic Disease: November 2007). See: http://www.fightchronicdisease.com/news/pfcd/pr12102007.cfm

The WSD project was established by the Department of Health in the UK and launched in May 2008. It represents the largest randomized control trial of telehealth and telecare services in the world. A total of 6,191 (3,030 of whom received telehealth devices) patients and 238 GP practices were involved across three UK sites. The two main goals of the WSD trial were to examine the effectiveness and cost effectiveness of (1) telehealth in managing patients with long-term illnesses and (2) telecare in the management of patients with social care needs; within the context of routine delivery of healthcare within the NHS [78]. Individuals were considered to have social care needs if they required night sitting, were receiving 10 or more hours per week of home care, had mobility difficulties, had fallen or were at risk of falling, were a live-in or nearby carer for someone or had cognitive impairment and had a live-in or nearby caregiver.

To date, published results from the WSD trial have focused on telehealth. The main findings, reported in [16] and summarized on the WSD website are listed below.

- A 45 % reduction in mortality rates
- A 20 % reduction in emergency admissions
- A 15 % reduction in accident and emergency (A&E) visits
- A 14 % reduction in elective admissions
- A 14 % reduction in bed days
- An 8 % reduction in tariff costs.

Following the WSD trial, the Department of Health in the UK believes that three million or more people around the UK with chronic conditions and/or social care needs could benefit from telehealth and telecare in their home. This led to the launch of the three millions lives project[8] in 2012 whose objectives over a 5-year period are for the NHS and industry to work together in developing the market for telehealth and telecare delivery, removing barriers to its uptake and to promote its benefits for patients and healthcare professionals alike.

Bardram et al. [79] have examined the transformations that occur in the patient-physician relationship when health monitoring moves into the home. They found that GPs having a much wealthier amount of data from the patient, providing a better statistical foundation for the patient's treatment and allowing them to quickly change medication if the home monitoring indicated this was required. Further, the patient becomes responsible for taking measurements accurately and regularly and they have much more detailed information to interpret and evaluate than when in their GP's office. This increased the patients' self-awareness of their condition and consequently increased their interest in managing it.

Home-based measurements could, in theory, provide more accurate measurements than those taken by a healthcare professional. For example, home-based measurement eliminates white coat syndrome. However, there are issues involving patients using the equipment correctly in the home. Participants in telehealth trials

---

[8] http://3millionlives.co.uk/

measuring blood pressure have reported being unsure of where to place the cuff, or how tight it should be [79].

A detailed White Paper, "Healthcare without Walls", considers how best the NHS should exploit the potential of telehealth [72] and provides an excellent, in-depth report on telehealth research.

Canada Health Infoway has also been actively developing telehealth solutions. In their 2011 analysis of benefits achieved though Telehealth [80], it was reported that Canada had 187,385 clinical telehealth sessions in Canada, with an additional 44,600 educational sessions and 27,538 administrative sessions. To a large extent, telehealth supported 21 % of the Canadian population that is located in rural and remote locations.

Ambient Assisted Living and Smart Homes

Ambient Assisted Living and Sensor Monitoring

Ambient Assisted Living (AAL) refers to noninvasive systems placed within people's homes to monitor their behavior and to facilitate independent living. AAL often consists of sensor systems that include presence/ movement Passive InfraRed (PIR) sensors, door and window latch sensors and resource usage sensors. A PIR sensor can be seen in Fig. 9.3. These sensors are very common in homes, as they are used in home security systems to detect intruders – simply, they detect movement in the home. The reason for choosing ambient sensors over body worn sensors, for example, is generally to reduce the impact of the sensing on peoples' lives, to remove the stigma of healthcare devices in the home and also to remove the poor compliance often associated with body worn sensors and pendent alarms. For example this poor compliance can often be due to the pendant alarm being left on a bed-post whilst taking a shower (a high falls risk scenario), but it can also be related to conditions such as dementia. The data recorded from ambient sensors in AAL is used to trigger alerts about either emergency scenarios in the person's home or to indicate changes in their regular patterns of behavior that might be indicative of a health decline. AAL makes this possible without the need for active input from the person.

While more detail is provided in Section "Case study – independent living in great northern haven" on how AAL sensing technology operates within an assisted living environment for older adults, we introduce here the types of activities that can be identified by such sensing, indicating the power of such inexpensive, unobtrusive technology. Figure 9.4 shows a visualization of data taken from the PIR sensors in one of the apartments in Great Northern Haven. The data is from a 60-day period and shows the older resident's movement/location within their home at certain times of the day. For example, we can see that they are typically in the bedroom between 10 at night and 9 in the morning. However, we can also see that this person sometimes moves around during the night, sometimes to use their en-suite bathroom and sometimes to go into the kitchen.

Fig. 9.3 Photo of a typical PIR sensor 2

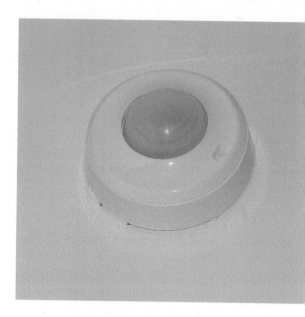

Fig. 9.4 Visualization older persons 90 days location. Visualization showing an older person's location in their home over a period of 60 days. Data taken from the apartment of one of the residents living in Great Northern Haven

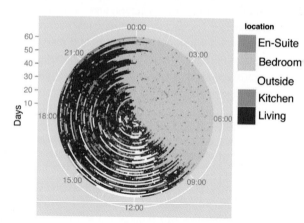

A second visualization showing data of a GNH resident's movement in their home is shown in Fig. 9.5. This image shows that this particular resident has very regular patterns of behavior – they typically go to bed at the same time each night and get up at the same time each morning. They have little movement outside their bedroom during the night.

The power of AAL and such sensing technology is the ability to detect changes to a person's normal behavior or activity that might be an indicator that something is wrong. For example, is a person begins to stay in bed much longer than they usually do, it could be an indicator of a number of things, such as illness or depression. In Great Northern Haven, one of the residents showed increased nighttime movement in the week, which led up to him being hospitalized for cardiac problems.

Fig. 9.5 One person
visualization GNH. Another
visualization showing a
person's location in the home
at various times of the day.
This data is taken from one
of the apartments in Great
Northern Haven and
highlights that people
typically have very regular
behavior patterns

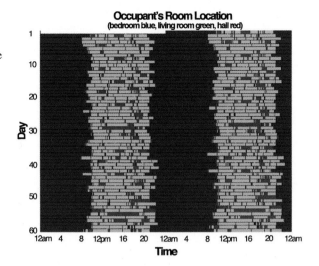

Automatic detection of such an event would trigger an alert to an appropriate person, such as a caregiver or clinician, who might then check on the person. Further detail on AAL sensor monitoring in GNH is presented in the section on "Case study – independent living in great northern haven."

Smart Homes

Smart Homes are domestic residences, augmented with AAL and ICT-based services that provide support to facilitate ageing-in-place [81, 82]. They can promote independent living and quality of life of older adults – particularly as they enable movement from a reactive to a more preventative model of healthcare. Smart homes that support longitudinal monitoring and behavior recognition enable a better understanding of the causes and the relative contributions and interactions between the different factors that contribute to illness. This is a pre-requisite for early detection, prevention and management and ultimately enables more individually tailored interventions that can be delivered in a timely fashion. This in turn results in a more individual patient-oriented treatment.

This section presents an overview of smart home initiatives, mostly aimed at enabling ageing-in-place, which have recorded data from residents living in their living labs over multiple weeks. Such studies range from a single highly sensed residence to a series of assisted living apartments kitted out with various unobtrusive activity detection technologies. Often these environments record the daily patterns and behaviors of its residents through a number of sensors, and intelligent algorithms have been created which automatically identify these behaviors. Significant research currently being undertaken is focusing on the extraction of activities of

Table 9.1 List of smart home initiatives and the type of sensing they support

	Tiger place	MavHome	GatorTech	Adaptive home	Aware home	House_n place	CASAS	Orca tech	GNH
Motion	yes		yes		yes	yes	yes	yes	yes
Contact sensors	yes		yes			yes	yes	yes	yes
Bed sensors	yes		yes			yes		yes	yes
Gait sensors	yes							yes	
Phone sensors	yes						yes	yes	
Vital signs sensors	yes	yes							yes
Food		yes	yes			yes	yes		
Cooking	yes					yes	yes		
Medication	yes	yes					yes	yes	
Lighting			yes						yes
Water usage		yes				yes	yes		yes
Electricity usage		yes				yes			yes
Heating				yes		yes			yes
Temperature				yes			yes		yes
Audio	yes				yes	yes			
Video	yes				yes	yes			

daily living (ADL) from such data, and most importantly in detecting deviations away from a person's normal activity patterns that might indicate the onset of poor health. Specific examples of ADL detection and possible interventions based on changes from usual behavior are presented in the case study in the section on "Case study – independent living in great northern haven".

A goal of much of the smart home research presented in this section is to integrate technologies that detect functional decline and/or alert care providers should an adverse event occur. Results from the analysis of this smart home data are mainly used to inform clinicians and care providers of changes in overall health status. Apart from Great Northern Haven (GNH) few support the provision of feedback to the older adult themselves, to support health self-management.

Table 9.1 provides an overview of smart home initiatives and highlights the type of monitoring they support. *TigerPlace* is a series of 32 private apartments designed to facilitate ageing-in-place [83]. The *Managing an Adaptive Versatile Home* (MavHome) project focuses on creating a smart home that maximizes comfort and minimizes cost through predicting the behavioral patterns of the inhabitant, the periodic monitoring of vital signs, water and device usage, use of food items, exercise regimen and medication intake [84–86]. The *GatorTech Smart House* is a smart home developed by the University of Florida [87]. The *Adaptive House* at the University of Colorado has been developed to dynamically predict future behavioral patterns of the use of lights, heating and temperature by its residents [88]. The *Aware Home* at Georgia Institute of Technology is a three story smart environment which investigates the design, development and evaluation of future domestic technologies with the overall aim of enhancing quality of life and lengthening lives [89, 90]. The MIT *House_n/PlaceLab* project investigated using a highly sensed smart apartment ADL detection, user prompting (for labelling of activities) and machine learning based inferencing engines [91–93]. The *CASAS Smart Home Project* at Washington State University is a three-bedroom apartment test bed whose priority is to improve the comfort, safety and/or productivity of the its resident(s) [81, 94, 95]. The *ORCATECH Living Lab* consists of a group of community dwelling older adults who have had unobtrusive monitoring technologies installed in their homes since 2006, who provide a test-bed for evaluating behavioral monitoring technology [96, 97].

Initiatives, such as those listed above, enable researchers to investigate the real-world living patterns of individuals over extended periods. The duration of time required to capture the overall variation in such behaviors and tasks is still unknown. Most of the studies collect data when people are staying temporarily in their living lab with the exception of ORCATECH, TigerPlace and GNH who are collecting real-world data from people living in their homes.

The remainder of this chapter describes Great Northern Haven, a series of 16 apartments managed by CASALA, where residents have been living since June 2010. One of the unique features of GNH is that information learned from ambient monitoring is returned to the resident themselves (rather than a solely carer or clinician) – empowering them to self-manage their wellness as well as their home's security and energy usage.

Case Study – Independent Living In Great Northern Haven

In an effort to prepare for the health-related challenges demographic change is going to bring about, new ways of monitoring health and wellbeing are being explored that will support people in living independently. Smart homes support the monitoring of older adults, with the potential to detect a wealth of information regarding the person's functional, cognitive, social and emotional wellbeing. Smart homes therefore have significant potential to enhance the lives of older adults, extending the period of healthy ageing, through monitoring their health and wellbeing, detecting decline and applying interventions to arrest this decline.

The Great Northern Haven is a series of 16 highly-sensed apartments located in Dundalk, Ireland. There are a total of 2,240 sensors and actuators throughout the GNH development, with approximately 100 sensors embedded within each home. The sensors include passive infra-red (PIR) sensors to detect motion; contact sensors on all windows; contact sensors on all exterior doors; contact sensors on three interior doors; sensors on all light switches; temperature sensors for each room; brightness sensors at three points in the homes; weather data including outside brightness, temperature, wind speed and rain alarm; sensors to detect power consumption and heating usage. In addition each home has a number of alarm cords and buttons, a home security system and a telecare device that links with a monitoring service.

Ambient sensor technology at GNH supports monitoring of patterns of behavior over extended periods of time, and more importantly deviations in normal patterns of behavior that might indicate the onset of illness, as described in Section "Ambient assisted living and sensor monitoring". To date, residents have been living in 15 of the GNH apartments since June 2010. Thus we have gathered large amounts of data from sensors in these apartments, and validation and analysis of the data has taken place. Models are being built to detect patterns in activities of daily living and health. GNH is a unique development in that it is not just a test bed for research. These are real peoples' homes and as such, the data we are collecting is extremely rich. One of the unique features of GNH is that information learned from ambient monitoring is returned to the resident themselves (rather than solely to a caregiver or clinician, which is the case with much of the smart home research presented in the section on "Smart homes") – empowering them to self-manage their wellness as well as their home's security and energy usage. Thus, we work very closely with GNH residents in determining their needs and they are very active co-designers in the research that takes place at CASALA and the Netwell Centre—they are not research volunteers, as is the case with most research projects, and this provides us with a unique setup. Furthermore, the residents represent a diverse cohort, ranging in age from early 60s to late 80s, representing varying levels of computer use and interest, and each with varying health conditions. We are currently beginning to feed the information that we are ambiently gathering back to residents to support them in managing their wellbeing and their homes—essentially closing the feedback loop in AAL [70]. This is achieved through interactive devices such as the iPad, hosting a suite of applications ranging from health and wellness, to home security and energy. Details of ongoing research at GNH can be found in [70, 98–102]. This section presents some of this work, outlining home automation and behavior recognition in GNH, as well as describing the type of feedback presented to residents to support them in self-management.

Home Automation

Some daily domestic tasks can become challenging in older age, perhaps due to the physical strength and/or the coordination required. Often products, furniture, and other household items are not designed for use by all, including older adults. For example, windows may be in locations that are difficult to reach, or doors may be too heavy (e.g. fire doors) to open easily. Home automation, or domotics, provides many options to allow individuals to regain complete autonomy of their environment. Some examples as implemented in the Great Northern Haven are described below and depicted in Fig. 9.6.

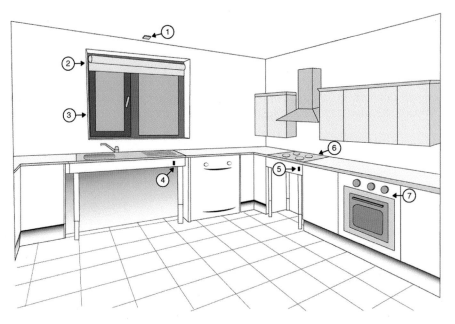

Fig. 9.6 Schematic Drawing Kitchen Great Northern Haven (GNH). A schematic drawing depicting the kitchen area of GNH apartments showing sensors (*1*), automatic window blind (*2*), automatic window (*3*), adjustable sink (*4*), adjustable range (*5*), induction range for safety (*6*), oven safety controls (*7*)

Automated Doors, Window and Blinds

Actuators fitted to doors, windows and blinds are beneficial to individuals with reduced physical functioning. Actuators are relatively small devices attached to the side of a door, window or blind that can open that window when a button is pressed. On/off switches are generally placed in convenient locations, in some cases a remote control may be used. For example, in the Great Northern Haven a remote control opens windows and blinds in places that are difficult to reach (e.g. over the kitchen sink) and a wall switch opens the heavy doors which residents may have difficulty with.

Adjustable Height of Kitchen Appliances

The kitchen sink and oven counter top range may be raised to different heights depending on the preference of the user. The ability to change this height is particularly applicable to residences with more than one occupant, however it also caters for the changing needs an individual may have over their life course (e.g. in cases where people become wheelchair users). In Great Northern Haven this is implemented using an up-down switch on the side of the kitchen sink and counter top stove; this is simple to use and understand, and also unobtrusive.

Safety Controls on Cooking Appliances

Confusion and forgetfulness, as seen in individuals with memory problems, may result in safety concerns particularly around cooking appliances. Induction stovetops are often used as they warm up and cool down quickly. Additionally, an induction hob will not heat up until the pot is placed on the hob. Timers are sometimes used on ovens to ensure they are not accidentally left turned on.

Environmental Sensing and Behaviour Recognition

Significant research into smart homes has focused upon extracting activities of daily living (ADL) and daily patterns of behavior using data collected from ambient, wearable and mobile devices. A tradeoff exists between the suitability for long-term deployment, and the ability and flexibility to accurately recognize certain activities and patterns. For example, (1) body-worn sensors may accurately measure gait speed and variability but may not be suitable for long-term data collection, (2) Cameras may be used to quantify and model an individual's pattern of movement or behavior throughout a house however many users find this very intrusive, and (3) ambient sensors alleviate many privacy concerns at the expense of a decreased specificity (e.g. the challenging task of distinguishing two users using ambient sensors).

Figure 9.7 shows the system architecture in GNH. The process begins with environmental sensing (through PIRs other sensors described above) and behavior recognition to detect certain behaviors and changes in behaviors. Ground truth data is also gathered

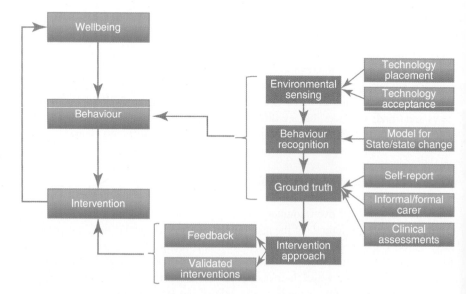

Fig. 9.7 Architecture Drawing Great Northern Haven (GNH) 2. Architecture diagram showing typical process of sensing, behaviour recognition and intervention approaches in GNH

directly from residents, in the form of quarterly clinically validated questionnaires and daily self-report data through an iPad application (described in the section on "Feedback to support self-management"). Such ground truth data is essential to help us understand and make sense of the ambient sensor data. Interventions are then deployed to residents of GNH based on assessments of their behavior. These may include interventions through devices such as iPads (described in the section on "Feedback to support self-management") or community-based interventions, such as recommending the person attend a falls clinic or a local class to encourage social interaction.

Activity and behavior recognition systems typically attempt to identify many different behaviors. These may range from recognizing whether the individual is sitting, standing or walking, performing specific tasks (such as leaving the house, sleeping, toileting, preparing breakfast, preparing dinner, eating, and showering), or at rest. Some of the information we are learning from ambient sensors in GNH is presented in the following subsections.

Residents' Movement Levels

Variations in resident's movement levels often reflect changes in a person's behavior. For example, in one instance an increase in resident's movement at nighttime was detected directly prior to hospitalization. Peaks in movement during the day may be indicative of a visitor being present. Decreases in movement while a person is in the home may indicate a decline in health or, alternatively, a change in the way a person uses their home. Feeding this data back to the resident can be useful in providing context to the changes that occur. An algorithm has been developed that measures the residents' movement per minute, hour and day.

Time Outside the Home

Time outside the home is important in considering the sociality of an individual. It may be calculated by subtracting the time a person closes an external door from the time they open an external door, providing no PIR inside the house has fired with a value of 1 during this period. While time outside the home isn't directly fed back to the resident, it is used in determining the resident's emotional wellbeing, further discussed below.

Location Mapping

A location-mapping algorithm has been developed to determine the location a person is in. Initially, the algorithm focused on using PIR motion sensors but was later extended to include adjacent rooms without PIR motion sensors through using light switch and contact sensors. A person is determined to be in an adjacent room if any of a subset of sensors within the adjacent room has fired. The location mapping algorithm is used in deriving various activity metrics, such as those relating to sleep and time outside the home and, as such, isn't fed back directly to the resident. Figure 9.8 shows location maps for one resident. For example, the dark blue areas represent when the resident is in the living room, while the red areas represent the bedroom. Two other examples of location mapping were depicted in Figs. 9.4 and 9.5.

Detecting Emotional Wellbeing

Emotional wellbeing is an important indicator of overall health in adults over 65. For some older people, age-related declines to physical, cognitive or social wellbeing can negatively impact on their emotional wellbeing, as can anxiety, loneliness

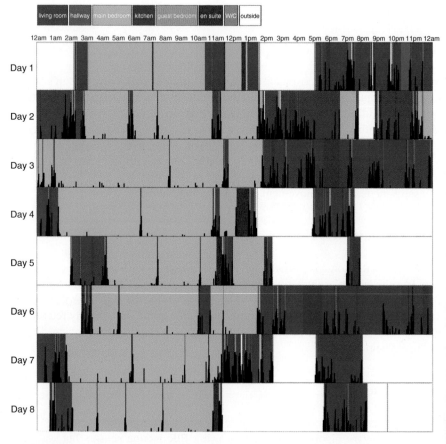

Fig. 9.8 Algorithm movement patterns. Location mapping algorithm identifies patterns, for examples how the resident moves around their house or the time they spend outside their house (often used as a proxy for sociality). The *light blue* represents the living room, purple is the hallway, *turquoise* is the main bedroom, *dark blue* is the kitchen, *green* is the guest bedroom, *red* is the ensuite bathroom, *orange* is the guest WC and *white* represents periods outside the home

and depression resulting from the notion of growing older, the loss of a spouse, a loss of sense of purpose or general worries about coping, becoming ill and/or death. It is estimated that up to 5 % of US citizens over the age of 65 living in the community have major depression compared with 13.5 % of those who require home health care and 11.5 % in nursing homes [103].

A person's emotional wellbeing state is typically assessed using clinically validated questionnaires such as the Center for Epidemiologic Studies Depression Scale (CES-D) or the Geriatric Depression Scale (GDS). The issue with such assessments in practice is that they are typically reliant on clinical professionals to administer them and thus are only delivered when a person visits their clinician. Developing mechanisms to shift aspects of these assessments, as well as treatment of emotional disorders from clinical settings to self-management in the home, and simultaneously providing continuous, in-depth, histories emotional wellbeing state changes between clinical visits is preferable.

Ambient sensing has the potential to support monitoring and prediction of changes to emotional state from within the home. We have recently begun to examine this within GNH. Figure 9.9 shows data for two GNH residents derived from the hallway PIR sensor and the front door contact sensor, to determine a person's time outside the house. To help visualize behavioral patterns the sensor data is represented on a spiral plot called a "last clock". These particular images represent data collected over a 5-month period. They show data on a 24- h clock with midnight at the top and spirals out from the centre. Each circuit represents a day. Complete circles indicate when a resident was away from the home, on holiday for example.

The clock plot in Fig. 9.9a shows data for an 'active' resident, while Fig. 9.9b shows the stark contrast of out-of-home behavior of an 'inactive' resident. From Fig. 9.9b, we can see that this resident typically leaves the home just before midday and returns by early afternoon. This data also shows that this resident became less active during winter. Baseline data gathered from this resident illustrates high levels

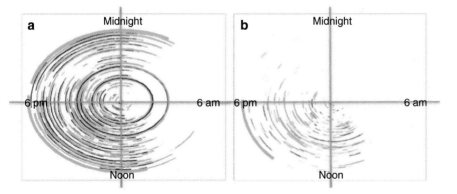

Fig. 9.9 (**a, b**) Two clock plots. Two clock plots show data for (**a**) an active resident and (**b**) an inactive resident in GNH. Data is derived by combining data from two sensors – the hallway PIR and the front door contact sensor – that indicate when a person has left the house

of depression. Interviews with this resident suggest that possible reasons behind the depression include worries about declining health but primarily a lack of social contact with others.

In contrast, the resident who's data is depicted in Fig. 9.9a is very active, spending much of their day outside the home, including at night time when this resident reports enjoying going out for a social drink with friends. Thus a visual comparison of these two clock plots provides us with a clear picture of the behavioral differences of someone who is potentially emotionally unwell compared with someone who is emotionally healthy.

What we are particularly interested in is looking for changes to a person's wellbeing state over time and intervening in a timely manner, to prevent a person from moving to an 'inactive' or unhealthy state of being.

Our next steps in ambiently assessing changes to emotional wellbeing involve integrating additional metrics that might be indicators of declining emotional wellbeing, including decreased or erratic movement levels and increased time in bed. Correlating these metrics with self-reported emotional wellbeing from the iPad wellness application [70] and our quarterly clinical questionnaires will allow us to determine the most effective measure of emotional state.

Detecting Sleep Patterns

Sleep is a fundamental physiological process with important restorative functions. Sleep disturbances may be indicative of poor health and functional deficits, especially in older adults [104, 105]. Total sleep time is reduced in the elderly and this is not due to a reduced need for sleep, but in a diminished ability to sleep [106]. Sleep complaints commonly reported by over 50 % of those aged 65 and older include getting less sleep, frequent awakenings, waking up too early, excessive daytime sleepiness, and napping during the day [103]. Sleeping difficulties have been associated with decreased quality of life, and higher rates of depression and anxiety, significant cognitive impairment, limited attention spans, and balance, ambulatory and visual problems [107, 108]. Additionally, the symptoms of various chronic conditions continue into the night and result in a disturbed sleep; these include movement disorders, neuromuscular diseases, depression, dementia, epilepsy, obesity and circadian rhythm disorders [109].

Traditional forms of sleep monitoring (e.g. polysomnography, wrist actigraphy or sleep diaries) are unsuitable for long-term deployments, particularly amongst certain populations, as they are labor intensive, costly, and/or require conscious and continued interaction with the user. Ongoing work is investigating whether longitudinally monitoring the relationship between sleep and health may provide scope for unobtrusive monitoring modalities. Recent advances in non-contact sleep monitoring include under mattress approaches [110], radar-based technologies (BiancaMed, NovaUCD, Dublin, Ireland), and smartphone applications (Sleep Cycle Alarm Clock, Maciek Drejek Labs, Sweden).

In Great Northern Haven recent work has focused on the extraction of daily rest/activity patterns using data collected from motion sensors, light switches, and contact sensors. Through identifying when an individual is at relative rest in their bedroom for a prolonged period at night (perhaps interspersed with toilet events), their *time-in-bed* can be estimated. A deeper understanding of a person's health may be quantified through longitudinally investigating the variance in a number of sleep metrics including *time-to-bed*, *time-in-bed*, number of bed exits, nocturnal restlessness, etc. For example, retrospective analysis found that an older adult's nocturnal movement levels increased greatly prior to a hospitalization, and subsequently returned to normal upon returning from hospital [97]. Similar findings have also been reported in other assisted living facilities (including Tiger Place, discussed in Section on "Smart homes"). Ongoing work is establishing normal longitudinal deviations in these metrics [111].

Feedback to Support Self-Management

The feedback provided to residents of GNH consists of an overview of one's wellbeing, trends over time and a series of educational messages aimed at increasing the resident' awareness of their wellbeing and supporting them in maintaining a healthy state of wellbeing. Such feedback is delivered on an iPad through the YourWellness application [70] (Figs. 9.10–9.12).

The YourWellness application asks GNH residents to self-report on their wellbeing on a daily basis, including their sleep, mood and social interactions. Residents also take their blood pressure and weight, both of which interface directly with the iPad. This information is analyzed, a wellness score is calculated

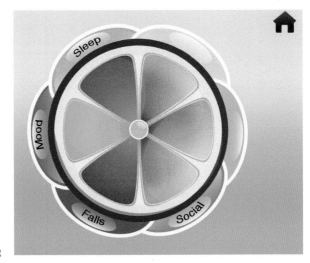

Fig. 9.10 Feedback wheel. The feedback wheel with each segment representing a particular aspect of wellbeing

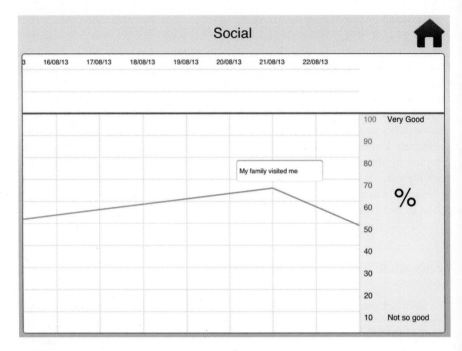

Fig. 9.11 Educational message example. Examples of educational/interventional messages delivered through the iPad to the resident

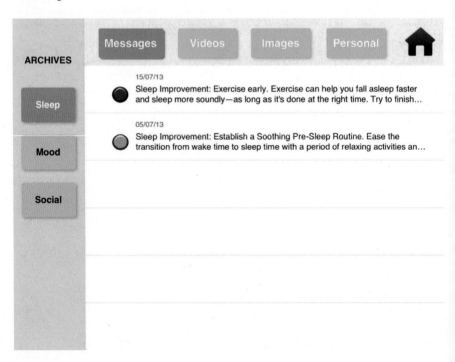

Fig. 9.12 Archive of interventional messages. Examples of the archived interventional messages delivered to the resident

for each category of wellbeing and this information is returned to the person as visual feedback. Key aspects of the design of feedback in YourWellness can be seen in Figs. 9.10–9.12. At the highest level, feedback is provided as a quick-glance overview of wellbeing. Based on feedback from participants, we have designed a feedback wheel to support this (Fig. 9.10). The wheel is divided into categories, based on what parameters of wellness are being monitored. The interior part of the segment is colored green if the individual is considered healthy, meaning they don't need to take any action regarding behavior change for that parameter of wellbeing. If the individual is scoring relatively low in a particular area of wellbeing, the segment is colored amber – indicating an orange alert and that some action should be undertaken to address this. A red segment means immediate action is required, and the individual will be alerted. The color of the segment is based on the person's past 7 days of data. In collaboration with clinical specialists and taking into account existing guidelines such as the NHS NICE guidelines (http://www.nice.org.uk/ including 'Treating Depression in Adults' and 'Mental Wellbeing and Older Adults'), we have determined a scoring algorithm that calculates a wellness score for determining whether a green, orange or red alert should be provided. This wellness score takes into account deviations from the individual's norm. For example, to set a baseline for blood pressure, we currently take 2 weeks of data from the person and then look at certain deviations away from their average or norm that may indicate abnormal bp (orange alert) or critical bp (red alert).

An individual can also click a particular segment of the overview feedback wheel to get further information, including their trending/historical data presented as a graph that will be made viewable as weekly or monthly data (Fig. 9.11). Educational and interventional content is also provided (Fig. 9.12). Such content has been defined for each type of alert in each category of wellbeing, in collaboration with clinicians and by examining existing guidelines. For example, if an individual is scoring in the orange zone for emotional wellbeing, feedback might include encouraging them to go for a regular walk. It might also involve asking additional questions to assess why the person is scoring low. The overall aim of such feedback is to help the individual to improve their wellbeing – to move from being in the red/orange zone to the green zone.

Summary/Discussion

Given current patterns of demographic ageing, the prevalence of health issues within older populations, and the effects of ageing on poor health outcomes, independent living technologies can impact the wellness and quality of life of older adults, extending healthy life years, or delaying the progression of decline. Through promoting independent living and shifting the locus of care from clinical settings to home-based self-management, such technologies can promote new systemic approaches, increasing the efficiency and sustainability of healthcare services directed at supporting older adults.

One of the most important aspects of independent living is that older people themselves are empowered to look after their health and wellbeing. It is therefore necessary to integrate feedback into independent living technologies – informing the person of their health status, educating them on how to look after their wellbeing and motivating them to adhere to healthy behaviors. People with specific illnesses, for example, must be provided with knowledge on how to deal with their condition and what to do if it begins to deteriorate.

While independent living applications tend to mostly be discussed within the context of supporting older adults to live longer, independence is also critical issue of those with disability or with chronic health problems who wish to retain a good quality of life whilst living at home.

While this chapter focused on technologies to support independent living, it is important to remember that technology should act as an enabler to healthy ageing rather than a replacement for current practice and service.

Downloads

Available from extras.springer.com:

Educational Template (PDF 98 kb)
Educational Template (PPTX 128 kb)

Acknowledgements We would like to acknowledge the team at CASALA and Netwell, all of whom have contributed to ongoing research there, including Rodd Bond, Andrew MacFarlane, Benjamin Knapp, Brian O'Mullane, Carl Flynn, John Loane and Andrea Kealy. CASALA is funded under Enterprise Ireland's Applied Research Enhancement Program with support from EU structural funds. Research at the Netwell Centre is supported by Atlantic Philanthropies.

References

1. Hayutin AM. How population aging differs across countries: a briefing on global demographics. Stanford Center on Longevity US. California: Stanford; 2007.
2. Kinsella K, Wan H. An ageing world: 2008. United States Census Bureau, International Population Reports P95/09-1 11; 2009.
3. CSO Ireland Ageing in Ireland Report. 2007. Available at: http://www.cso.ie/en/media/csoie/releasespublications/documents/otherreleases/2007/ageinginireland.pdf.
4. US Census Bureau. An aging world. 2008. Available at: https://www.census.gov/prod/2009pubs/p95-09-1.pdf.
5. Centers for Disease Control and Prevention. Health, United States. Hyattsville: National Center for Health Statistics; 2011.
6. European Commission. Major and chronic diseases executive summary. European Commission. Belgium: Brussels; 2007.

7. Turner K, Arnott A, Gray PD, Renals S, et al. Grand challenge in assisted living – home care technologies. Match Consortium, UKCRC Grand Challenges in Computing Research. Edinburgh, 2010.
8. DeFrances CJ, Hall MJ, Podgornik MN. 2003 national hospital discharge survey. Advance data from vital and health statistics, 359. Hyattsville: National Center for Health Statistics; 2005.
9. Jencks SF, Williams MV, Coleman EA. Rehospitalizations among patients in the Medicare fee-for-service program. N Engl J Med. 2008;360:1418–28.
10. Dewsbury G, Clarke K, Rouncefield M, Sommerville I. Depending on digital design: extending inclusivity. Housing Stud. 2004;19(5):811–25.
11. Koch S. Home tele-health current state and future trends. Int J Med Inform. 2006;75: 565–76.
12. Magnusson L, Hanson E, Borg M. A literature review study of information and communication technology as a support for frail older people living at home and their family carers. Technol Disabil. 2004;16:223–35.
13. Brennan PF, Moore SM, Smyth KA. Computer link: electronic support for the home caregiver. ANS Adv Nurs Sci. 1991;13(4):14–27.
14. Brennan PF, Moore S, Bjomsdottir G, Jones J, Visovsky C, Rogers M. HeartCare: an internet-based information and support system for patient home recovery after coronary artery bypass graft (CABG) surgery. J Adv Nurs. 2001;35(5):699–708.
15. Cooper R. Wheeled mobility and manipulation technologies. The Bridge: Linking Engineering and Society; 2009.
16. Steventon A, Bardsley M, Billings J, Dixon J, et al. Effect of telehealth on use of secondary care and mortality: findings from the Whole System Demonstrator cluster randomised trial. BMJ. 2012;344:e3874.
17. Czaja S, Charness N, Fisk A, Hertzog C, Nair S, Rogers W, Sharit J. Factors predicting the use of technology: findings from the Center for Research and Education on Aging and Technology Enhancement (CREATE). Psychol Aging. 2006;21(2):333–52.
18. Hawthorn D. Possible implications of aging for interface designers. Interacting Comput. 2000;12:507–28.
19. Salces FS, Baskett M, LLewelyn-Jones D, England D. Ambient interfaces for elderly people at home. Ambient Intelligence in Everyday Life. Lecture notes in computer science 2864. 2006. pp. 256–84.
20. Gardner D, Helmes E. Locus of control and self-directed learning as predictors of well-being in the elderly. Aust Psychol. 1999;34(2):99–103.
21. Melenhorst AS, Rogers W, Caylor E. The use of communication technologies by older adults: exploring the benefits from the user's perspective. Human factors and ergonomics society 45th annual meeting. Minneapolis, USA; 2001.
22. Davis F. A Technology acceptance model for empirically testing new end-user information systems: theory and results. Unpublished doctoral thesis, MIT Sloan School of Management, Cambridge, MA, 1985.
23. Oppenauer C. Motivation and needs for technology use in old age. Gerontechnology. 2009; 8(2):82–7.
24. Wilkowska W, Ziefle M. Which factors form older adults' acceptance of mobile information and communication technologies? In: Proceedings of HCI and usability for E-Inclusion, USAB, Linz: Springer LNCS; 9–10 Nov 2009. pp. 81–101.
25. Umemuro H. Computer attitudes, cognitive abilities and technology usage among Japanese older adults. Gerontechnology. 2004;3(2):64–76.
26. Alm M, Gregor P, Newell AF. Older people and information technology are ideal partners. In: Proceedings of the international conference on for universal design (UD 2002), Yokohama, 2002.

27. Carmichael A, Rice M, MacMillan F, Kirk A. Investigating a DTV-based physical activity application to facilitate wellbeing in older adults. In: Proceedings of HCI conference on people and computers XXIV (HCI 2010), Dundee, 2010. pp. 278–88.

28. Doyle J, Skrba Z, McDonnell R, Arent B. Designing a touch screen communication device to support social interaction amongst older adults. In: Proceedings of HCI conference on people and computers XXIV (HCI 2010), Dundee, 2010. pp. 177–85.

29. Jones C, Winegarden C, Rogers W. Supporting healthy aging with new technologies. ACM Interactions. 2009;16(4):48–51.

30. Bieber G, Koldrack P, Sablowski C, Peter C, Urban B. Mobile physical activity recognition of stand-up and sit-down transitions for user behaviour analysis. In: Proceedings of 3rd international conference on PErvasive technologies related to assistive environments, Samos, 23–25 June 2010.

31. Lorenz A, Mielke S, Oppermann R, Zahl L. Personalised mobile health monitoring for elderly. In: Proceedings of 9th international conference on Human Computer Interaction with Mobile Devices and Services (Mobile HCI), Singapore, 11–14 Sept 2007. pp. 297–304.

32. Doyle J, Bailey C, Dromey B, Ni Scanaill C. BASE – an interactive technology solution to deliver balance and strength exercises to older adults. In: Proceedings of 4th international conference on Pervasive Computing Technologies for Healthcare, Munich, 22–25 Mar 2010. pp. 1–5.

33. Tinetti M, Williams C. The effect of falls and fall injuries on functioning in community-dwelling older persons. J Gerontol A Biol Sci Med Sci. 1998;53(2):M112–9.

34. Chang JT, Morton SC, Rubenstein LZ, Mojica WA, et al. Interventions for the prevention of falls in older adults: systematic review and meta-analysis of randomized clinical trials. BMJ. 2004;328:680–3.

35. Gannon B, O'Shea E, Hudson E. Economic cost of falls and fractures among older people in Ireland. Ir Med J. 2008;101(6):170–3.

36. Kerse N, Flicker L, Plaff JJ, et al. Falls, depression and antidepressants in later life: a large primary care appraisal. PLoS One. 2008;3(6):e2423.

37. Stevens JA, Corso PS, Finkelstein EA, Miller TR. The cost of fatal and non-fatal falls among older adults. Inj Prev. 2006;12:290–5.

38. Rockwood K, Mitnitski A. Frailty in relation to the accumulation of deficits. J Gerontol A Biol Sci Med Sci. 2007;62:722–7.

39. Bandeen-Roche K, Xue QL, Ferrucci L, et al. Phenotype of frailty: characterisation in the women's health and aging studies. J Gerontol A Biol Sci Med Sci. 2006;61A:262–6.

40. Santos-Eggiman B, Cuenod P, Spagnoli J, Junod J. Prevalence of frailty in middle-aged and older community-dwelling Europeans living in 10 countries. J Gerontol A Biol Sci Med Sci. 2009;64(6):675–81.

41. Smit E, Winters-Stone KM, Loprinzi PD, Tang AM, Crespo C. Lower nutritional status and higher food insufficiency in frail older US adults. Br J Nutr. 2013;110(1):172–8.

42. Fillit H, Butler RN. The frailty identity crisis. J Am Geriatr Soc. 2009;57:348–53.

43. SilverFit. http://www.silverfit.nl/en/index.htm. Accessed Feb 2014.

44. Egglestone SR, Axelrod L, Nind T et al. A design framework for a home-based stroke rehabilitation system: identifying the key components. In: Proceedings of 3rd international conference on Pervasive Computing Technologies for Healthcare, London, 1–3 Apr 2009. pp. 1–8.

45. Campbell AJ, Robertson MC, Gardner MM, et al. Randomised control trial of a general practice programme of home based exercise to prevent falls in elderly women. BMJ. 1997;315:1065–9.

46. Hawkley LC, Preacher KJ, Cacioppo JT. Loneliness impairs daytime functioning but not sleep duration. Health Psychol. 2010;29:124–9.

47. Hawkley LC, Thisted RA, Masi CM, Cacioppo JT. Loneliness predicts increased blood pressure: five-year cross-lagged analyses in middle-aged and older adults. Psychol Aging. 2010;25:132–41.

48. Tilvis RS, Kahonen-Vare MH, Jolkkonen J, Valvanne J, Pitkala KH, Strandberg TE. Predictors of cognitive decline and mortality of aged people over a 10-year period. J Gerontol A Biol Sci Med Sci. 2004;59:268–74.

49. Patterson AC, Veenstra G. Loneliness and risk of mortality: a longitudinal investigation in Alameda County, California. Soc Sci Med. 2010;71:181–6.
50. Czaja S, Guerrier J, Nair S, Landauer T. Computer communication as an aid to independence for older adults. Behav Inform Technol. 1993;12(4):197–207.
51. Dalsgaard T, Skov M, Thomassen B. eKiss: sharing experiences in families through a picture blog. In: Proceedings of HCI conference on People and Computers XXI (HCI 2007), Lancaster, 3–7 Sept 2007. pp. 67–75.
52. Sokoler T, Svensson MS. Presence remote: embracing ambiguity in the design of social TV for senior citizens. In: Changing television environments – 6th European conference EUROITV. Salzburg, Austria; 2008. pp. 158–62.
53. Riche Y, Mackay W. PeerCare: supporting awareness of rhythms and routines for better aging in place. Comput Supported Coop Work. 2010;19(1):73–104.
54. Ferri CP, Prince M, Brayne C, Brodaty H, Fratiglioni L, Ganguli M, et al. Global prevalence of dementia: a Delphi consensus study. Lancet. 2005;366(9503):2112–7.
55. Astell A, Alm N, Gowans G, Ellis M, Dye R, Vaughan P. Involving older people with dementia and their carers in designing computer based support systems: some methodological considerations. Universal Access in the Information Society. 2009;8(1)49–58.
56. Arnott J, Alm N, Waller A. Cognitive prostheses: communication, rehabilitation and beyond. In: Proceedings of IEEE system man and cybernetics conference, 1999. pp. 346–51.
57. Kautz H, Arnstein L, Borriello G, Etzioni O, Fox D. An overview of the assisted cognition project. In: AAAI-2002 workshop on automation as Caregiver: the role of intelligent technology in elder care. Edmonton, AB, Canada; 2002.
58. Wherton J, Monk AF. Problems people with dementia have with kitchen tasks: the challenge for pervasive computing. Interacting Comput. 2010;22(4):253–66.
59. Wherton J, Monk AF. Technological opportunities for supporting people with dementia who are living at home. Int J Hum Comput Stud. 2008;66:571–86.
60. Woods B, Spector A, Jones C, Orrell M, Davies S. Reminiscence therapy for dementia. Cochrane Database Syst Rev. 2005;(2):CD001120.
61. Sarne-Fleischmann V, Tractinsky N, Dwolatzky T, Rief I. Personalized reminiscence therapy for patients with Alzheimer's disease using a computerized system. In: Proceedings of the 4th international conference on Pervasive Technologies Related to Assistive Environments (PETRA '11), 2011.
62. Kikhia B, Hallberg J, Synnes K, Sani Z. Context-aware life-logging for persons with mild dementia. Conf Proc IEEE Eng Med Biol Soc. 2009;2009:6183–6. doi: 10.1109/IEMBS.2009.5334509.
63. Dem@Care EU Project. http://www.demcare.eu/.
64. McHugh JE, Wherton JP, Prendergast DK, Lawlor BA. Teleconferencing as a source of social support for older spousal caregivers: initial explorations and recommendations for future research. Am J Alzheimers Dis Other Demen. 2012;27(6):381–7.
65. McHugh JE, Wherton JP, Prendergast DK, Lawlor BA. Identifying opportunities for supporting caregivers of persons with dementia through information and communication technology. Gerontechnology. 2012;10(4):220–30.
66. Discover for Carers EU Project. http://www.discover4carers.eu/.
67. Vurgun S, Philipose M, Pavel M. A statistical reasoning system for medication prompting. In: Proceedings of UbiComp. Innsbruck, Austria; 2007. pp. 1–18.
68. Consolvo S, Landay JA. Designing for behaviour change in everyday life. IEEE Comput. 2009;42(6):86–9.
69. Lane ND, Mohammod M, Lin M et al. BeWell: a smartphone application to monitor, model and promote wellbeing. In: Proceedings of 5th international conference on Pervasive Computing Technologies for Healthcare, Dublin, 23–26 May 2011.
70. Doyle J, O'Mullane B, McGee S, Knapp B. YourWellness: designing an application to support positive emotional wellbeing in older adults. In: Proceedings of HCI conference on People and Computers XXVI (HCI 2012), Birmingham, 12–14 Sept 2012.
71. Marcu G, Bardram JE, Gabrielli S. A framework for overcoming challenges in designing persuasive monitoring and feedback systems for mental illness. In: Proceedings of 5th international conference on Pervasive Computing Technologies for Healthcare, Dublin, 23–26 May 2011.

72. Cruickshank J, Beer G, Winpenny E, Manning J. Healthcare without walls: a framework for delivering telehealth at scale. 2010. Available at http://www.2020health.org/2020health/Publication-2012/NHSit/telehealth.html.

73. McLean A, Protti D, Sheikh A. Telehealth for long term conditions. BMJ. 2011;342:d120.

74. Farmer A, Gibson O, Tarassenko L, Neil A. A systematic review of telemedicine interventions to support blood glucose self-monitoring in diabetes. Diabet Med. 2005;22:1372–8.

75. Martinez A, Everss E, Rojo-Alvarez J, Figal D, Garcia-Alberola A. A systematic review of the literature on home monitoring for patients with heart failure. J Telemed Telecare. 2006;12:234–41.

76. Barlow J, Singh D, Bayer C, Curry R. A systematic review of the benefits of home telecare for frail elderly people and those with long-term conditions. J Telemed Telecare. 2007;13:172–9.

77. Canadian Health Infoway Collaboration and communication for Chronic Disease Patients. Available at: http://www.youtube.com/watch?v=9ICjviv1_-8.

78. Bower P, Cartwright M, Hirani SP, Barlow J, et al. A comprehensive evaluation of the impact of telemonitoring in patients with long-term conditions and social care needs: protocol for the whole systems demonstrator cluster randomised trial. BMC Health Serv Res. 2011;11:184.

79. Bardram JE, Bossen C, Thomsen A. Designing for transformations in collaboration – a study of the deployment of homecare technology. In: Proceedings of GROUP '05. Sanibel Island, FL, USA; 2005.

80. Canada Health Infoway Telehealth Benefits and Adoption: Connecting People and Providers Across Canada. 2011. Available at: https://www.infoway-inforoute.ca/index.php/resources/toolkits/knowing-is-better-for-clinicians/index.php?searchword=benefits+of+telehealth&ordering=newest&searchphrase=all&areas%5B%5D=docman&limit=5&option=com_search&Itemid=736. Accessed 12 Feb 2014.

81. Cook D, Hagras H, Callaghan V, Helal A. Making our environments intelligent. J Pervasive Mobile Comput. 2009;5:556–7.

82. Cook D, Schmitter-Edgecombe M, Crandall A, Sanders C, Thomas B. Collecting and disseminating smart home sensor data in the CASAS project. In: Proceedings of the CHI workshop on developing shared home behavior datasets to advance HCI and ubiquitous computing research. Boston, MA, USA; 2009.

83. Skubic M, Guevara R, Rantz M. Testing classifiers for embedded health assessment. Impact analysis of solutions for chronic disease prevention and management. In: Icost 2012, LNCS 7251, 2012. pp 198–205 Springer-Verlag, Berlin Heidelberg.

84. Bhattacharya A, Das SK. LeZi-Update: an information-theoretic approach to track mobile users in PCS networks. In: Proceedings of the 5th annual ACM/IEEE international conference on Mobile Computing and Networking (MobiCom'99). Seattle, WA, USA; 1999.

85. Das SK, Cook DJ, Bhattacharya A, Heierman EO, Lin TY. The role of prediction algorithm in the MavHome smart home architecture. IEEE Wireless Commun. 2002;9(6):77–84.

86. Jain G, Cook D, Jakkula V, Monitoring health by detecting drifts and outliers for a smart environment inhabitant. In: Proceedings of the international conference on smart homes and health telematics (I-COST), Northern Ireland, 2006. pp. 114–21.

87. Helal S, Mann W, El-Zabadani H, King J, Kaddoura Y, Jansen E. The gator tech smart house: a programmable pervasive space. Computer. 2005;38(3):50–60.

88. Mozer MC. The neural network house: an environment that's adapts to its inhabitants. In: Proceedings of the AAAI spring symposium on intelligent environments, technical report SS-98-02. Palo Alto, CA, USA; 1998. pp.110–4.

89. Kidd CD, Orr R, Abowd GD, Atkeson CG, Essa IA, MacIntyre B, Mynatt ED, Starner T, Newstetter W. The aware home: a living laboratory for ubiquitous computing research. In: Proceedings of the second international workshop on Cooperative Buildings, Integrating Information, Organization, and Architecture (CoBuild '99). Pittsburgh, PA, USA; 1999. pp. 191–8.

90. Kientz JA, Patel SN, Jones B, Price E, Mynatt ED, Abowd GD, The Georgia Tech aware home. In: Proceedings of CHI '08 Extended Abstracts on Human Factors in Computing Systems (CHI EA '08). Florence, Italy; 2008. pp. 3675–80.

91. Intille SS. Designing a home of the future. IEEE Pervasive Comput. 2002;1(2):76–82.

92. Logan B, Healey J, Philipose M, Tapia EM, Intille S. A long-term evaluation of sensing modalities for activity recognition. In: Proceedings of the 9th international conference on Ubiquitous Computing (UbiComp '07). Innsbruck, Austria; 2007. pp. 483–500.
93. Tapia EM, Intille SS, Larson K. Activity recognition in the home setting using simple and ubiquitous sensors. In: Proceedings of PERVASIVE. Vienna, Austria; 2004. pp. 158–75.
94. Chen C, Das B, Cook D. A data mining framework for activity recognition in smart environments. In: Proceedings of the international conference on Intelligent Environments. Kuala Lumpur, Malaysia; 2010.
95. Rashidi P, Cook DJ, Holder LB, Schmitter-Edgecombe M. Discovering activities to recognize and track in a smart environment. IEEE Trans Knowl Data Eng. 2011;23(4): 527–39.
96. Jimison H, Bajcsy R. Integrated communications and inference systems for continuous coordinated care of older adults in the home. NSF Collaborative Research Grant. http://www. orcatech.org/research/studies/integrated-communications-and-inference-systems-for-continuous-coordinated-care-of-older-adults-in-the-home. Accessed Feb 2014.
97. Kaye JA, Maxwell SA, Mattek N, Hayes T, Dodge H, Pavel M, Jimison H, Wild K, Boise KL, Zitzelberger T. Intelligent systems for assessing aging changes: home-based, unobtrusive and continuous assessment of aging. J Gerontol Psychol Sci. 2011;66B:i180–90.
98. O'Brien A, McDaid K, Loane J, Doyle J, Walsh L. Visualisation of movement of older adults within their homes based on PIR sensor data. In: Proceedings of PERVASENSE, workshop at pervasive health'12, San Diego, 2012.
99. Loane J, O' Mullane B, Bortz B, Knapp B. Looking for similarities in movement between and within homes using cluster analysis. Health Informatics J. 2012;18(3):202–11.
100. O'Mullane B, Knapp B, O'Hanlon A, Loane J, Bortz B. Comparison of health measures to movement data in aware homes. In: AmI'll Proceedings of the second international conference on Ambient Intelligence, Amsterdam, 2011. pp. 290–4.
101. Doyle J, O'Mullane B, O'Hanlon A, Knapp B. Requirements gathering for the delivery of healthcare data in aware homes. In: 5th Intl conference on pervasive computing technologies for healthcare, Dublin, 2011.
102. Doyle J, Kealy A, Loane J, Walsh L, et al. An integrated home-based self-management system to support the wellbeing of older adults. Accepted for publication in Journal of Ambient Intelligence and Smart Environments (JAISE); 2014;6(4):359–83.
103. Hybels CF, Blazer DG. Epidemiology of late-life mental disorders. Clin Geriatr Med. 2003;19(4):48–51.
104. Manabe T, Matsui M, Yamaya T, Sato-Nakagawa N, Okamura H, Arai H, Sasaki H. Sleep patterns and mortality among elderly patients in a geriatric hospital. Gerontology. 2000;46(6):318–22.
105. Miles LE, Dement WC. Sleep and aging. Sleep. 1980;3(3):119–220.
106. Ancoli-Israil S. Sleep problems in older adults: putting myths to bed. Geriatrics. 1997;52(1):20–9.
107. Barbar SI, Enright PL, Boyle P, Foley D, Sharp S, Petrovitch H, Quan SF. Sleep disturbances and their correlates in elderly Japanese American men residing in Hawaii. J Gerontol A Biol Sci Med Sci. 2000;55(7):406–11.
108. Brassington GS, King AC, Bliwise DL. Sleep problems as a risk factor for falls in a sample of community-dwelling adults aged 64-99 years. J Am Geriatr Soc. 2000;48(10): 1234–40.
109. Happe S. Excessive daytime sleepiness and sleep disturbances in patients with neurological diseases. Drugs. 2003;63(24):2725–37.
110. Walsh L, Moloney E and McLoone S. Identification of nocturnal movements during sleep using non-contact under mattress bed sensor. In: Proceedings of 33rd annual international conference of the IEEE Engineering in Medicine and Biology Society (EMBC'11), Boston, 2011.
111. Kealy A, McDaid K, Loane J, Walsh L, Doyle J. Derivation of night time behaviour metrics using ambient sensors. In: Proceedings of 7th international conference on pervasive computing technologies for healthcare (Pervasive Health'13), Venice, 5–8 May 2013.

Part III
Administration

Chapter 10
Administration Applications

Hélène Clément

Abstract Healthcare administrators face a variety of demands such as program planning, resource management, financial management, organizational reporting, and quality improvements. Consequently, administrators have a need for accurate, timely information to support decision-making, as well as tools to support the communication of such decisions. Information and data are considered corporate assets, in that they provide the foundation for informed decisions. This chapter covers both management information systems – those solutions that collect, synthesize and present information and data to support decision making, and the office automation systems which assist administrators communicate their decisions.

Keywords eHealth • Nursing informatics • Quality management • Nursing workload measurement systems • Case costing • Nursing Systems

Key Concepts

eHealth
Nursing informatics
Informatics Standards
Nursing Systems

Introduction

Managers and caregivers throughout the healthcare system are constantly working to increase the efficiency and effectiveness of patient care while simultaneously reducing or at least maintaining existing levels of resource consumption (Fig. 10.1). A principal strategy being used to achieve these goals is to consider and use information as a corporate strategic resource and provide enhanced information

---

Supplementary material is available in the online version of this chapter at 10.1007/978-1-4471-2999-8_10. Videos can also be accessed at http://www.springerimages.com/videos/978-1-4471-2998-1.

H. Clément, RN, BScN, MHA, CPHIMS-CA
Independant Health Informatics Executive, Richmond Hill, ON, Canada
e-mail: HClement@rogers.com

© Springer-Verlag London 2015   215
K.J. Hannah et al. (eds.), *Introduction to Nursing Informatics*,
Health Informatics, DOI 10.1007/978-1-4471-2999-8_10

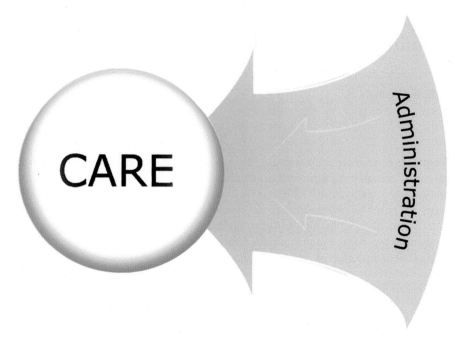

Fig. 10.1 CARE graphic 3: administration

management methods and tools to caregivers and managers across the health sector. The idea is to use information to help managers utilize available resources most effectively.

Administrative uses of information systems can be classified in two ways: those that provide managers with information for decision making and those that help managers communicate the decisions. In this chapter, the administrative uses of information systems that help managers with decision making are called "management information systems." Those applications of information systems in nursing administration that help managers communicate their decisions are called "office automation systems." This chapter defines management information systems and describes the information needs related to the management of clinical settings providing care to patients and clients. This chapter concludes with the nursing role in the management of information and obstacles and issues in management information systems.

Definition of Management Information Systems

The idea of management information systems was developed in the business and industrial sectors. It has been studied, analyzed, and evaluated in detail by management scientists for decades. In those sectors, there are many definitions of the concept of management information systems (MISs). Some definitions place an emphasis on the physical elements and design of the system, while others focus on the function of a MIS in an organization. In this book, MIS is a "general term for information system that supports operations, management, analysis and decision-making functions within an organization; involves the use of computer hardware and software, data and databases, and decision making" [1]. The Health Information and Management Systems Society [2] definition of MIS "refers to either a class of software that provides management with tools for organizing and evaluating their department, or the staff that supports information systems". Although these definitions could include both manual and computerized systems, we will only discuss computerized MISs in this book.

Information Needs for the Management of Patient Care

Organizational information needs, as represented by its managers, are targeted to fulfill that aspect of the mission related to the provision of patient or client care, regardless of the healthcare setting where services are being delivered. Management information systems help nursing in the areas of quality management, unit staffing, and ongoing reporting. Such systems also support managers in their responsibilities for allocation and utilization of the following resources required to deliver healthcare services in the patient/client care environments: human resources, fiscal resources (including payroll, supplies, and materiel), and physical resources (including physical facilities, equipment, and furniture) [3].

Patient care delivery can occur in many different healthcare settings. This includes hospitals, long term care, health centres, community care centres, home care, primary care (physicians' and nurse practitioners' offices), educational settings, correctional facilities, and other community-based service agencies. As such, clinicians regardless of the physical setting where they work, must have access to information for managing patient care. As patient care is being delivered and documented electronically, data is being collected. This data can be transformed, providing information that was previously not easily available in a paper environment. As more technologies are made available at point of care, the data collected during the delivery of services will provide a wealth of information and knowledge. This will allow for secondary use of data for other purposes such as more customized health care delivery, quality management, system planning, human resources planning, just to name a few. The use of data to demonstrate the value and use of information in the continuum of care can be viewed in the attached documentation from the Canadian Institute for Health Information (CIHI). Other examples of use of information can be found on the Canada Health Infoway website (see http://www.infoway-inforoute.ca/index.php?option=com_googlesearchcse&n=30&Itemid=1307&cx=004947342097296117226%3A3cbkgdvxvm8&cof=FORID%3A11&ie=ISO-8859-1&q=HSU+initiatives&sa=Search&hl=en&siteurl=https%3A%2F%2Fwww.infoway-inforoute.ca%2F).

Quality Management

Total quality management (TQM) and continuous quality improvement (CQI) continue to be commonly encountered approaches to quality management and improvement [4]. TQM is an important process for staff nurses and administrators alike. It is useful to staff nurses in two ways: it provides them with feedback about the nature of their individual practice and provides them with opportunity to influence patient care in their organization. Administrators use it to assess the general quality of patient care provided within their organizations and as a process to receive and communicate opportunities to enhance patient care and organizational effectiveness.

A process of establishing and maintaining organizational effectiveness (i.e., the quality of care provided to patients), TQM is an institutional plan of action to empower staff to influence corporate achievement of the highest possible standards for patient care. The delivery of patient care is monitored by all staff to ensure that established standards are met or surpassed. Implicit in the concept of TQM is the ongoing evaluation of the standards themselves, thus ensuring that they reflect current norms and practices in healthcare. Organizations use a variety of formal and informal means to gather information to evaluate the quality of care provided to patients. The formal means are encompassed in a quality assurance program. Information needs associated with quality assurance might include patient care databases, patient evaluations of care received, nurses' notes on the chart, patient care plans, performance appraisals, and incident reports. These sources of information are reviewed by either a concurrent or retrospective audit. Concurrent nursing audits occur during the patient's stay in the hospital, whereas retrospective nursing audits occur after the patient leaves the hospital. Audit reviews are a major tool for any TQM program.

The literature referring to the development of quality in healthcare ranges from 30 years to 3,000 years as identified by historians. The impetus for the establishment of quality assurance programs emerged during the 1970s as the result of rising consumer awareness, increasing healthcare costs, and the growing professionalism of nursing [5]. An additional factor was the desire of governments to monitor the cost and quality of care associated with its healthcare programs. Almost simultaneously, three things happened: professional standards review organizations were established in a number of countries such as the United States, Canada, and Australia (as available at organizations including the Canadian Nurses Association www.cna-aiic.ca, Nursing World www.nursingworld.org, or the Australian Nursing & Midwifery Federation www.anf.org.au), standards of practice were developed and published by nursing organizations, and accreditation organizations were created. For example, the American Joint Commission on Accreditation for Hospitals established the requirement for medical and nursing audits. This resulted in organizations requiring the collection of massive amounts of data. Transforming this data into information for multiple purposes added pressure to the entire quality assurance process, which became dependant on the timely processing and review of this data, in turn consuming enormous amounts of nursing time. As these audits were done, healthcare professionals gained an increased awareness of the variability in documentation practices and its link to data quality. This resulted in improved documentation in the form of nursing care plans and patient records, and further increased the volume of information to be reviewed and evaluated in the nursing audits.

As the pressure continued to increase regarding enhanced data quality, documentation comprehensiveness and the need for timely health information to assist clinicians in delivering healthcare, integrated hospital information systems made their entry into the healthcare delivery system. Quality assurance/improvement programs in nursing needed two things to succeed: standardized terminology and standardized care plans. These two elements were also required if information systems were to be any help to nurses in providing nursing care regardless of the health care setting while ensuring seamless delivery of care across the continuum of care. The standardization of terminology required for computerized documentation of nurses' notes, and the development of standardized care plans, coincided with the need for standardized terminology, development of patient care standards and quality improvement programs (see Chap. 7). Quality assurance or quality improvement programs are now implemented in most healthcare organizations and are key for management at all organizational levels.

Health information terminology for clinical documentation is an important component of the EHR [6]. One implementation aspect of these terminology standards is the development and use of minimum data sets (MDS). MDS have been developed and used to document clinical information across all health care settings and specialities. The Resident Assessment is an example of a minimum data set standardized tool. These Resident Assessments have been developed to collect assessment information in different clinical settings such as long term care, nursing home, rehabilitation, complex continuing, and mental health. The report "Highlight of 2012–2011 Inpatient Hospitalizations and Emergency Department Visits" published by the Canadian Institute for Health Information (CIHI) is an example on how data can be used [7]. In Canada, the Data Set C-HOBIC (Canadian Health Outcomes for Better Information and Care) includes standardized terms and concepts linking nursing practice and patient outcomes in the EHR (see the Canada Health Infoway, https://www.infoway-inforoute.ca/index.php/programs-services/standards-collaborative/pan-canadian-standards/canadian-outcomes-for-better-information-and-care-c-hobic and C-HOBIC, http://c-hobic.cna-aiic.ca/default.aspx websites).

The ability of a computer to retrieve, summarize, and compare large volumes of information rapidly has proven useful for managers charged with the responsibility of implementing quality assurance programs. The first obstacle to using computers for this purpose was the lack of widespread availability of integrated hospital information systems. The second obstacle was the lack of a widely implemented common nursing vocabulary and methods of coding nursing diagnoses and interventions (see Chap. 7). Both obstacles are being overcome with the integration of sophisticated information systems. Taxonomies for nursing diagnoses, interventions, and contributions to patient care outcomes have been developed [8]. Some of the taxonomies include NANDA (www.nanda.org), Nursing Intervention Classification (NIC), and Nursing Outcomes Classification (NOC). (For more information, see the

following website: http://www.nasn.org/PolicyAdvocacy/PositionPapersandReports/
NASNPositionStatementsFullView/tabid/462/ArticleId/48/Standardized-Nursing-
Languages-Revised-June-2012). Unfortunately, much of this work has not yet
received widespread implementation in the nursing profession and its different practice settings. It is only starting to be incorporated as a framework for the organization
of nursing databases by developers of information systems.

Another challenge associated with computerized quality assurance programs is
the limitations of the data entry tools. Consequently, much effort has been focused on
the process aspects incorporated in the TQM concept. Unfortunately, the vendors of
computer software have not given high priority to the information needs related to
TQM or the development of clinical software packages for healthcare organizations.
This situation has created a major barrier to the effective, widespread use of information systems for quality monitoring in hospitals. Several organizations have developed TQM programs that incorporate procedures for conducting concurrent chart
audits. These organizations use a manual concurrent audit conducted by staff nurses
with special training in concurrent clinical auditing during the delivery of health care
services (www.currentnursing.com) on the patient care units. The data from the completed audit forms are then put into the computer for tabulation, summarization, and
analysis. This combination of manual and computer methods partially reduces the
labour-intensive process associated with totally manual audits. As healthcare technologies and standards are being deployed in healthcare organizations, this is assisting managers to support quality improvement processes. The data collected, when
transformed into information, has provided valuable insight in use of services within
health care organizations. The reports "Highlights of 2010–2011 Selected Indicators
Describing the Birthing Process in Canada" and "Highlight of 2010–2011 Inpatient
Hospitalizations and Emergency Departments Visits" published by the Canadian
Institute for Health Information (CIHI) are examples of how data can be used.

There is a growing emphasis on patient care outcomes as the major focus of nursing TQM programs. Similarly, there is a growing trend away from the problem resolution model to a planning model as the major criterion for measuring quality
assurance. Simultaneously, there is an increasing demand from the public for better
resource management in the healthcare sector, and the public has an increasing
awareness of quality as a cost component of healthcare. As nursing leaders, we need
to process, analyze, and make timely decisions ranging from practice to management and planning perspectives. These factors are creating a demand for more
sophisticated computerized information systems that are able to handle and process
data which can be transformed into information to will support decision making.

Patient Classification, Workload Measurement, and Patient Care Unit Staffing

In the past, innumerable nurse leaders and supervisors in healthcare organizations and
agencies around the world spent countless hours each day "doing the time." Even
when master rotation plans were used, manual scheduling of personnel work rotations

could not eliminate all the problems, such as vulnerability to accusations of bias when assigning days off or shift rotation, difficulty establishing minimum staffing to avoid wasting manpower, and dependence on an individual's memory in the nursing administrative structure. Consequently, automated staff scheduling is a highly desired component of a management information system for patient care administration. Frequently, when an organization has limited resources and limited computerized patient management information system, it mobilizes resources to set up a computerized staffing system. This is becoming more critical as managers must plan for services that include not only nursing but other healthcare professionals for the delivery of comprehensive patient care in many different healthcare settings such as hospitals, long term care, community care centres, home care, or anywhere where services are provided.

Researchers at many healthcare organizations have developed diverse systems for personnel time assignment. The complexity of these systems varies greatly. Some merely use the computer to print names into what was formerly a manual master rotation schedule; others adjust staffing interactively and dynamically on a shift-to-shift basis by considering patient acuity, workload levels for one or more healthcare discipline, and the expertise of available personnel. To develop complex, sophisticated systems for automated personnel scheduling, a great deal of planning and data gathering is required: the workload must be identified in the organization; the different healthcare professionals delivering services must be identified; the various levels of expertise of staff members must be categorized and documented; criteria for determining patient acuity and nursing workload must be established; personnel policies must be clearly defined; and the elements of union contracts must be summarized. When all this information is available, a computer program is designed to schedule clinical staff (nursing, physiotherapy, respiratory therapy, etc.) on patient care units. The capacity of the computer to manipulate large numbers of variables consistently and quickly makes personnel time assignment an excellent use of this technology.

Documented advantages of automated scheduling of personnel include the following.

- Easier recruitment and increased job satisfaction because schedules are known well in advance
- Less time spent on manual scheduling, thereby providing more time for nurse managers to carry out other duties
- Advance notice of staff shortages requiring temporary replacements
- Unbiased assignment of days off and shift rotation
- More effective utilization and distribution of personnel throughout the institution or agency
- Capacity to document the effect of staff size on quality of care
- Ability to relate quantity and quality of nursing staff to patient acuity.

Workload measurement systems function with automated scheduling. Nursing workload measurement systems (NWMSs), sometimes called patient classification systems (PCSs) are tools that measure the number of direct, indirect, and nonclinical patient care hours by patient acuity on a daily basis [9, 10]. PCSs and NWMSs have evolved to focus on providing uniform, reliable productivity information to help with staffing, budgeting, planning, and quality assurance. NWMS have become a valuable management tool for managers, department heads, senior management, and governments alike. As healthcare costs and demands continue to escalate, the appropriate and effective utilization of scarce human resources becomes increasingly onerous. There are many PCSs and NWMSs available commercially [11]. All differ in one or many respects, and the criteria used to choose such a system ultimately depend on the specific organization's needs. The different workload measurement systems can not only measure nursing care requirements but also patient care requirements delivered by a number of healthcare disciplines. Hence, some healthcare organizations are now referring to workload as an interdisciplinary workload measurement system. These workload systems can capture information in a wide variety of settings such as hospitals, health centres, community care centres, home care, correctional facilities, and other community based service agencies where healthcare is provided. (For more information, see the following website; http://www.healthleadersmedia.com/page-1/TEC-266546/Patient-Classification-Systems-Address-Nurse-Staffing-Balance)

Some workload measurement systems are able to capture both prospective and retrospective workload information. A prospective workload measurement system captures patient requirements for the next 24 hour period providing managers with data to plan resources requirements for the delivery of services. A retrospective workload measurement system captures resources used by patients often by being integrated with a clinical documentation system or through data entry in the workload measurement system. In healthcare organizations where both prospective and retrospective workload measurement systems are implemented, managers are able to compare patient care projected against the patient care services delivered. This information has provided managers with valuable data for quality improvement, planning and other opportunities for innovations in patient care delivery. In some healthcare organisations, workload measurement systems have been interfaced to case costing systems, providing organizations with valuable information about cost associated with each patient visit or encounter.

Increased job satisfaction, easier recruitment of staff, unbiased rotation assignment, workstation printouts, and advance notice of temporary shortages—all contribute to improved staff morale and thus indirectly result in better patient care. Administrative time saved and more effective utilization and distribution of personnel have also been suggested as factors influencing quality of patient care within the agency or organization. Documentation of the relationship between staffing and quality of patient care gives the manager strong data to justify staffing requests and decisions to the senior management team within their healthcare organization.

Case Costing

Case costing systems or cost accounting systems provide information on the cost of delivering healthcare to an individual patient within a clinical service area. These systems can receive data from different systems within the organization such as financial, payroll, scheduling, workload measurement, documentation systems.

The information that is generated from case costing systems can be used to support management activities, strategic planning and present different perspectives for the analysis of financial information.

There are many case costing systems on the market which differ in one or many respects. The choice of systems by the healthcare organization ultimately are driven by specific organizational needs. The system can provide valuable data by identifying costs associated with program realignment, determining potential costs associated with new programs, identifying opportunities for improve resource utilization, to name a few. Organizations have been able to use case costing information for different purposes, such as to identify costs associated with an outbreak in the facility, to expand or add new programs, to evaluate change in practice, to determine the financial impact of healthcare service being delivered in an outpatient rather than an inpatient setting, and to perform "what if" scenarios and forecasting. (For additional information on the costs of services, see http://ourhealthsystem.ca). The data collected will provide valuable information about the cost associated with service delivery. Case costing initiatives are being implemented in Canada in a number of organizations. (For additional information, see http://www.cdha.nshealth.ca/search/apachesolr_search/case costing http://www.occp.com/mainPage.htm).

Reporting

In most hospitals, nursing costs represent a large portion of the entire hospital budget. For other healthcare organizations, nursing and other clinical professional costs also represent a large percentage of budget allocation. Management information systems collect, summarize, and format data for use in administrative decision making related to the nursing component of the hospital budget. Managers are familiar with periodically produced budget summaries that allow monitoring of the budget, adjustments between over-committed and under-committed categories and help when forecasting the following year's budget. Decision support systems have been designed and are being refined to provide similar decision-making support in a variety of areas ranging from the nosocomial infection rate to resources utilisation. Other systems such as human resources systems are able to collect information and track different indicators ranging from illness and absenteeism to expertise and experience of staff members. The emphasis in these reports is on graphic displays such as histograms, time series charts, and map plots.

Organizations have many choices in regards to the types of administrative solutions available commercially. The following video clip presents an example of a popular administrative solution used for workload management (Video 10.1).

Detailed and comprehensive reporting is critical both at the organization level, health system level, and government level. Managers need timely information that can be retrieved, compiled, summarized, and presented in a meaningful and comprehensive format for different levels of reporting. Another major advantage is the ability to tailor reports to each manager's information needs. In addition, managers are often responsible for healthcare delivery provided by different healthcare disciplines. A comprehensive system not only provides healthcare discipline focus, but also an integrated picture of services delivery within their areas of responsibilities. Furthermore, sharing data and developing knowledge of clinical staff at all levels not only improves data quality but also assists in more effective and efficient use of the data included in reports for decision-making. This facilitates the ongoing monitoring of activities within the organization and the preparation of reports by the manager to senior management or government agencies. As services are delivered within the community by different groups and agencies, integration of this information is critical for monitoring and planning purposes [12].

Human Resource Management

Management of people on a patient care unit is a complex, time-consuming task. In the increasingly decentralized administrative structures that characterize healthcare organizations, managers need information related to all aspects of the allocation and utilization of staff on patient care units. For example, the manager must have immediate access to such information as the following.

- Skills and education of all employees
- Job classification and salary level for all staff on the unit
- Dates for performance reviews
- Dates for recertification of medically delegated and transferred functions, other professional delegated activities
- Dates for annual education and ongoing educational sessions, whether required by contract, by organizational policy, or by accreditation standards (e.g., back care, cardiopulmonary resuscitation, fire and disaster response, restraints)
- Annual vacation schedule summary for the unit
- Statutory holiday schedules
- Labor relationships contracts for all collective bargaining units representing employees employed on the unit, including grievance procedures
- Sick time records for each employee
- Seniority level
- Union requirements

Through access to the information systems using different platforms and databases, the manager is quickly able to obtain the necessary information without the need to maintain duplicate records in different formats. The Canadian Institute for Health Information (CIHI) has published a number of reports that outline trends in human resources. An example of human resources reports can be found at https://secure.cihi.ca/estore/productFamily.htm?locale=en&pf=PFC1661.

Fiscal Resources

Healthcare organizations are implementing "line of business" oriented management information systems. These systems identify, define, collect, process, and report the information necessary for the planning, budgeting, operating, and controlling aspects of the management function. The current demands for fiscal responsibility in healthcare organizations exceed all previous experience in the healthcare sector. Increasingly, managers are expected to understand the contextual challenges of their organizational environment and the health system. To respond to internal and external factors influencing the corporate environment in which they function, managers must do many things such as:

- Understand their fiscal responsibilities, situation and challenges
- Identify the issues, opportunities for innovation and process improvement
- Generate innovative solutions and opportunities
- Monitor progress toward departmental, organization and health system goals
- Evaluate the effectiveness of the solutions or the achievement of goals and objectives
- Link data with process improvement and best practice in a cost-efficient model.

These activities require the management of financial and statistical data. The MIS Standards developed by the Canadian Institute for Health Information (CIHI) provide the framework for data collection from different healthcare organizations and allow for comparisons among peer groups (www.cihi.ca). The ultimate objective is to relate the cost of resources consumed to patient outcomes and when possible, to health system outcomes. To effectively manage the information related to their responsibilities for fiscal accountability, managers require financial information (including payroll, supplies/materiel, and services) and statistical information (e.g., patient length of stay, nursing hours per patient-day, other healthcare professionals' hours per patient-day, and other assessment tools). This information must be timely, accurate, relevant, comprehensive, complete, consistent, concise, sensitive, and comparable. The manager needs to be able to present this information in different formats and views for senior management, health system and governmental reporting [13]. When the financial information is combined with clinical data, this can provide valuable insight on the costs of services being delivered.

A number of reports have been published by the Canadian Institute for Health Information (CIHI) on expenditures that illustrate the use of data when it is transformed into information, and can be found at https://secure.cihi.ca/estore/productFamily.htm?locale=en&pf=PFC1671.

Physical Resources

Managers are also responsible for overseeing the care and maintenance of the physical facilities of their patient care unit/service area. They are responsible for equipment and furniture on their units/service area and ensuring that it is in good working order. Although the actual inventory is often the responsibility of another department (such as materiel management), managers are accountable for budgeting, ordering, and retaining capital assets on their units/service area and for initiating maintenance or replacement procedures. Consequently, managers need access to capital asset inventory for their unit. In addition, they should conduct regular systematic inspections of the workplace for physical hazards such as faulty electrical equipment or loose floor tiles. These inspections must document identified hazards, the date on which corrective action was requested or initiated, and the date that the hazard was resolved. Such information must be stored in an easily retrievable format with a calendar to bring forward reminders of follow-up items. For managers working in community care, the service areas can be comprised of a multitude of locations spread over large geographic setting. The systems managing physical resources must allow for this level of complexity.

Office Automation

Office automation is the integrated electronic technology distributed throughout the administrative office and supporting managers at all levels and different organization settings. The purposes of office automation are to improve effectiveness, efficiency, and control of operations. This technology can have application in nursing administration, nursing education, continuing nursing education, and nursing research. Office automation affects the filing and retrieval of documents, text processing, telephone communications, management of calendars, and meetings. Office management activities require broad skills including document management, preparation of presentation material, spreadsheets, electronic correspondence, archiving, marketing to name a few. The sophistication of applications used to support office management continues to increase exponentially and requires advanced computer skills.

Nursing's Role in Managing Information in Healthcare Organizations

In most healthcare organizations, the manager is responsible for a program that may include a number of patient care units, nursing and different healthcare professionals. The healthcare organizations are as varied as the settings where services are provided, and can include hospitals, long term care, health centres, community care centres, home care, primary care (physicians' and nurse practitioners' offices), educational settings, correctional facilities, and other community based service agencies. In some healthcare settings, nurse clinicians are responsible for the clinical practice and nursing process components, allowing the manager to focus on the administrative and management components of the program/patient care units within the organization. Therefore, nursing's role in the management of information generally has been considered to include the information necessary to manage nursing care using the nursing process and the information necessary for managing patient care units in the organization (e.g., resource allocation and utilization, personnel management, planning and policymaking, decision support). As the role of nurses in organizational governance and decision making diversifies, their role and responsibility for information management to support these decision-making responsibilities continues to evolve. Information related to organizational management, planning and policies, as well as resource allocation and utilization, widely available to nursing staff, supports these roles and responsibilities.

During the last decade, we have seen nursing involvement increase in the Health Information Management field. Clinical expertise combined with knowledge of the health care environment and its intricacies have provided nurses with diverse employment opportunities such as with software development companies, consulting firms implementing clinical systems, in change management, project management and other transformational roles. COACH, Canada's Health Informatics Association has developed a career matrix that depicts the key role played by clinicians in the health informatics field (www.coachorg.com). As a result, clinical use of technologies for service delivery, management, planning and other key components are an integral part of Health Informatics Associations around the world. These include associations such as the Health Informatics Society of Australia (www.hisa.org.au), COACH Canada's Health Informatics Association (www.COACHorg.com), the American Medical Informatics Association (www.Amia.org), the Healthcare Information and Management Systems Society (www.HIMSS.org) and the Health Informatics Society of Ireland (www.hisi.ie).

Obstacles to Effective Nursing Management of Information

In most hospitals, the major obstacles to more effective nursing management of information are the sheer volume of information, the lack of access to information-handling techniques and equipment, and the inadequate information management infrastructure. As noted in the preceding sections, the volume of information that nurses manage on a daily basis for patient care purposes or organizational management purposes, is enormous and continues to grow. Nurses continue to respond to this growth with incredible mental agility. However, humans do have limits, and one of the major sources of job dissatisfaction among nurses is information overload, resulting in information-induced job stress.

Manual information systems (e.g., handwriting of orders, requisitions, medication records, and a kardex entry for each intervention or medication) and outdated information transfer facilities (e.g., nurses hand-carrying requisitions and specimens for stat blood work to the laboratory) are information-redundant and labor-intensive processes, to say nothing of an inappropriate use of an expensive human resources. Electronic information transfer and communication systems and networks have allowed for timely and accurate transfer of information to various departments and diagnostic service areas [13, 14].

The lack or limited access to software and hardware for electronic communication is only one aspect inhibiting the development of an information infrastructure. This is not as prevalent in large healthcare organizations and hospitals, but it is a key concern for the community sector that is providing health care services over large geographic areas. Another major aspect lacking in most healthcare organizations and again more noticeable in the community sector is the appropriate support staff to facilitate information management. Information systems support staff require preparation in health information science to gain expertise in both information systems and a solid understanding of the functioning of the healthcare system, and its organizations. Similarly, financial and statistical support personal are necessary to help managers appropriately interpret information. The different privacy and security regulations relating to the maintenance, dissemination, handling and all aspects related to personal information and personal health information require skills not only in hospitals, but within all healthcare settings where services are being delivered [15, 16].

Issues Related to Effective Nursing Management of Information

Primary among the nursing issues regarding information management is the lack of adequate educational programs in information management techniques and strategies for managers. Educational programs have started to include the health informatics in their educational offerings, however availability of such courses is highly variable and frequently educational institutions lack qualified faculty to develop and deliver such specialized content. These programs are continuously evolving, but the rapid changes in the management of information are an ongoing challenge for organizations. Some of the programs offer health informatics as elective instead of a compulsory program. At a minimum, the programs offered should include advanced study of information management techniques, strategies for information analysis, advanced used of databases, applications of informatics for clinicians and other basic management information elements. Ideally, health informatics courses would also introduce concepts and provide hands-on experience related to the use of patient care information systems.

Clinicians' knowledge about health informatics is essential as systems are being introduced in the work environment. Clinical involvement and participation in the requirements definition, selection and implementation of patient care information systems and financial management systems is imperative. Regrettably, many senior managers fail to recognize the importance of this activity and opt out of the process. They subsequently complain when the systems do not meet the needs of nursing and other healthcare professionals. Senior management must recognize the importance of allocating staff and financial resources to participate in the strategic planning process for the planning and implementation of information systems in their organizations. In any hospital, nurses are the single largest group of professionals using a patient care system, and nursing represents the largest part of the budget requiring financial management. Nursing, therefore, represents the single largest stakeholder group related to either a patient care information system or an enterprise health information system.

The final major issue that nursing must address regarding information management in hospitals is the hospital patient discharge abstract. The patient discharge abstracts prepared by the health records departments across Canada and the United

States currently contain little if any nursing care and other healthcare professional delivery information. Therefore, the abstracts fail to acknowledge the contribution of nursing and other clinical professionals during the patient's stay in the hospital. This is important because the abstracts are used by many agencies for a variety of statistical purposes including funding allocation. Presently, much valuable information is being lost and not communicated in a timely manner to healthcare providers in the community. With early patient discharge and the increase of healthcare provision within the community sector, the availability of this information to primary care, nurse practitioners, and other healthcare providers becomes critical. The patient discharge abstract information is important for determining hospitalization costs and the effectiveness of patient care. As the importance of national health databases increases, it is imperative that a minimum number of essential nursing elements be included in that database. Such a set of data elements would be similar to the nursing minimum data set or the core set of data elements identified by the nursing profession as essential to nursing documentation. Such data are required to allow description of the health status of populations with relation to nursing care needs, establish outcome measures for nursing care, and investigate the use and cost of nursing resources. The nursing profession must provide leadership when defining appropriate nursing and other clinical data elements that must be included in the patient discharge abstract.

Summary

Management information systems and office automation systems enable the manager to contribute to organizational efforts to increase the efficiency and effectiveness of patient care and program planning while simultaneously reducing or at least maintaining levels of resource consumption. This can be accomplished in part by considering *information* as a corporate strategic resource and thinking of the clinical managers' *use* of information as a management method and tool, thereby empowering the clinical managers to utilize available resources most effectively.

Suggested Websites

Canada Institute for Health Information, www.cihi.ca
Healthcare Information and Management Systems Society (HIMSS), www.himss.org
American Nurses Association, www.nursingworld.org
Canadian Nurses Association, www.cna-aiic.ca
Australian Nursing Federation, www.anf.org.au
Society for Quality Assurance, www.sqa.org
Current nursing, www.currentnursing.com
NANDA www.nanda.org

Downloads

Available from extras.springer.com:

Educational Template (PDF 97 kb)

Educational Template (PPTX 115 kb)

Video 10.1 GRASP (Grace Reynolds Application and Study of PETO). An example of a popular administrative solution used for workload management. With permission from GRASP Systems International, Inc (MP4 50378 kb)

References

1. Healthcare Information and Management Systems Society HIMSS. HIMSS dictionary of healthcare information technology terms, acronyms and organizations. Chicago: Healthcare Information and Management Systems Society (HIMSS); 2010.
2. Canadian Healthcare Association. Fundamentals of health information management. Ottawa: Canadian Healthcare Association; 2009.
3. Hannah KJ, Ball MJ, Edwards MJA. Introduction to nursing informatics. 3rd ed. New York: Springer; 2006.
4. Shojania KG, Grimshaw JM. Evidence-based quality improvement: the state of the science. Health Aff. 2006;24(1):138–51.
5. Graham NO, editor. Quality in health care, theory, application, and evolution. Gaithersburg: Aspen; 1995.
6. Weaver CA, Delaney CW, Weber P, Carr RL. Nursing and informatics for the 21st century. Chicago: Healthcare Information and Management Systems Society (HIMSS); 2010.
7. Canadian Institute of Health Information Highlight of the 2011–2012 Inpatient Hospitalizations and Emergency Department Visits. 2013. From https://secure.cihi.ca/free_products/DAD-NACRS_Quick%20Stats_Highlights_2011-2012_EN_web.pdf. Retrieved 21 Jan 2014.
8. Lunney M, Delaney C, Duffy M, Moorhead S, Welton J. Advocating for standardized nursing languages in electronic health records. J Nurs Adm. 2005;35(1):1–3.
9. Hall LM, Doran D, Laschinger HS, et al. A balanced scorecard approach for nursing report card development. Outcomes Manag. 2003;7(1):17–22.
10. Seago JA. A comparison of two patient classification instruments in an acute care hospital. J Nurs Adm. 2002;32(5):243–9.
11. Harper K, McCully C. Acuity systems dialogue and patient classification system essentials. Nurs Adm Q. 2007;31(4):284–99.
12. McKinney C, Hess R, Whitecar M. Implementing business intelligence in your healthcare organization. Chicago: Healthcare Information and Management Systems Society (HIMSS); 2012.
13. Langabeer II, James R. Performance improvement in hospitals and health systems. Chicago: Healthcare Information and Management Systems Society (HIMSS); 2009.
14. Wager KA, Lee GW, Glaser JP. Health care information systems, a practical approach for health care management. Chicago: Healthcare Information and Management Systems Society (HIMSS); 2009.
15. Gensinger Jr RA. Introduction to healthcare information enabling technologies. Chicago: Healthcare Information and Management Systems Society (HIMSS); 2010.
16. Bergeron BP. Performance management in healthcare: from key performance indicators to balanced scorecard. Chicago: Healthcare Information and Management Systems Society (HIMSS); 2006.

Chapter 11
Data Privacy and Security

Ross Fraser

Abstract The concept of privacy is complex and it is common to think of privacy as interchangeable with security. In fact, this is not true and this chapter will introduce readers to the definition of privacy. The concept of personal health information (PHI) is explored in relation to collection, use, disclosure, and retention. Additionally, the rationale for privacy, implicit and deemed consent, and revoking consent are presented. Other approaches to protecting privacy include developing a privacy policy, designating a privacy officer, de-identification and pseudomization, and the list to privacy. The chapter closes by exploring how nurses can contribute to the protection of privacy.

Keywords Privacy • Security • Consent • Health information custodian • Data steward • De-identification • Pseudonymization • User enrolment • User authentication • Audit

Key Concepts

Privacy
Security
Consent
Health information custodian
Data steward
De-identification
Pseudonymization
User enrolment
User authentication
Audit

The online version of this chapter (doi:10.1007/978-1-4471-2999-8_11) contains supplementary material, which is available to authorized users.

R. Fraser, CISSP, ISSAP
Sextant Corporation, Toronto, ON, Canada
e-mail: Ross.Fraser@sextantsoftware.com

Introduction

Informational privacy is best thought of as a human right. While laws and customs in most jurisdictions do not yet afford personal health information the same level of protection as is accorded to rights such as security of the person, freedom from arbitrary search and seizure, or the right to vote, an increasing body of law of law and jurisprudence in western democracies recognizes the importance of ensuring that individuals have basic rights in relation to their own personal information.

As has been discussed in previous chapters, the provision of modern healthcare is a multidisciplinary endeavour. Perforce, such provision therefore requires the exchange of patient information among the members of the patient's healthcare team (see Chap. 6 for a discussion of document exchange). Nurses ask patients to share information about their health, their work, their home, their social life, their sex life, and their emotional state. Patients comply with the implicit assumption that the information will remain confidential; i.e., that it will be shared with a limited audience and only for certain purposes related to healthcare.

This chapter includes a brief overview of how thinking about privacy has evolved since the 1970s and how societies have come to view privacy and the protection of personal information, including personal health information. It defines some common terms used in contemporary discussions of patient privacy and describes the basic privacy principles that underpin contemporary thinking about informational privacy. Since health records are increasingly stored electronically rather than on paper, we survey the techniques used to secure personal health information and discuss some issues that arise from the computer technology now in use. We also discuss the challenges to healthcare providers in maintaining the privacy and security of personal health information. Finally, we discuss the role of nurses in maintaining the privacy and security of personal health information.

Throughout this chapter, the discussion will focus almost exclusively on the protection of personal information, especially personal health information. This type of protection complements, but is distinct from, maintaining privacy of the person. The latter issue is important to healthcare providers, since the cultural norms that inform a patient about what constitutes invasion of personal privacy may be very different from those informing the healthcare providers treating the patient. While most cultures place special emphasis on privacy of the person in respect to the genitals, there is wider variation in the emphasis given to privacy of buttocks or breasts, and great variation in the cultural significance attached to viewing a woman's face. Healthcare providers are usually sensitive to such issues—traditional hospital gowns notwithstanding. In any event, the relevant issues are typically dealt with effectively by ensuring that physical examinations are conducted in private and by respecting a patient's wishes about the gender of the examining healthcare provider or about the additional presence of a person of specified gender to act as witness or chaperone. Protecting the confidentiality of personal health information is a much more complex undertaking than protecting privacy of the person. As we shall see below, the definition of what constitutes personal health information can itself be the subject of debate, the technical challenges involved in maintaining the confidentiality and availability of the information may be daunting, and the information collected may need to be securely protected for decades. The focus of the rest of the chapter will therefore be on informational privacy: i.e., the protection of personal information. Yet the reader must remain aware that however much patients may care about the confidentiality of their records, they care just as much—if not more—about the privacy and sanctity of their own persons.

Why Patient Privacy Matters

For an effective relationship to exist between healthcare providers and their patients, patients must believe that the information they provide will remain confidential. Patients may otherwise withhold information critical to their treatment and care. Ask yourself the following questions:

1. Given that men with paedophile tendencies make up 4 % or more of the adult male population [1, 2], do you believe that men with paedophilic urges should seek counselling and treatment before those urges overwhelm them? Or are the risks entailed by such secret desires becoming public knowledge so great that such men should never discuss them with a healthcare provider and hence never obtain treatment?
2. Given that alcohol and drug abuse affects as much as 15 % of the adult workforce [3] and that functioning alcoholics and individuals struggling with drug addiction may hold senior positions in corporations, government, and the military, which society would you feel safer living in: one in which such individuals continue to work and live without recourse to effective treatments because disclosure of their condition might irreparably harm their careers? Or one in which such individuals seek out treatment, secure in the knowledge that their drug or alcohol problems will not become public knowledge?
3. Given that more than 2.7 million people become newly infected with AIDS each year [4], should adults and teens be able to openly discuss HIV/AIDS prevention strategies with their healthcare providers, even if it means discussing intimate details of their sexuality, or should they instead avoid such discussions on the assumption that such details might become publicly known and hope instead that they'll be able to get all of the information they need from the Internet?

Privacy may not matter to every patient, but as the questions above indicate, it matters a great deal to patients whose treatment and care impact the health of an entire society. How healthcare providers handle patient privacy can therefore play an important role in shaping the kind of society in which we live. As healthcare providers with extended access to patients, nurses have a vital role to play in building trust, encouraging patients to be entirely forthcoming about healthcare issues that concern them, and reassuring those patients that their healthcare information will remain confidential.

While the need to assure patients that their privacy would be protected existed long before the computerization of health records, the introduction of electronic health records has considerably increased public concern about the confidentiality of personal health information. There are several reasons for this. Firstly, there is truth in the old adage that 'to err is human but to really screw things up requires a computer.' Computerization has allowed losses of confidentiality to occur on an industrial scale. Whereas loss of paper records rarely involved more than a few thousand records, privacy breaches involving electronic records routinely involve tens of thousands of records in a single breach. The list of incidents over the last two decades is long and dishonourable and the reasons for the breaches are diverse:

- **Inadvertent loss** – dozens of hospitals across the US lost access to electronic medical records for 5 hours during a computer outage in 2012 that was caused by human error [5]. Within minutes of the outage, doctors and nurses reverted to writing orders and notes by hand, but in many cases no longer had access to patient information previously saved in electronic records, potentially compromising patient care.
- **Technical failures** – patient records at the University of Michigan Medical Center were left exposed on the Internet because the center thought that they were on a server protected with a password [6]
- **Failure to adequately dispose of paper records** – the United Kingdom Information Commissioner's Office (ICO) ordered Belfast Health and Social Care Trust to pay a £225,000 fine after determining that the organization had breached the UK Data Protection Act by closing a hospital in 2006 and leaving behind patient medical records, X-rays, scans, lab results, and unopened pay-slips; all abandoned in the empty hospital building [7]. On several occasions, trespassers subsequently gained access to the site and took photographs of the records and posted them online.
- **Failure to adequately dispose of electronic records** – The UK ICO fined Brighton and Sussex University Hospitals £325,000 after highly sensitive personal data belonging to tens of thousands of patients and staff was stolen and sold on eBay [8]. The data, including some relating to HIV and genito-urinary patients as well as information referring to criminal convictions and suspected offences, had been stored on hard drives sold on an Internet auction site in October and November 2010.
- **Failure to comply with established policies** – personal health data of tens of thousands, possibly hundreds of thousands of Canadians were accessed without proper authorization, including information on the mental, physical and sexual health of individuals, as well as lifestyle and use of health services. In the most serious cases, the British Columbia provincial government notified 38,486 individuals of the breaches by letter [9]. In three separate instances in 2010 and 2012, health information was saved on USB sticks and shared with researchers at the universities of B.C. and Victoria or with contractors. Proper permissions had not been obtained and suitable procedural protocols had not been devised.

- **Staff misconduct** – a state public health worker in Florida sent the names of 4,000 HIV positive patients to two Florida newspapers [10, 11]
- **Computer hacking** – in 2009, a computer hacker successfully compromised a health database used by pharmacies and doctors to track narcotics and painkiller prescriptions and stole records of more than eight million patients [12]. The hacker then demanded a $10 million ransom from the state of Virginia, which the state government refused to pay. Russian hackers held an Australian medical centre to ransom in 2012 after encrypting thousands of patient health records and then demanding $4,000 to decrypt them [13].

If the recent past is any indication, patient privacy and the confidentiality of personal health records will remain in the news and hence in the public's awareness for many years to come.

There is a final argument that is sometimes made to minimize the importance of privacy: that inter-generational shifts in attitudes have taken place and young people are not concerned about their privacy (or at least less concerned than their parents' generation). The evidence for such statements is equivocal. Certainly, societal attitudes shift over time in regard to what one might normally consider confidential. In 1968, Canadian gay men and lesbians were still subject to criminal prosecution for having consensual sex with their partners. Thirty-five years later, such couples could legally marry anywhere in Canada. This shift in societal attitudes in that country has had an obvious impact on the importance placed on the confidentiality of sexual orientation as recorded in personal health records.

Definitions

Some terms are inevitably encountered in any robust discussion of privacy and information security and they are included in the discussion that follows. While nearly all of these terms are also used outside of healthcare, some have special meaning for healthcare providers. Where this is the case, additional discussion is provided on the use of these terms in healthcare settings.

Participants in a nursing informatics conference in Toronto in 2013 were asked to provide a definition of **privacy**. After much lively discussion, they defined it as the right of individuals and organizations to decide for themselves when, how, and to what extent information about them is transmitted to others. It is as good a definition as can be found in many privacy-related discussions, and more relevant to nursing than most.

Consent is an agreement, approval, or permission given voluntarily by a competent person that permits some act(s) for some stated purpose(s) [14]. For example, a patient may consent to having their personal health information collected by a clinic or consent to its disclosure to a third party (e.g., an insurance provider). Note that in this chapter, consent will always be used to refer to informational consent (i.e., consent to share or disclose information) as opposed to consent to treatment and care. Although consent for treatment and consent to collect, use or disclose health information are sometimes bundled together on the same patient consent form, they are distinct concepts. A patient may consent to an abortion but not consent to her personal health information being disclosed or used outside the clinic: indeed, she may insist that it not be. Conversely, a patient may consent to participation in a medical research project on sexual practices and sexually transmitted diseases without consenting to (or having any expectation of receiving) treatment.

Patient consent can take one of several forms. **Express consent** is an explicit (usually written) instruction from the patient – a voluntary agreement regarding what is being done or proposed that is unequivocal and does not require any inference or assumptions on the part of the healthcare organization or healthcare provider seeking consent. **Implied consent** is a voluntary agreement that can be reasonably determined through the actions or inactions of the patient. For example, if a patient voluntarily provides a urine sample to a diagnostic laboratory for the purpose of performing a lab test requested by the patient's healthcare provider, it can reasonably be inferred that the patient has consented to information related to the test being disclosed by the lab to the healthcare provider (otherwise, why bother to provide the urine sample and perform the tests?) In most jurisdictions, implied consent is sufficient for the collection, use and (limited) disclosure of personal health information.

Some jurisdictions have statutory provisions for **deemed consent**: under certain stated conditions, the law permits organizations to act as if the patient has consented, regardless of whether or not the patient has actually done so; the patient has no right to withdraw or withhold consent. This may include disclosures of personal health information for the purpose of mandatory reporting of certain infectious diseases, or to allow healthcare providers to comply with certain professional ethical practices.

A patient may **withhold consent** by expressly stating that s/he does not consent to a particular activity. A patient may also **withdraw consent** previously given (also referred to as a patient **revoking consent**). Withholding consent occurs when a patient indicates that s/he does not consent to the sharing of personal health information previously collected. Withdrawing or revoking consent occurs when a patient who has expressly provided consent or where consent has previously been implied revokes that consent at some later date.

A patient's **circle of care** refers to the persons participating in, and the activities related to, the provision of health care to the patient. This includes healthcare providers involved with necessary but incidental activities such as laboratory work or professional consultation. The term is sometimes used in privacy discussions and even privacy policies of healthcare organizations; e.g., when promising not to share a patient's personal information outside their circle of care without the patient's express consent.

A **health information custodian** (sometimes called a **data steward**) is an individual or organization that collects, uses, or discloses personal health information for the purposes of patient treatment and care, medical billing, health system planning and management, or health research. Depending on a jurisdiction's law or policy, any of the following entities may be considered a health information custodian:

- healthcare providers, i.e., professionals licensed or registered to provide health services
- Ministries or Departments of Health for a country, state, province, municipality or other governmental jurisdiction
- regional health authorities (where such entities exist)
- hospitals, nursing homes or other identified health care facilities
- pharmacies (and pharmacists, who are included above under healthcare providers)
- boards of health, agencies, committees and other organisations identified in jurisdictional regulations (e.g., a mental health board, cancer care board, etc.) and
- ambulance operators and paramedics.

Not every jurisdiction has privacy laws protecting personal health information. Where law and policy do not clearly outline custodial responsibilities in the collection, use and disclosure of personal health information, healthcare providers may need to look to their professional associations, licencing bodies, or colleges for guidance about their professional responsibilities.

A **privacy officer** is an individual who oversees activities related to the development, implementation, maintenance of, and adherence to an organization's policies and procedures covering the privacy, confidentiality and sometimes security of personal information. In many jurisdictions, it is now standard practice for large healthcare organizations such as hospitals to have a designated privacy officer. Privacy officers oversee access to personal health information by patients and their families. They also ensure patients are notified of their privacy rights. They educate staff about privacy responsibilities and provide privacy oversight and review of the organisation's information handling practices. They also respond to questions and complaints from patients and the public concerning the organization's information privacy practices. Privacy officers may also be required to periodically review and revise organizational privacy policies and practices in order to ensure currency with industry best practices and legislative developments.

Anonymity allows the subjects in a database to remain nameless and unidentified. Patient anonymity is frequently found in research databases and in data that consists of statistical summaries.

If data is anonymised, the data subject(s) cannot be identified by the recipients of the data. The process of anonymising data involves removing any information that identifies the patient or any information that could be utilized, either alone or with other information, to identify the patient. This process of **de-identification** is typically a non-trivial undertaking: it consists of taking steps necessary to ensure that the anonymised data cannot be utilized, either alone or with other information, to identify a patient. A variety of statistical techniques may need to be employed to ensure successful de-identification: i.e., to ensure that the risk of re-identification has been reduced to an acceptably low level.

Anonymity can also apply to users of information systems. Truly anonymous access to an online service is only obtained when each individual instance of system access cannot be linked over time to later access to the same or other online services (i.e., users are not asked to register or log in to such systems and repeated access over time by a user is not tracked by means of web browser cookies or other such technical means).

Pseudonymity allows the subjects in a database to be tracked over time while at the same time remaining nameless. Pseudonyms (e.g., patient X, patient Y, etc.) are attached to records instead of names, addresses and other public identifiers. Users of online services can also be given pseudonyms (or choose their own) during user registration, thereby allowing them to maintain a consistent (pseudonymous) presence from one online encounter to another. Facebook and many other Internet services allow users to remain pseudonymous. Note that much discussion of anonymity is actually a discussion of pseudonymity and many users claiming to want online anonymity actually want online pseudonymity (e.g.: blogs, Facebook, Twitter…).

The terms anonymous and anonymity are often used when the terms pseudonymous and pseudonymity should be used instead. Truly anonymous patient data is typically useless in a long-term longitudinal study, as new data collected on a given patient cannot be matched up with data collected on the same patient the previous year or the year before (all the patients are anonymous). Rather, such databases are typically pseudonymous: data collected last year on patient 13,786 is linked to new data collected from patient 13,786. Such schemes require some trusted party or methodology to reliably and consistently derive the pseudonym (13,786) from personal identifiers such as patient name, address, birthdate, etc. This process of **pseudonymization** is said to be **irreversible** if, after identifiable data have been processed to produce pseudonymous data, it is computationally infeasible to trace back to the original identifier from the pseudonym.

Every information system used in healthcare requires that users be identified, registered as new users, and authorized to access various types of data (e.g., patient demographics, billing data, or lab test results) or to perform various types of services (registering a new patient, writing a prescription, or ordering a lab test). **User identification** (sometimes referred to as **user identity verification**) is done once during **user registration** prior to allowing an individual to access an information system. Identification answers the question "who are you?" and is an essential part of the user registration process.

User enrolment is done once for each online service or computer program within an organization that a registered user is authorized to access. User enrolment answers questions such as: "what information repositories do you need to access?" and "do you need to edit records as well as view them?" Once enrolled, a user has the **authorization** to access the relevant data or services.

User authentication is done each time a user logs into a computer system or program. User authorization attempts to securely answer the question "is the person logging into the system really you?"

Auditing is done by keeping **audit log** files (sometimes referred to as an **audit trail**) that record *which* users have done *what* and *when*. An audit log answers, for each user, the questions "what information have you accessed?", "what changes to information have you made?", "what actions have you performed? (printing records, transferring records, merging records, etc.)" and "when were these actions performed?"

What Constitutes Personal Health Information?

Personal health information is information about an identifiable individual that relates to the physical or mental health of the individual, or provision of health services to the individual. It may include:

- information about registration of the individual for the provision of health services, including name, address, phone numbers and other contact details, and other demographic information such as birthdate
- information about payments or eligibility for heath care insurance,
- a number, symbol or particular reference assigned to an individual to uniquely identify the individual for health care purposes,
- information about the individual that is collected in the course of the providing the individual with health services,
- information derived from the testing or examination of a body part or bodily substance, or
- identification of healthcare providers involved in the provision of healthcare to the individual [15].

Personal health information does not include information that is anonymised, either by itself or when combined with other available information (see above for a discussion of anonymity).

What Determines the Sensitivity of Personal Health Information?

In the past, there has been a tendency to treat certain types of clinical information as more or less sensitive than other types. For example, tests revealing HIV status have been considered more sensitive than other lab test results. Encounter records have been thought more sensitive than demographic data and mental health records have been felt to be more sensitive than other encounter records. Such attempts to build a hierarchy of sensitivity levels within personal health information are fraught with challenges. Firstly, the patient ultimately decides which data is most sensitive. To a woman escaping an abusive partner, the confidentiality of information about the treatment of her broken arm may be of little concern, but the confidentiality her new address at a women's shelter may be of vital importance. Someone treated for a drinking problem may consider a list of allergies to be of no consequence but would consider a disulfiram prescription in the medication history to be highly confidential. The mere presence of a patient's name in the registry of a cancer clinic would indicate to others that the patient had cancer – an inference that the patient may not want anyone outside the circle of care to make.

The belief that personal health information admits of degrees ('not confidential,' 'somewhat confidential,' 'highly confidential') and that these can be determined beforehand by information system designers is largely a myth. Personal health information – all of it – should be treated as confidential, not shared outside the patient's circle of care without the patient's express consent except where permitted or required by law. It must be protected by reasonable technical and administrative safeguards throughout its entire useful lifetime, and then securely disposed of when no longer needed.

A Brief History of Informational Privacy

Fair Information Practice was a term initially proposed in a report prepared in 1973 on behalf of the US Secretary of Health [16]. The report was written in response to the growing use of data processing systems containing information about individuals. Its lasting contribution to privacy was the development of a code of fair information practices for record-keeping organizations collecting personal data. By contemporary standards, these practices are straightforward: that there be no databases containing personal information whose very existence is secret; that individuals have the right to find out what type of information is held about them and what it is used for; that personal information collected for one purpose must not be subsequently used for another purpose without obtaining the individual's consent; that there be some procedure allowing an individual to correct or amend a record of personal information about that individual; and that organizations creating, using, maintaining or disseminating records of identifiable personal data must assure the reliability of the data for their intended use and must take reasonable steps to prevent misuse of the data [17]. These recommendations subsequently provided the foundation for the US Federal Privacy Act of 1974.

In 1980, the Council of Europe adopted a *Convention for the Protection of Individuals with Regard to Automatic Processing of Personal Data* [18]. It extended somewhat the Fair Information Practice core principles and included (modest) special provisions for "personal data concerning health or sexual life." [19] In the same year, the Organisation for Economic Cooperation and Development (OECD) proposed *Guidelines on the Protection of Privacy and Transborder Flows of Personal Data* [20]. These OECD Guidelines, the Council of Europe Convention, and the 1995 European Union Data Protection Directive [21] all built upon the Fair Information Practices as core principles, revising and extending the original concepts. The OECD guidelines influenced subsequent privacy law and policy in many countries, including Canada [22], Australia [23], the UK [24], and others. Contemporary approaches to patient privacy continue to evolve.

Privacy Principles

While the OECD *Guidelines on the Protection of Privacy and Transborder Flows of Personal Data* have influenced both law and policy on the protection of personal information, the eight principles in the *Guidelines* have been further elaborated upon in several countries to incorporate nuances that were not explicit in the original. Below we will examine the ten privacy principles in the *Model Code for the Protection of Personal Information* [25], published by the Canadian Standards Association in 1996 and later incorporated into Canadian laws that protect personal health information. With minor variations, these principles can also be seen in the laws in Europe, Australia, New Zealand, and other countries. Some aspects of these principals can also be seen in the US Health Insurance Portability and Accountability Act of 1996 [26]. As core principles, they facilitate an easily recognisable and principled approach to data protection. The ten principles are stated below in a form that emphasizes their relation to personal health information:

1. **Accountability for information**: Organizations that collect, use or disclose PHI are responsible for the personal health information in their custody or care.
   A named individual within the organization should be responsible for facilitating organizational compliance with applicable data protection legislation and organizational privacy policies.
2. **Identifying purposes for collection, use and disclosure of information**: To allow patients to make appropriate decisions about their PHI, it is important that they be made aware of the purposes for which this information is being collected, used, and disclosed.
   There are many legitimate purposes for collecting personal health information; indeed, an international standard classification of such purposes has been developed [27]. These purposes include:

- providing clinical care to an individual
- providing emergency care to an individual
- supporting care activities for the individual within the healthcare organisation
- enabling medical billing (and/or permissions from a funding party for providing health care services to the patient)
- health service management and quality assurance
- education for health care professionals
- public health surveillance and disease control (i.e., monitoring populations for significant health events and then intervening to provide health care or preventive care to relevant individuals)

- public safety emergency (i.e., protecting the public in a situation in which there is significant risk that is possibly not health-related)
- population health management (i.e., monitoring populations for health events, trends or outcomes in order to inform strategy and policy)
- research
- market studies to support the discovery of product-specific knowledge
- law enforcement (enforcing jurisdictional legislation or assisting forensic investigation)
- patient use (in support of the patient's own interests)

Personal health information collected for the purposes of treatment and care cannot generally be used for unrelated purposes (e.g., for clinical research) unless the patient consented to these additional purposes at the time of collection. Specific jurisdictions may have exceptions in law or regulation that permit such secondary uses without obtaining express consent from each patient.

3. **Consent**: An organisation should be able to demonstrate that it is in compliance with applicable laws and that the patient can reasonably be expected to know that information about them was going to be collected and used for defined purposes. In order for an instance of consent to be valid, it must:

- be given by the individual to whom the information relates if she or he is capable of consenting at the time of consenting or by a substitute decision-maker;
- relate to the information in question;
- not be obtained through deception or coercion;
- be knowledgeable (i.e. it must be reasonable in the circumstances to believe that the patient knows the purposes for which the information is being collected, used, or disclosed, that the patient has had the opportunity to withhold consent – if that is what the patient wants – and that the patient has been informed of the reasonable consequences of such action).

The latter point deserves elaboration. A balance needs to be found between either demanding blanket access to all available personal health information, versus allowing patient consent restrictions to stand in the way of effective treatment. Patients need to understand that restrictions they place on the disclosure of their personal health information may impact the quality of their care. Healthcare providers, for their part, need to understand that refusing to treat a patient unless the patient allows the unrestricted collection, use and disclosure of his/her personal health information not only shows disrespect for patient privacy but also holds patients to ransom ("give use all your data or we won't treat you.") The cost of striking the necessary balance need not be burdensome: a brief but well-written notice to patients (e.g., posted in waiting rooms) can go far towards streamlining the administration of patient consent while at the same time enhancing patient trust.

4. **Limiting collection**: Organisations should limit collection of personal health information to that which is necessary for the identified purposes; i.e. personal health information should not be collected indiscriminately.

Historically, many fields of data (e.g., religion and race) were collected in patient records, even in cases where they had little or no bearing on treatment and care. While there may be jurisdictional laws that mandate the collection of certain information (e.g., race) for statistical and public health surveillance purposes, designers and implementers of electronic health record systems need to carefully review the relevance of the data collected and limit collection to what is needed.

5. **Limiting use, disclosure and retention**: Once organisations identify the purposes for which they collect personal and seek consent, as appropriate, from patients to collect information for these purposes, the organization should then only use, disclose and retain information for these purposes.

   Personal health information should not be collected for one purpose (e.g., treatment and care), and then used for another (e.g., research) without first obtaining the consent of the patient for the new use. When a later use is found for data, this new use is sometimes called a **secondary use**. Secondary uses usually require express patient consent, but there may be certain exemptions in local laws or regulations.

6. **Accuracy**: The need for accuracy as a fair information practice is particularly relevant in the delivery of healthcare. Patients are typically aware of the need to provide accurate information in order to ensure that healthcare is delivered in a safe, efficient and effective way. Personal health information needs to be sufficiently accurate, complete and up-to-date to minimize the possibility that inappropriate information is being used to make a decision about a patient. Of particular concern to healthcare organizations is ensuring that patients are properly identified and that the subject of the data is actually the patient in question.

7. **Safeguards**: By implementing information security safeguards, organisations protect personal health information against loss and theft, as well as unauthorised access, disclosure, copying, use, and modification. These safeguards are discussed further in the section below.

8. **Openness**: It should be possible for concerned patients to know the purposes for which information about them is collected, used, and disclosed. Also, they should have access to an overview of the technical and administrative safeguards that are in place to ensure the confidentiality of that information. At a minimum, the organizations' privacy policy should be available to patients.

9. **Individual access**: Patients should have the right to access their own personal health information so that they can assure its accuracy, and amend inaccurate or incomplete information. This may require mediated access: i.e., patients may need to go over their record with a healthcare provider to understand the meaning of the information contained therein. Patients may also need counselling, as appropriate, to ensure that potentially disturbing information is reviewed appropriately and sensitively. Nurses are sometimes called upon to perform this counselling function.

10. **Challenging compliance**: The right of a patient to lodge a privacy complaint against an organization was first articulated when the *Fair Information Practices* were promulgated more than 40 years ago [28].

Privacy Policy

It has become common for organizations to formulate a privacy policy and make it available to the public. Healthcare organizations are active participants in this trend. Even where nurses are not involved in the development of the policy, they, like all staff, should be familiar with it.

There is no universally agreed-upon format or outline for an organizational privacy policy in healthcare. Good policies typically contain most or all of the following components:

- a broad description of the types of personal information held – but not an exhaustive list of data fields (e.g., contact information, diagnostic test data, or lists of currently active prescriptions)
- a description of the purposes for which the information is collected, used, and disclosed (e.g., treatment and care, fundraising, clinical research)
- a statement about how the information is used (e.g., during patient consultation and diagnosis)
- a commitment to maintain the confidentiality of the information (e.g., an assurance that the organization is committed to respecting personal privacy, safeguarding confidential information and ensuring the security of personal health information within its custody)
- a non-technical description of the security steps taken to protect confidential information when it is stored or transmitted
- a description of the circumstances under which personal information will be disclosed to third parties (e.g., to an IT service provider securely hosting the data on a central server or providing external processing),
- a description of the circumstances under which data is depersonalized or aggregated (e.g., for the purpose of gathering and reporting healthcare statistics) and
- contact information and procedures to follow for individuals who have questions about the privacy of their data or who have a complaint.

Information Security Principles

Maintaining the confidentiality of information is one of three primary goals of information security. The other two goals are maintaining the integrity of data (i.e., preventing information from being corrupted, either unintentionally or maliciously) and maintaining the availability of information systems and data in the face of environmental disasters such as equipment failures, fires, floods, or power outages; or denial of service attacks on systems by Internet hackers or disgruntled employees. Information security specialists typically pursue all three goals in tandem.

Effective information security is a chain with many links: many separate safeguards are required to ensure that the confidentiality of data is maintained. The resulting security is only as good as the weakest link(s) in the chain. There are so many links in the information security chain that a series of international standards was developed to catalogue them and describe their effective use. The best known of these standards are ISO 27001 (*Information technology – Security techniques – Information security management systems – Requirements*) [29] and ISO 27002 (*Information technology – Security techniques – Code of practice for information security management*) [30], published by the International Organization for Standardization. While these standards are not specific to any particular industrial sector, a healthcare-specific guideline for information security, ISO 27799, was developed in 2006. All of these standards break down the task of providing information security into 11 specific areas. Each is described below.

1. **Information Security Policy**: Every organization collecting, using, or storing personal health information should have a security policy, appropriate to the jurisdiction in which the organization operates. Security is far too complex—and security incidents can unfold far too quickly—for staff to make up procedures as they go along. A robust security policy deals with all of the areas below that are relevant to the organization's operations.
2. **Organizing Information Security**: Like the first privacy principle above (accountability for information), good information security requires that there be a named individual responsible for security (sometimes called a chief information security officer) within any organization that hosts an electronic health record system or other large repository of personal health information. Reporting responsibilities for security incidents also need to be clear and unambiguous.
3. **Asset Management**: Organizations need to be aware of all their information assets, including not only databases but the systems, software and hardware on which they run. When faced with the Y2K bug in the late 1990s, many healthcare organizations realized that they did not have an adequate inventory of system and data repositories – even when such systems and data were critical to patient treatment and care.
4. **Human Resources Security**: Organizations need to ensure that staff members: are aware of information security threats and concerns; prevent damage from security incidents and malfunctions caused by human error; and reduce the risks to information security from theft, fraud or misuse of facilities.
5. **Physical and Environmental Security**: Physical security prevents unauthorised access, damage and theft of equipment or information storage media. Environmental security protects against damage or compromise of assets and interruption to business activities from fires, floods, and other environmental disasters.
6. **Communications and Operational Security**: Communications security aims to protect (principally via encryption) the confidentiality and integrity of data and messages transmitted from, or to, or within an organization. Operational security ensures the correct and secure operation of information processing facilities; protects the integrity of software and information; maintains the integrity and availability of information processing; minimizes the risk of

systems failures; safeguards information in databases and supporting infra-structures; prevents damage to information assets; and prevents loss, modification or misuse of information or documents exchanged between organisations. Data security aims to protect the confidentiality, integrity and availability of all data stored in data repositories.

7. **Access Control**: This includes the identification of users during user registration, the assignment of access privileges that determine which information resources and services these users can access, their subsequent authentication during log in, and their authorisation prior to being granted access to specific services and data. Access control is intended to prevent unauthorised access to information systems as well as to ensure information security when users are accessing data via mobile computing and networking facilities.

8. **Information Systems Acquisition, Development and Maintenance**: Information systems need to be developed with security in mind: security must be an integral component of information systems: baked-in like the flour in a cake, not layered on later, like icing. If security is an afterthought, the information system will not be robustly secure.

9. **Security Incident Handling**: Security incident management builds an organizational infrastructure for reporting security incidents and suspected weaknesses and in doing so, minimizes the damage from security incidents and malfunctions. Security incidents within healthcare organizations need to be managed effectively and improvements need to be implemented to prevent future occurrences. Like all healthcare providers, nurses have an important role to play in reporting (suspected) security breaches.

10. **Business Continuity**: The demands placed on healthcare organizations can be onerous: environmental problems such as hurricanes that are notorious for sharply increasing the demand for emergency medical services are the at the same time tests of the ability of information systems to remain operational in adverse circumstances. Components of disaster recovery such as data backup can entail unique information security challenges: copies of backed-up data, for example, are just as confidential as the original data.

11. **Compliance**: Organizations must comply with the laws of their jurisdiction that protect personal health information. An important component of information security is ensuring that the steps taken to secure the collection, use, disclosure, and retention of personal health information meet the minimum requirements set out by law and regulation.

Limits to Privacy

Maintaining the implied trust that exists between patients and their healthcare providers requires that the reasonable expectations of both groups to be met. It is reasonable for a gynaecologist to ask a patient whether an abortion had previously been carried out. It is almost entirely unreasonable that this question be posed by a dentist. What, then, constitutes a reasonable request for personal health information? For patients, such privacy-related assessments are often founded on the patient's perception of a need-to-know. Will surrendering personal information help my healthcare provider make a more accurate diagnosis? Is the information needed to allow better decisions to be made about my treatment? Will it help my care team assess the outcome? To the extent that patients believe the answer is "yes", they are more likely to comply with attempts to collect such information.

Patient perceptions of the healthcare provider's need-to-know may therefore need to be addressed in the structuring of intake procedures and the related forms that gather needed personal information. Nurses involved in intake play an important role in reassuring patients that requests for personal information are reasonable; i.e., that the information requested is needed by healthcare providers to perform the tasks of assessment, diagnosis, or treatment—tasks that will directly benefit the patient. Conversely, "just fill in the form" is never a good answer to the question "why are you asking me these personal questions"?

Not all patient privacy concerns can be addressed realistically. A common concern of patients is whether a friend, neighbour, or relative who works as a healthcare provider will be able to access the patient's personal health data [31]. When the healthcare provider in question is also a staff member of the facility collecting the information, it may be difficult to place restrictions on their access to such data. An important role is played in this situation by the operation of an audit log that records all accesses to all records by all users of an electronic medical record system. Regular review of audit logs goes far towards eliminating the problem of inappropriate access to records, and it thus helps in the enforcement of professional standards.

Finally, patients may have unrealistic expectations about the granularity or grouping of data fields in the their records. They may naively assume that information about a specific condition such as HIV/AIDS can be easily masked ("don't disclose the AIDS flag") whereas the information they are concerned about may be evident from many data sources (e.g., treatment for HIV/AIDS may be evident from summary care records, diagnostic test results, prescription medications, and counselling records, among others). Moreover, most medical record systems cannot block access to data on a field-by-field basis. Patients need to be informed about both the extent and the format of the information they are concerned about so that their privacy concerns can be realistically assessed.

Privacy of Healthcare Providers

While the focus of this chapter has been on patient privacy, healthcare providers also have legitimate privacy concerns. Perhaps primary among those concerns is whether data collected for one purpose (e.g., patient wait-time management) can later be used for a different purpose (e.g., ranking healthcare providers as identifiable professionals on their timely delivery of healthcare services)? In some jurisdictions, data collected on healthcare professionals by healthcare organizations is explicitly excluded from consideration as personal information. In others, the distinct is not clear-cut.

Nurses, like other healthcare professionals, are also patients. Most healthcare professional associations demand a clear delineation between data collected on healthcare providers as professionals rendering healthcare services, and data collected on healthcare providers as patients undergoing treatment. Organizations must be careful to ensure that the rights of nurses and other healthcare professionals as patients are not compromised by their involvement as professionals and staff in the very organizations responsible for their treatment.

The Role of Nurses In Maintaining the Privacy and Security of Personal Health Information

This chapter has discussed several areas of privacy administration in which nurses can fulfil an important role:

- In the formation and review of institutional privacy policies: healthcare institutional policies need to accommodate the work flow of all healthcare providers, not just those of physicians. Nurses need to ensure that privacy policies are both robust and practicable. They should be empowered to provide appropriate feedback when this is not the case.
- During patient admission and at other times during the course of treatment and care when information is elicited from patients: patients need trustworthy advice about what types of personal information will be collected from them, and for what purpose and uses. How long will this information be retained? How will its confidentiality be protected? To whom will it be disclosed and why? These questions deserve informed answers and nurses should be prepared to provide them.
- In the creation of patient education materials that clearly explain how personal health information is collected, used, retained and disclosed, and how that information is protected while being held.
- In inculcating patient trust: nurses can provide a supportive atmosphere in which patients can disclose deeply personal information that is sometimes painful to divulge. This is arguably the most important activity that nurses carry out in relation to an individual patient's privacy. It is a task for which nurses are perhaps most uniquely suited.

By diligently carrying out these activities when assigned, nurses maintain a venerable tradition. The oldest ethical guide for the nursing profession was provided by Canadian-born Lyster Gretter in 1893 and known as the Florence Nightingale pledge: "… I will do all in my power to maintain and elevate the standard of my profession, and will hold in confidence all personal matters committed to my keeping and all family affairs coming to my knowledge in the practice of my profession. …" [32] One hundred and twenty years later, there is nothing much more that need be said.

Downloads

Available from extras.springer.com:
Educational Template (PDF 98 kb)
Educational Template (PPTX 114 kb)

References

1. Hall, et al. Sexual arousal and arousability to pedophilic stimuli in a community sample of normal men. Behav Ther. 1995;26:681–94.
2. Cloud J. Pedophilia. Time Magazine, 29 Apr 2002.
3. Frone MR. Prevalence and distribution of alcohol use and impairment in the workplace: a U.S. national survey. J Stud Alcohol. 2006;67:147–56.
4. McNeil DG, Jr., New cases of AIDS hit plateau, New York Times, 21 Nov 2011.
5. Terhune C. Patient data outage exposes risks of electronic medical records, Los Angeles Times, 3 Aug 2012.
6. Carter M. Integrated electronic health records and patient privacy: possible benefits but real dangers. Med J Aust. 2000;172:28–30.
7. Information Commissioner's Office (United Kingdom). Belfast trust fined £225,000 after leaving thousands of patient records in disused hospital, News release, 19 June 2012.
8. Information Commissioner's Office (United Kingdom). NHS rust fined £325,000 following data breach affecting thousands of patients and staff, News release, 1 June 2012.
9. Canadian Broadcasting Corporation. B.C. privacy breach shows millions affected, CBC News, 14 Jan 2013.
10. Stein L. The electronic medical record: promises and threats; web security: a matter of trust. Web J. 1997;2(33): http://oreilly.com/catalog/wjsum97/excerpt/.
11. Jurgens R. HIV testing and confidentiality: final report. Canadian HIV/AIDS Legal Network & Canadian AIDS Society. 2001. http://www.aidslaw.ca/publications/publicationsdocEN.php?ref=282.
12. Krebs B. Hackers break into virginia health professions database, demand ransom, Washington Post, 4 May 2009.
13. Hicks S. Russian hackers hold Gold Coast doctors to ransom, ABC News, 11 Dec 2012.
14. Adapted from Black's Law Dictionary. 9th ed. 2009. ISBN-13: 9780314199492.
15. Adapted from the definition of personal health information in: Health Canada Advisory Committee on Information and Emerging Technologies (ACIET), Pan-Canadian Health Information Privacy and Confidentiality Framework, 6 Jan 2005.
16. Hare WH. Records, Computers and the Rights of Citizens, Rand Corporation, 1973.
17. Hare WH. Records, Computers and the Rights of Citizens, Rand Corporation, 1973, p. 3.
18. Council of Europe. Convention for the protection of individuals with regard to automatic processing of personal data. Strasbourg; 28 Jan 1981.
19. Council of Europe. Convention for the protection of individuals with regard to automatic processing of personal data. Strasbourg; 28 Jan 1981, article 6.
20. Organization for Economic Co-Operation and Development. Guidelines on the protection of privacy and transborder flows of personal data. last modified Jan 1999.
21. European Union. Data Protection Directive (95/46/EC), 1995.
22. Holmes N. The right to privacy and parliament, Library of Parliament (Canada), Feb 2006.
23. Clarke R. Beyond the OECD guidelines: privacy protection for the 21st century, Cyber Security and Information Systems Information Analysis Center (CSIAC), Rolling Meadows, IL: Jan 2000.

24. Smith GK. Privacy in the information age, De Montfort University, Apr 1994.
25. Canadian Standards Association. Model code for the protection of personal information (CAN/CSA-Q830-96). 1996.
26. US Government Printing Office. Health insurance portability and accountability act. 1996.
27. ISO/TS 14265: Health informatics – classification of purposes for processing personal health information. International Organization for Standardization; 2011.
28. Federal Trade Commission. Fair Information Practice Principles (FIPs), 5. Enforcement/ Redress. Washington, DC.
29. ISO 27001: Information technology – security techniques – information security management systems – requirements. International Organization for Standardization; 2005.
30. ISO 27002: Information technology – security techniques – code of practice for information security management. International Organization for Standardization; 2005.
31. Gostin LO. National health information privacy regulations under the Health Insurance Portability and Accountability Act. JAMA. 2001;285(23):3015–21. doi:10.1001/jama.285.23.3015.
32. Cabrera E, Papaevangelou H, Mcparland J. Patient's autonomy, privacy and informed consent. IOS Press, 2000. ISBN 1586030396, 9781586030391.

Chapter 12
The Role of the Informatics Nurse

Lynn M. Nagle

Abstract In the last decade, the scope of practice for nurses in informatics roles has been evolving and shifting in response to the needs of health care organizations. While the informatician's practice has been seldom consistently defined or circumscribed in terms of role responsibilities and scope, they have been significant contributors to the evolution and dissemination of information and communication technology (ICT) across the globe. Further the advent of formalized education in nursing and health informatics has led to the establishment of associated credentials and situated informatics as a specialty within the nursing profession. In this chapter, the author will review the types of informatics roles that have been assumed by nurses working in the field of informatics, key role functions, and a perspective on the essential leadership roles and possible directions for the next generation of nurse informaticians.

Keywords Nurse informatician • Informatics role • Informatics specialist • Informatics competencies • Information and communication technology • Health informatics • Clinical intelligence • Business intelligence

Key Concepts

Nurse informatician
Scope of practice
Role functions
Competencies
Information and communication technology
Health informatics
Clinical intelligence
Business intelligence

The online version of this chapter (doi:10.1007/978-1-4471-2999-8_12) contains supplementary material, which is available to authorized users.

L.M. Nagle, RN, BN, MScN, PhD
Lawrence S. Bloomberg, Faculty of Nursing, University of Toronto, Toronto, ON, Canada
e-mail: lynn.nagle@utoronto.ca

© Springer-Verlag London 2015   251
K.J. Hannah et al. (eds.), *Introduction to Nursing Informatics*,
Health Informatics, DOI 10.1007/978-1-4471-2999-8_12

Introduction

The various roles, practice and competencies of nurses in informatics have been evolving for several decades. Similarly, academic opportunities and credentials in the field have become increasingly available and sought after by nurses. In the early years, information and communication technology (ICT), initiatives in health care organizations were almost exclusively led by traditional information technology (IT) and or telecommunications departments. When deemed necessary, clinicians, including nurses, were typically seconded for short or long term stints to bring a clinical perspective to the table. Anecdotally, these positions were largely time limited and focused mostly on system implementation and the training of users. These incidental assignments often came with the designation of *IT nurse* as the titles nurse informatician, informatics specialist or informaticist were uncommon until the emergence of formal programs of study and opportunities to obtain formal certification. More often than not, nurses were engaged after ICT choices and designs were finalized, with little consideration for the potential impacts on the daily work of the largest group of health care providers, nurses.

Today a majority of healthcare organizations recognize that successful implementation and adoption of ICT necessitates the inclusion of clinician perspectives beyond those of physicians. Furthermore, studies are demonstrating that organizations with the foresight to involve nurses and other clinicians at the outset of ICT initiatives, including the acquisition and design phases, are more likely to achieve success in adoption and use [1–5].

While a wide variety of "informatics" positions are commonly filled by nurses, consistency and clarity of what constitutes the *work* of these positions is lacking. Over the years, many unique position descriptions have been created with an array of titles, roles and responsibilities. Nursing positions in informatics run the gamut from the unit-based "*nurse super user*" to the organizational executive level, "*Chief Information Officer*" (CIO) or nurse executive position of "*Chief Nursing Informatics Officer*" (CNIO). Accompanying the work variability is a range of requisite experience, education and associated competencies even for those with similar titles. However, the finding of variability in the work of informatics' nurses is not unique to nursing and has been recognized as an area in need of greater specificity and uniformity in health informatics' practice in general [6–8].

In this chapter, the author provides an overview of informatics as a nursing specialty, nurses' work in informatics, roles, responsibilities, and associated activities. The title *nurse informatician* will be used as the default reference to nurses working in informatics in order to provide illustrations within the context of this chapter. Additionally, speculation on directions for future informatics roles for nurses is offered for the reader's consideration.

Informatics as a Specialty

...a specialty that integrates nursing science, computer science, and information science to manage and communicate data, information, and knowledge in nursing practice. Nursing informatics facilitates the integration of data, information, and knowledge to support patients, nurses, and other providers in their decision-making in all roles and settings. This support is accomplished through the use of information structures, information processes, and information technology [9].

Small groups of nurses interested in informatics and its potential application to practice, education, administration and research began organizing on an international scale as far back as the 1960's. Organized international and national gatherings of nurses occurred over many years in several nations long before nursing informatics became formally recognized as a specialty [10]. In the early years, a contingent of nurses organized as a special interest group of the International Medical Informatics Association (IMIA) and became established as the Nursing Informatics Special Interest Group (IMIA NI-SIG). The IMIA NI-SIG currently serves as a unifying body supporting networking and collaboration among nurse informaticians around the globe, while also advancing the practice and research of informatics. Table 12.1 reflects the current goals and objectives of the NI-SIG which are each supported by specific activities and challenges to the community.

In 1992, the American Nurses Association (ANA) recognized the specialty of nursing informatics, publishing *The Scope of Practice for Nursing Informatics* [11] and *The Standards of Practice for Nursing Informatics* [12]. These were subsequently revised into a single publication in 2008 to reflect the scope and standards of practice and professional performance for the informatics nurse specialist [13]. See Table 12.2 for the overarching dimensions of the ANA nurse informatics specialist standards for practice and professional performance.

In the late 1980's, Canadian nurses working in informatics were initially organized as the Nursing Informatics – Special Interest Group (SIG) of the Canadian Organization for the Advancement of Computers in Health (COACH). Disbanded in 2001, this group was reconstituted in 2002 as an independent corporate entity, the Canadian Nursing Informatics Association (CNIA). A year later, the CNIA was granted Affiliate Group status with the Canadian Nurses Association (CNA), formally recognizing the specialty within the Canadian nursing community. Shortly thereafter, the CNIA became the COACH nominee to the represent Canadian nurses on the IMIA NI-SIG. During the last decade, although CNIA members have been invited to participate in international initiatives, they have been most active in the development of national health data standards, core informatics competencies for basic nursing curricula, resources for nurse educators and formal education and certification programs in Canada.

Although beyond the scope of this chapter, nurses working in informatics have continued to organize worldwide and are convening regularly to network and

Table 12.1 IMIA Special Interest Group – Nursing Informatics Goals & Objectives

Goals and Objectives
The focus of IMIA-NI is to foster collaboration among nurses and others who are interested in Nursing Informatics to facilitate development in the field. We aim to share knowledge, experience and ideas with nurses and healthcare providers worldwide about the practice of Nursing Informatics and the benefits of enhanced information management.
Specific Objectives
Explore the scope of Nursing Informatics and its implication for health policy and information handling activities associated with evidence based nursing practice, nursing management, nursing research, nursing education, standards and patient (or client) decision making and the various relationships with other health care informatics entities.
Identify priorities or gaps and make recommendations for future developments in Nursing Informatics
Support the development of Nursing Informatics in member countries and promote Nursing Informatics worldwide.
Promote linkages and collaborative activities with national and international nursing and healthcare informatics groups and nursing and health care organisations globally.
Provide, promote and support informatics meetings, conferences, and electronic communication forums to enable opportunities for the sharing of ideas, developments and knowledge.
To participate in IMIA working groups and special interest groups to present a nursing perspective.
Develop recommendations, guidelines, tools and courses related to Nursing Informatics.
Encourage the publication and dissemination of research and development materials in the field of Nursing Informatics
To support and work with patients, families, communities and societies to adopt and manage informatics approaches to healthcare.
Ensure the group is more visible by providing up to date information on the web site enabling external groups e.g. WHO, ICN to access as required.

Last updated: 07 Dec 2012; Accessed 1 Mar 2013 at: http://www.imia-medinfo.org/new2/node/151
IMIA-NI International Medical Informatics Association – Nursing Informatics

address shared issues and challenges at national and international meetings and conferences. IMIA member and non-member countries are invited to participate in a number of scientific meetings (e.g., Medinfo, International Nursing Informatics Congress, European Federation for Medical Informatics), which take place every 2–3 years in a variety of locales. In the early days, these forums were commonly the venue by which a majority of nurses obtained the foundations of their training and education in informatics. This is likely still the case for nurses from countries in which other informatics learning options are non-existent.

Specialty Preparation and Certification

In conjunction with the recognition of nursing informatics as a specialty, numerous college and university based programs were launched in the early 90's, offering individuals an opportunity to obtain a wide variety of certificates, diplomas and undergraduate and graduate degrees. Existing programs are varied in their focus,

Table 12.2 Informatics nurse specialist standards of practice and professional performance

Standards of Practice
1. Assessment
2. Problem and issues identification
3. Outcomes identification
4. Planning
5. Implementation
5a. Co-ordination of activities
5b. Health teaching and health promotion and education
5c. Consultation
6. Evaluation
Standards of Professional Performance
7. Education
8. Professional practice evaluation
9. Quality of practice
10. Collegiality
11. Collaboration
12. Ethics
13. Research
14. Resource utilization
15. Advocacy
16. Leadership

Adapted from: American Nurses Association (ANA) [13]

duration and completion credential but are intended to provide nurses and others with the specialized knowledge and skills needed to become effective informaticians. Over the last 10 years, many online program offerings have also been developed further extending the reach of continuing education opportunities. The American Medical Informatics Association (AMIA) maintains a comprehensive inventory of US and internationally based informatics program and course offerings on their website [14]. Similarly, the Canadian health informatics association, COACH, maintains a listing of educational opportunities targeting individuals with technical and/or clinical backgrounds [15]. In addition to these education offerings, there are now a number of professional journals that have a specific focus on issues of practice and research in nursing informatics including: (a) *CIN: Computers, Informatics, Nursing* and (b) the *Online Journal of Nursing Informatics*. Although the publication of nurse informaticians' work is not limited to these journals, they do offer nurses opportunities to publish their experiences and learnings from practice, education and research with a nursing audience in mind.

In addition to formal programs of study, those with health informatics expertise may realise a nationally recognized professional designation upon successful completion of national certification examinations. Among these is the Health Information Management Systems Society (HIMSS) designation of Certified Professional in Healthcare Information and Management Systems [16, 17]. A Canadian variation, CPHIMS-CA, on this credential is also offered for interested individuals with clinical or technology backgrounds. Upon successful completion of the certification exam, individuals receive a credential signifying that they have the health informatics "skills, knowledge and abilities to perform safely and effectively in a broad range of practice settings" [15]. While the ANA has afforded nurses the option of securing a Board certification in nursing informatics for several years now [18] this type of nursing specific professional certification is not widely available to nurses in other countries. In addition to nursing and informatics education credentials, many nurses have also completed a course of study and exam to achieve a Project Management Professional® (PMP) certification in response to the demand for project leadership skills within healthcare settings.

With the establishment of nursing informatics organizations and the creation of opportunities to complete formal informatics education offerings, informatics has achieved recognition as a specialty within nursing [5, 7, 17, 19–21]. Nonetheless many nurses remain unaware of the potential opportunities in the field and often encounter these by chance rather than design. Until core informatics competencies become integrated into the curricula of all entry level nursing programs, informatics may not even be on the radar as a specialty option for a majority of nurses. Increasing awareness and knowledge of informatics within the broader nursing community continues to be a key area of focus for many nursing informatics specialty groups.

Current Nursing Informatics Workforce

According to McLane and Turley [7], *"informaticians are prepared to influence, contribute to, and mold the realization of an organization's vision for knowledge management"* (p. 30). Today many individuals throughout North America, including nurses, have attained credentials that denote their knowledge, expertise and experience in the field of health informatics. Over the years, many nurses have moved into senior executive positions including the role of Chief Information Officer; some of the challenges for nurses in this role have been described previously [22]. Roles for nurses have actually evolved to the extent that executive positions with the designation of CNIO have been established in some health care organizations. Nevertheless public advocacy for more positions of this ilk continues [20, 23–25]. It is most common to find nurses specializing in the field of informatics referred to as informaticists, informaticians, informatics nurse specialists and/or clinical informatics specialists, sometimes but not always, denoting that they have advanced training or a credential in informatics. However, despite the emergence of informatics specific educational offerings and positions, many nurses do not have formalized training and often find themselves in informatics roles for which they are ill-prepared. And as was found in a recent HIMSS survey, a majority of nurse informaticians continue to derive their knowledge and experience through on-the-job training [17]. Some additional findings from this survey are provided to provide the reader with a sense of the current context of nurses' work in informatics at least within North America albeit primarily within the United States.

Work Location and Reporting

Of the 660 survey participants, 48 % reported working in a hospital, 20 % working in the corporate offices of a healthcare system, 9 % in an academic setting and 5 % for a consulting firm or vendor, with the remainder working in a variety of other settings. Most of the respondents (52 %) indicated that they report to an information systems department, reflecting an increase (2 %) from the previous survey in 2007. Those individuals reporting to a nursing department dropped from 38 to 32 % in the same time period with a slight shift in reporting to administration. Sixty-one percent indicated that they had no direct or indirect staff reports suggesting that a majority do not have management positions [17].

Years of Experience, Credentials, and Titles

Forty-nine percent reported years of informatics experience as 7 or more and 56 % reported being in their current position for more than 3 years. While 20 % reported being currently enrolled in an informatics program (bachelors, certificate, masters/ PhD), another 40 % reported receiving a formal credential in 2011. A majority (58 %) reported that they did not have any type of informatics certification (e.g., ANCC, CPHIMS) [16, 18], but 56 % indicated their intent to obtain one in the future. When asked about their job titles, 20 % indicated that they have a title of nursing informatics specialist and 10 % are referred to as clinical specialists. The title of nursing informatics specialist was more common than previously reported and 37 % indicated that their title clearly denoted the informatics nature of their work [17].

Position Responsibilities

The respondents' top three areas of job responsibility were reported in the following areas (shown by top eight areas identified):

- Systems implementation (57 %)
- Systems development (53 %)
- Quality initiative (31 %)
- Informatics education (23 %)
- Liaison (23 %)
- Strategic planning (16 %)
- Nursing education (11 %)
- Operations (10 %)

Systems implementation and development activities included: user preparation, training, support and system customization or updating. Ranked third, the focus on quality improvement activities including: problem-solving, issues of patient safety and system evaluation, reflecting a promising 10 % increase when compared to the previous survey in 2007 [17]. The applications reported to be the most often the focus of the respondents' development and implementation activities included the following (shown by top nine areas identified):

- Nursing clinical documentation (77 %)
- Electronic Medical Record/Electronic Health Record (62 %)
- Computerized Provider Order Entry (CPOE) (60 %)
- Clinical Information Systems (58 %)
- Non-nursing Clinical Documentation (56 %)
- Electronic Medication Administration Record (48 %)
- Bar Coded Medication Management (41 %)
- Point-of-care Decision Support (33 %)
- Quality Improvement/Risk (30 %)

Respondents reported that they also had the most experience with these applications and systems. These findings are not surprising in light of the current investments and emphasis on clinical information system deployments throughout the United States and beyond. In particular, the focus on clinical documentation and CPOE reflects the current state of EHR maturity within a majority of health care organizations throughout North America. The survey respondents were found to be least likely involved in activities associated with utilization review, voice communications, practice management, and remote monitoring [17]. Since only 4 % of the respondents came from outside of the United States, it is difficult to generalize the findings of the HIMSS 2011 nursing informatics workforce survey to other countries. However, the results do offer some interesting insights into the evolution of nursing informatics within a developed nation, especially one in which it has been recognized as a specialty for more than two decades.

Nurse informaticians can be found working within health care organizations, leading and participating in ICT initiatives. Others have secured roles working in government and legislative bodies, advancing standards, policy and strategic initiatives. In academic settings, nurses are advancing informatics education and research and informing innovations in teaching and learning. And still others have been recruited by ICT software and hardware developers and suppliers to bring their expertise to bear on the evolution of technology solutions to support clinical care delivery. The evolution of nurse informatician roles has occurred as a direct result of the need to converge nursing expertise with the knowledge of informatics to better inform systems design, implementation, education, and evaluation. Nurses knowledge and skills have been acknowledged as integral to the effective implementation of ICT as well as effective information and knowledge management [5, 7, 8].

Domains of Nurse Informatician Work

Informatics roles in practice settings have been widely varied in their scope and function but have largely focused on components of the system lifecycle (e.g., design, implementation, training, and evaluation). Hersh [6] underscored the ill-defined relationship between the practice of informaticians and job titles. A recent publication by McLane and Turley [7] offers perspectives on the keys areas in which the nurse informatician can play a role within healthcare organizations. They also highlight the intricacy and complexity of the knowledge and skills required by organizations endeavouring to deliver on an ICT agenda that will lead to safer, more effective care and also support clinical practice.

Although there continues to be a lack of clarity and consistency in defining the roles and responsibilities of nurses in informatics, the following discussion provides a broad categorization of major domains of informatics practice. Table 12.3 provides a synthesis of the seven domains of work and common areas of work focus within each (Audio 12.1, 12.2, 12.3, and 12.4):

1. Leadership
2. ICT Life Cycle Management
3. Health System Use
4. Entrepreneurship
5. Vendor Support
6. Education
7. Research

Leadership

Notwithstanding the fact that all informatics roles require an element of leadership capacity, for the purpose of this discussion, the domain is applied to those roles that are typically senior positions within healthcare organizations, ICT companies or government. These individuals typically provide strategic or operational oversight of organizational, regional and national ICT solutions. They may provide expert consultation on issues of ICT strategy, including support for the processes of acquisition, deployment, implementation, evaluation and education. Some nurses in these senior roles may focus on issues of advocacy or political action to drive broad ICT or health and professional policy directions. To date, the number of nurses recognized for their informatics expertise at government and policy tables has been limited but there is clearly an opportunity and need for the voice of nurses to be heard.

The concept of *change leadership* is an essential role function for the senior nurse informatician such that the ICT vision, strategy and solutions, management teams and supporting actors and activities are provided with explicit and committed executive support. Titles such as Chief Information Officer, CNIO, Vice-President or Director of Nursing Informatics, Nurse Informatics Consultant or Advocate are most commonly used to designate these positions.

ICT Life Cycle Management

Smith and Tyler [21]; p78] described the system development life cycle (SDLC) as comprised of five phases: initiation, analysis, design, implementation, and continuous improvement or support (Fig. 12.1). Further they illustrated the alignment of the

Table 12.3 Domains and areas of focus for nurse informaticians

Domain	Areas of focus
Leadership	Strategy
	Strategic planning
	Change leadership
	Consultation
	Advocacy
	Political action
	Health policy
	Customer relations
ICT life cycle management	Systems analyses
	Workflow
	Process improvement
	Usability
	Ergonomics
	Socio-cultural
	Functional specification
	Acquisition
	Application design
	Data representation
	Terminology
	Standards development
	Interoperability/integration
	Implementation
	Change management
	Education
	Competency assessment
	Training & education
	Evaluation
	Formative
	Summative
	Systems support
Health system use	Data analytics
	Aggregate reporting
	Utilization management
	Decision support
	Generation of new knowledge
	Use of data, information, and knowledge
	Outcomes Management
	Quality Improvement
	Ethical use
	Protection of privacy
Entrepreneurship	Software/hardware solution development
	Consulting

Table 12.3 (continued)

Domain	Areas of focus
Vendor support	Product development
	Sales
	Customer support
Education	Curriculum/course development & delivery
	Competency assessment
	ICT innovation in education
Research	Conduct of research focused on applications of informatics in practice, education, and/or administration

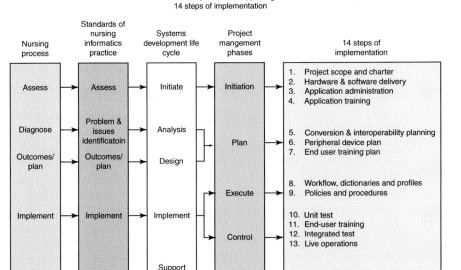

Fig. 12.1 Standard processes supporting 14 steps of implementation (With permission © McGraw Hill)

SDLC with the standards of nursing informatics practice (see Fig 12.1), the project management process and the nursing process. The roles encompassed within this domain constitute by far, a majority of positions currently filled by nurse informaticians. Given the breadth and depth of activities needed to manage the ICT life cycle, these roles typically vary widely in title, scope of responsibility and employers' requisite qualifications. The work of nurses in this area may include:

(a) providing oversight (e.g., project management) or hands-on involvement in the tasks of information gathering and analyses to inform ICT functional specifications for solution acquisitions and designs;

(b) process mapping and analyses of current and desired future states;

(c) supporting or engaging in application design and build activities;
(d) assuring the use of data and interoperability standards;
(e) usability testing
(f) ergonomic evaluation;
(g) developing methods and tools for initial and ongoing user support, training and education;
(h) leading and supporting evaluation activities, formative and summative;
(i) reviewing, revising, and developing relevant practice related ICT policies.

These work efforts are largely focused on getting the solution functionality and supporting processes and infrastructure designed as well as possible to achieve successful clinician adoption and integration into practice. Each of the core work elements requires oversight, expertise, and iterative engagement of the targeted user community. To this end, project management, clinical expertise, and skilled change management are necessary ingredients to success. Not all nurse informaticians will have the experience, skill, and knowledge to contribute to all aspects of the ICT lifecycle, but in the course of time and experiential practise, it is likely that most will garner exposure and an understanding of each dimension.

The work of systems analyses is typically undertaken by a combination of technical and clinical experts. Nurse analysts will generally focus on the clinical systems pre- and post-ICT, starting with activities to inform the solution acquisition through to understanding the chosen solution's impact on clinical and associated business processes. The work usually encompasses the capture and documentation of clinical operations in the context of specific settings and is inclusive of all clinicians and non-clinicians for whom a new technology will potentially change or impact the flow of their day to day activities.

Expertise in the areas of data standards, terminologies, and systems interoperability (See Chaps. 1, 6, and 7) is of utmost importance but as yet not well understood by many clinicians. The adoption and use of clinical data standards among nurses are particularly challenging as the use of standardized language is a foreign concept to most. Perhaps the most universally understood and applied standard is the rubric of the nursing process, but the standardized terminologies that underpin the documentation of the steps are less so (e.g., nursing diagnosis, interventions, outcomes). The integration nursing data standards and codification of these in electronic health records is an area needing the engagement of many more nurse informaticians, given that a future which includes comparable, analyzable and reportable nursing relevant metrics depends upon it.

The area of human factors addresses a myriad of socio-technical issues not the least of which is the usability of ICT solutions. As a division of cognitive psychology, in the context of informatics human factors is largely concerned with human-machine or human-computer (i.e., devices and applications) interactions. The emphasis on human factors has emerged in recent years as a consideration that is germane to the ultimate success of ICT deployment. Nurses working in this area will concern themselves not only with the cognitive impact of ICT solutions on nurses' and others' work but also with the physical or ergonomic design issues (e.g., workstation height, lighting).

Role designations such as Project Manager, Data/Terminology/Standards Specialist, Application Specialist, Nurse Informatics Specialist, Clinical Informatics Specialist, Business/Clinical Process Analyst, Usability Specialist, Nurse Ergonomist, ICT Policy and Procedure Manager are examples of some of the commonly used titles associated with these responsibilities.

Health System Use

The area of health system use is emerging to likely be the most important focus of health informaticians' work in the years ahead. Health system use reflects the shift from the investment and development in information systems to the analysis and use of data to inform business and clinical decisions. Health data analytics may inform or drive reactive, proactive or retrospective actions or decisions. The increasing sophistication of health information systems is affording decision-makers, managers, and clinicians the capacity to make better informed decisions to achieve both short and long term outcomes. In addition to the phrase health system use, the terms business intelligence and clinical intelligence are being increasingly applied to describe the processes and outputs of this work. The outputs may be driven by specific business, clinical or research questions, focused on specific financial or clinical performance metrics and outcomes, and often encompass the provision of benchmarking and performance measurement reports. In its most basic application, health information use can occur at the patient/client, unit/program, or organizational level. In this regard, one might deem the staff nurse or nurse manager as the first level of user, focused on the use of clinical data, information and knowledge to inform clinical or management practice decisions respectively.

Although it is still early days for ICT supported clinical decision-making, nurses have been using tools such as nursing workload management systems for more than three decades. Originally designed to support staffing decisions based upon patient acuity scores, these tools became pervasive in healthcare during the 1980's and 90's. (For additional information about these systems, refer to Chap. 10) While not commonly used to adjust daily staffing levels, the data from these systems have been used to track patient acuity, as a proxy for the costs of nursing care, and often to guide organizational decisions about issues such as staff mix. Nurses supporting the implementation and use of these systems were typically designated as the *vendor name* (e.g., Medicus™, GRASP™), *workload* or *systems* nurse. Commonplace among the nursing workforce, these were likely the first informatics nurses found in clinical settings, but the position titles did not denote the importance of their activities as data managers and custodians, assuring data quality, reliability and completeness of workload data. These roles continue to exist in many health care organizations today, but as clinical system vendors are beginning to design tools to generate nursing workload and patient acuity as bi-products of clinical documentation, they may well become unnecessary in the future and subsumed by the work of the nurse informatician.

At local levels, many health care provider organizations have acquired business analytic software tools that support the mining and analysis of data to inform business and clinical decisions. Considering broader levels of system use, data and information from health information systems can support program quality and safety improvements, planning and resource allocation, clinical utilization review, and management of public health issues and substantially support health services research. At present, these are the most common applications to which the term health system use is being applied. Health system use analyses are being conducted at regional, national and international levels to inform funding directions, health policy, and overall health system improvements. In some countries, national data repositories have been created to house data for these purposes (e.g., Canadian Institute of Health Information [CIHI], National Database of Nursing Quality Indicators® [NDNQI®], Institute for Clinical Evaluative Sciences [ICES]). For examples of national reports being generated by CIHI go to Chap. 10. While not necessarily staffed by nurse informaticians, many health care organizations have dedicated departments doing this type of work. The supporting roles are commonly referred to by titles such as Decision Support Analyst, Business Analyst, Clinical Decision Support Analyst and Quality and Safety Improvement Officer.

Vendor Support

In recent years, vendors, particularly those developing software solutions to support clinical care, have begun to recognize the invaluable perspectives and knowledge of nurses to inform the design of tools that are deemed to be useful in support of clinical practice. Nurses working for software and hardware companies often find themselves attending sales meetings and informatics conferences, conducting product demonstrations for prospective clients, and supporting healthcare customers post-sales. Others have assumed roles focused on product design, development and functional evaluation activities. Positions such as Nursing Product Consultant, Sales Representative, Application Specialist and, in some large software organizations, senior level positions (e.g., Chief Nursing Officer or VP Nursing) are not uncommon.

Education

Nurse educators have been introducing the concepts of informatics to students in undergraduate and graduate programs for many years. Despite many faculty early adopters in this area, a majority of nursing schools still have limited or no informatics content in the undergraduate nursing curricula.

Whether recognized or not, in today's world, informatics is simply a part of every faculty member's tool kit. Therefore, it should not be offered or developed as a separate course. Rather it should be integrated with approaches to the theoretical and practical teachings in every course. [26, p24]

Typically offered as a single course, elective or required, the need to integrate informatics content as a thread throughout entry level nursing programs remains significant. Because of its niche nature to date, there are a limited number of nursing faculty who have a comfort level with the delivery of informatics content. Despite many informatics concepts being central to basic nursing practice (e.g., evidence-informed decision-making), it would seem that many educators see informatics as a wholly separate area of expertise. Albeit the practice of a nurse informatician is quite different from that of a bedside nurse, they are conceptually and practically interconnected. But until informatics becomes explicit and integral to the work of practitioners and educators, it is likely that the number of nurse informatician educators in schools of nursing will remain few in number. See Chaps. 15 and 16 for a detailed discussion on informatics and education.

In practice settings however, the role of the nursing informatician in educating and training clinicians in the use of ICT solutions is much more common. In many settings, the assumption of these responsibilities by clinical nurse educators is currently not viewed as being part of their work. Rather ICT education and training is seen to be separate and within the sole purview of Systems Nurses or other designated individuals with or without clinical backgrounds. These educators typically report to the IT or informatics department. In addition to these roles, it is common for unit-based or program-based nurses to be designated as "super users" to provide staff with ongoing support following the implementation of a new solution. These are often nurses who have expressed an affinity for technology but not always; at times individuals are conscripted into these roles – not usually a successful strategy.

Research

Over the years, nurse researchers have committed entire careers studying the concepts and practice of informatics in nursing (See Chap. 13 for more on research in nursing informatics). Relative to other areas of nursing research, the extent of informatics nursing research being conducted world-wide is limited. Indeed there is a need for considerably more research in the field and additional evidence to advance our informatics knowledge base. In particular, within each of the domains of *Leadership, ICT Life Cycle Management, and Health System Use* as highlighted in Table 12.3, there are as yet many unanswered questions regarding ICT effectiveness, efficiency, outcomes and overall benefits to nursing and the health care system as a whole. The future development of researchers in the field will be largely dependent upon there being an increased recognition of informatics within the academic arena. Budding researchers will need the guidance and mentoring of nurse educators with informatics and research expertise.

Entrepreneurship

Over the years, many enterprising nurses have undertaken to create independent business operations with an informatics focus. The scope of these businesses has encompassed the provision of expertise to support any of the previously described domains of informatics work. Most commonly nursing informatics consultants have supported the work of ICT vendors and health care organizations lacking the requisite knowledge and experience to successfully execute an ICT acquisition, deployment and/or evaluation. The nurse informatics consultant is typically a seasoned practitioner who has an established track record in the field and viewed by actual and prospective clients as a valuable and trusted advisor. As previously discussed, nurses working solo or in partnership with other companies, have also led or contributed to the design, development, and distribution of proprietary software products to support the clinical, administrative, research and educational work of other nurses (e.g., GRASP™, Emerald Health Information Systems).

In this section, the key domains that may provide the focus of a nurse informatician's work have been broadly described and summarized. Table 12.4 provides the reader with a further synthesis of various role functions, position titles and some of the activities associated with each. Although the delineation and separation of some role functions may not be consistent within or among health care organizations, this discussion is intended provide a simplified framework of the types of work that the nurse informatician may undertake. Neither the position titles nor designated activities are meant to be authoritative or prescriptive, but representative of a specialty that is in evolution.

Nurse Informatician Roles for the Future

Across the globe, the healthcare industry continues to wrestle with clinician acceptance and full integration of ICT solutions into the processes of care delivery. Although seemingly protracted, the duration of this journey is not surprising and the evolution of systems will continue for many years to come. However, at this juncture it is important to rethink the role of nurse informaticians for the next decade. Some organizations have created formal informatics leadership positions and to a lesser extent informatics departments, but most continue to designate a small number of willing individuals to represent the clinical perspective within ICT initiatives. Additionally, a majority of nurses continue to derive their knowledge and expertise via the school of hard knocks as the *informatics* or *IT nurse* within an organization. Until the core concepts and competencies of informatics become embedded within the undergraduate curricula of the health professions and recognized as this landscape is unlikely to change. The specialty has been recognized within the profession for more than two decades, but the essential nature of these roles in all domains has to be widely recognized and embraced by academia and healthcare organizations.

Table 12.4 Role focus, position titles and activities of nurse informaticians

Role focus	Position titles	Activities
Change leadership	Chief information officer	Strategic planning
	Chief nursing informatics	Innovation
	Officer	Sponsorship
	Director nursing	Team building
	Informatics	System acquisition and funding
	Consultant	Health policy & political action
	Advocate	
Change management	Project manager	Operational management
	Informatics nurse specialist	Problem-solving
	Informatician	Budget management
	Informaticist	Team building
		User relationship management
		Vendor management
Systems analyses	Clinical analyst	Process analysis
	Business analyst	Standards
	Application specialist	System acquisition
	Usability specialist	Application design & build
	Nurse ergonomist	Human factors testing
	Data standards specialist	Ergonomics
	Interoperability specialist	Evaluation
Implementation	Informatics nurse	User support
	Application support specialist	Application support
		Device support
Education	Systems educator/trainer	Education
	Nurse educator	Training
		Support
		Orientation
Evaluation	Informatics researcher	Pilot testing
	System user	Interative design/usability testing
	Informatics specialist	Formative/summative
Systems support	Informatics nurse	Ongoing support in use of ICT
	Nurse educator	Program/department/unit based
	Nurse super user	
	Application support	
System use	**Nurse as:**	Nurse as knowledge worker
	Data gatherer	Outcomes management
	Information user	Evidence-based practice
	Knowledge user	
	Knowledge generator	

(continued)

Table 12.4 (continued)

Role focus	Position titles	Activities
Data analyses	Business analyst	Data mining and analytics
	Decision support analyst	Benchmarking
	Quality improvement	Outcomes monitoring
	Clinical intelligence co-ordinator	Quality and risk management
	Nurse clinical safety officer	Appropriate access & use
	Clinical utilization manager	
Vendor product development	Informatics specialist	Customer engagement and support
Sales & support	Informatics nurse	
	VP CNO	
Consultation	Informatics consultant	Support for any of the above

"There are two roles in informatics: the informatics specialist and the clinician who must use health information technology. This means in essence that every nurse has a role in informatics" [27], p4].

Heightened concerns for safety and quality have been directly linked to the need for timely access to information and evidence to support optimal clinical decision-making. In the context of increasingly ICT enabled clinical environments that equip nurses with advanced informational support, there is a place for informatics in the work of all nurses [28]. However, in contemplating future roles for nurse informaticians, it is important to consider that the evolving context of ICT use in healthcare delivery organizations (see Chaps. 2, 5, 7, and 10) will likely include:

(a) organizations and providers reaching greater levels of maturity in their use of systems, necessitating an enhanced understanding of meaningful use among clinicians;
(b) increased integration of ICTs across care sectors (e.g., acute care, primary care, long-term care, home care)
(c) citizens taking an increasingly active role in managing their health and health information;
(d) expanded virtualization of health service delivery (e.g., telehomecare, mobile health, telehealth, cloud computing);
(e) increased emphasis on cost containment to assure that services are accessible and affordable;
(f) genomic information as core data within electronic health records will introduce new ethical issues.

These emerging contexts will necessitate the evolution of new nurse informatician roles to contend with new challenges that will surely arise. Envision the nurse informatician who specializes in the virtualization of care, nurse genomic ethicist, personal health record nurse specialist, health data integration and continuum of care and cost management expert, to mention but a few. Imagining the world beyond that which we experience today – consider the implications of the possibilities associated with the advanced simulation, the need for robotics nurse experts, and expertise to manage and optimize health information technologies that extend health care information and services beyond regions and countries to address the needs of developing nations and underserved communities. In the current context of health care services in the developed world, and in considering the possibilities for the future, the nurse informatician is well situated to fulfill critical role for many years to come. Chap. 17 presents a vision of the future and how nursing informatics will support professional practice, advocacy, and the delivery of optimal client care.

Downloads

Available from extras.springer.com:

Educational Template (PDF 103 kb)

Educational Template (PPTX 123 kb)

Audio 12.1. The role of the informatics nurse by Roy Simpson, RN, C, CMAC, FNAP, FAAN, current role vice president, nursing informatics, at Cerner Corporation

Audio 12.2. The role of the informatics nurse by Cheryl Stephens-Lee, RN, BScN, MScNI, Clinical Applications Consultant, Markham Stouffville Hospital, Markham, Ontario, Canada

Audio 12.3. The role of the informatics nurse by Suzanne Brown, RGN, RM, BNs, MScHealth Informatics, Assistant Nurse Coordinator Computer Services, Mater Misericordiae University Hospital, Information Management Services Department, Dublin, Ireland.

Audio 12.4. The role of the informatics nurse by Dairin Hines, RGN, RCN, BSc, HSM, MScHealth Informatics, Clinical Informatics Manager, Temple Street Children's University Hospital, ICT Department, Dublin, Ireland.

Audio 12.3 Transcript (PDF 300 kb)

Audio 12.4 Transcript (PDF 37 kb)

References

1. Ash JS, Stavri PZ, Dykstra R. Implementing computerized physician order entry: the importance of special people. Int J Med Inform. 2003;69:235–50.
2. Ash JS, Bates DW. Factors and forces affecting EHR system adoption: report of a 2004 ACMI discussion. J Am Med Inform Assoc. 2005;12:8–12.
3. Leatt P, Shea C, Studer M, Wang V. IT solutions for patient safety: best practices for successful implementation in healthcare. Healthc Q. 2006;9(1):94–104.
4. Studer M. The effect of organizational factors on the effectiveness of EMR system implementation: what have we learned? Healthc Q. 2005;8(4):92–8.

5. Warm D, Thomas B. A review of the effectiveness of the clinical informaticist role. Nurs Stand. 2011;25(44):35–8.
6. Hersh W. Who are the informaticians? What we know and should know. J Am Med Inform Assoc. 2006;13(2):166–70.
7. McLane S, Turley J. Informaticians: how they may benefit your healthcare organization. J Nurs Adm. 2011;41(1):29–35.
8. Smith SE, Drake LE, Harris J-G, Watson K, Pohlner PG. Clinical informatics: a workforce priority for 21st century healthcare. Aust Health Rev. 2011;35:130–5.
9. Staggers N, Thompson CB. The evolution of definitions for nursing informatics: a critical analysis and revised definition. J Am Med Inform Assoc. 2002;9(3):255–61.
10. Scholes M, Tallberg MA, Pluyter-Wenting E. International nursing informatics: a history of the first forty years: 1960–2000. London: British Computer Society; 2002.
11. American Nurses Association. Scope of practice for nursing informatics. Washington, DC: ANA; 1994.
12. American Nurses Association. Standards of practice for nursing informatics. Washington, DC: ANA; 1995.
13. American Nurses Association (ANA). Nursing informatics: scope and standards of practice. Silver Spring: Nursesbooks.Org; 2008. At: http://www.nursingworld.org/HomepageCategory/NursingInsider/Archive_1/2008NI/Jan08NI/RevisedNursingInformaticsPracticeScopeandStandardsofPractice.html. Accessed 19 Feb 2013.
14. American Medical Informatics Association. Academic informatics programs. 2013. Accessed at: http://www.amia.org/education/programs-and-courses. 25 Feb 2013.
15. COACH. Health informatics education. 2013. At: http://coachorg.com/en/healthinformatics/healthinformaticseducation.asp. Accessed 25 Feb 2013.
16. Health Information Management Systems Society (HIMSS). Health IT certifications. 2013. At: http://www.himss.org/health-it-certification?navItemNumber=13588. Accessed 25 Feb 2013.
17. Health Information Management Systems Society (HIMSS). HIMSS 2011 nursing informatics workforce survey. 2011. At: http://www.himss.org/ResourceLibrary/ResourceDetail.aspx?ItemNumber=11587. Accessed 25 Feb 2013.
18. American Nurses Credentialing Center (ANCC) (nd). Nursing informatics. At: http://www.nursecredentialing.org/Certification/NurseSpecialties/Informatics.html. Accessed 25 Feb 2013.
19. Huryk L. Interview with an informaticist. Nurs Manage. 2011;42(11):45–8.
20. Murphy J. The nursing informatics workforce: who are they and what do they do? Nurs Econ. 2011;29(3):150–3.
21. Smith K, Tyler DD. Systems life cycle: planning and analysis. In: Saba VK, McCormick KA, editors. Essentials of nursing informatics. 5th ed. New York: McGraw-Hill; 2011. p. 77–92.
22. Nagle LM. Nurses *Carpe Diem*. In: One step beyond: the evolution of technology and nursing. Proceedings of 7th International Congress Nursing Informatics Conference on CD, Auckland, 2000.
23. Remus S, Kennedy M. Innovation in transformative nursing leadership: nursing informatics competencies and roles. Can J Nurs Leadersh. 2012;25(4):14–26.
24. Simpson R. Why not just any nurse can be a nurse informatician. Can J Nurs Leadersh. 2012;25(4):27–8.
25. Swindle CG, Bradley VM. The newest O in the C-Suite: CNIO. Nurse Leader. 2010;8(3):28–30.
26. Nagle LM. Everything I know about informatics, I didn't learn in nursing school. Can J Nurs Leadersh. 2007;20(3):22–5.
27. Sewell J, Thede L. Informatics and nursing: opportunities and challenges. 4th ed. Philadelphia: Wolters Kluwer – Lippincott Williams & Wilkin; 2010.
28. Pringle D, Nagle LM. Leadership for the information age: the time for action is now. Can J Nurs Leadersh. 2009;22(1):1–6.

Part IV
Research

Chapter 13
Research Applications

Kathryn Momtahan

Abstract Nursing research is a vital part of nursing professional practice, whether the activity is reading and critiquing research in order to use evidence in nursing practice, participate in research, or lead research. This chapter reviews the nursing research process and describes the types of technology available to conduct research with examples of recent research using the technology. Areas covered include idea generation, literature search and review, data collection and analysis tools for quantitative, qualitative, and mixed methods research, data and visualization tools. The ethical implications of using new technology for nursing research are briefly discussed and an example area of nursing informatics research is provided.

Keywords Nursing research • Qualitative research • Quantitative research • Mixed methods research • Data collection • Data analysis • Knowledge translation • Time-motion studies • Informatics

Key Concepts

Clinical intelligence
Nursing research
Qualitative research
Quantitative research
Mixed methods research
Data collection
Data analysis
Knowledge transition
Time-motion studies

The online version of this chapter (doi:10.1007/978-1-4471-2999-8_13) contains supplementary material, which is available to authorized users.

K. Momtahan, RN, PhD
Nursing Professional Practice, The Ottawa Hospital and the
Ottawa Hospital Research Institute, Ottawa, ON, Canada
e-mail: kmomtahan@ottawahospital.on.ca

© Springer-Verlag London 2015   273
K.J. Hannah et al. (eds.), *Introduction to Nursing Informatics*,
Health Informatics, DOI 10.1007/978-1-4471-2999-8_13

Introduction

Information and communication systems, the Internet, the World Wide Web, mobile computing, social networking, Web 2.0, and the subsequent proliferation of web applications, have changed how researchers conduct everything from literature searches to data analysis and publishing of research results. Since the last chapter on research applications in the 3rd edition of this book published in 2006 [1], ubiquitous computing has become a reality with the prevalence of reasonably-priced lightweight laptop computers, smartphones, and tablet computers.

Ubiquitous computing refers to a form of human-computer interaction that can be performed on many different devices in a fairly seamless way.

Technology that Supports Nursing Research Activities

What Is 'Nursing Research'?

Often people wonder what the difference is between 'research' and 'nursing research'. Polit and Beck [2] define research as a "systematic inquiry that uses disciplined methods to answer questions or solve problems", adding that "[t]he ultimate goal of research is to develop, refine, and expand knowledge". The authors define *nursing research* as the "systematic inquiry designed to develop trustworthy evidence about issues of importance to the nursing profession, including nursing practice, education, administration, and informatics" (Pg 3).

Regardless of whether you call the type of research you are engaged in 'nursing research', 'clinical research', 'informatics research', or something else, the processes you engage in are the same:

1. Idea generation
2. Literature search
3. Literature review
4. Forming a research team
5. Synthesis of the literature
6. Choosing a theoretical framework
7. Developing a methodology
8. Developing a proposal
9. Determining available resources
10. Submitting your proposal to the appropriate Research Ethics Board (REB)
11. Data collection

12. Data analysis
13. Writing
14. Knowledge translation (KT) activities such as submitting a manuscript and/or presenting at conferences

The position of the items on the above list may differ from study to study based on researcher preference, and some of the items may occur more than once in the research process. In all stages of the process, however, there is information technology to support the activity. A set of excellent articles written by Dr. Diane Wink, sometimes co-authored with Elizabeth Killingsworth, review topics such as digital books [3], optimizing use of library technology [4], cloud computing [5], and how to use free Google tools [6]. Although these articles are geared towards nursing education activities in general rather than focusing on research, the reviews are also very useful for the nurse researcher.

The goal of this chapter is to review the technology supports available to nurse researchers but it does not attempt to provide a comprehensive overview of the nursing research process and nursing research methods. These topics are covered in detail by Polit and Beck [2] and Wood and Ross-Kerr [7] as well as many others.

Idea Generation

In nursing, ideas are often generated from clinical experience combined with continuous reading in your area of expertise. Best Practice Guidelines are based on research evidence so a good understanding of Best Practice Guidelines that apply to your clinical area is a good start. The Registered Nurses of Ontario (RNAO) has many nursing best practice guidelines. Type 'nursing best practice guidelines' into a search engine such as Google, and you will find them (http://rnao.ca/bpg). You can also check the national nursing organizations in your country to discover more information about the best practice guidelines promoted for use within specific countries.

Literature Search

Historically, librarians were the 'go-to' professionals for literature searches. They still are! Nurse researchers might choose to perform a preliminary literature search when starting a project. Very experienced, very skilled researchers may even do all of their own literature searches. Despite the internet and publically available databases such as PubMed, librarians are still the experts in this area because of their educational background in library science and the constant professional work that they do. Librarians who specialize in healthcare are familiar with the healthcare-related literature, how it is indexed, and how best to access the information.

A literature search and a literature review (critical assessment of the literature) can be done to help develop research ideas or can be done once the research idea has been developed. The literature review helps you and your research team develop an overall picture of the current knowledge about your research topic. It can be valuable to help identify gaps in the literature, areas that need more research, and types of tools that can be used in your research.

It has become common practice in journal articles to report the "search strategy" used (i.e. which databases were searched, over what period of time and which subject headings or keywords were used for the literature review). It is often very useful to start by looking for a systematic review on a topic. For instance, Cochrane Reviews are considered to be the gold standard of literature reviews. If the topic of interest is "improving efficiency of nursing documentation", entering 'nursing documentation' into the search field in the Cochrane Database of Systematic Reviews would reveal the following record:

Nursing Record Systems: Effects on Nursing Practice and Healthcare Outcomes

The systematic review by Urquhart et al. [8] provides a great deal of information on previous studies in the area and would reveal that 'nursing record systems' would be a good keyword phrase to use when continuing with your literature search. By entering 'nursing record systems' into the PubMed database, several articles are revealed.

What is a database? A database is an organized collection of data. A database like PubMed contains systematically organized information (records) about journal articles, books or other types of literature. Literature (records) are organized into broad topics such as 'healthcare', 'education', or 'engineering', which are searchable to enable finding relevant information on a topic. The following list of common databases, the steps in developing a search strategy, and the description of MeSH terms were obtained from our hospital's Library Services department.

Common databases to search for healthcare-related literature:

- **CINAHL:** the Cumulative Index to Nursing and Allied Health Literature contains nursing and allied health literature.
- **EBM Reviews:** Cochrane Database of Systematic Reviews explores the evidence for and against the effectiveness and appropriateness of treatments/interventions in specific circumstances.
- **EBSCO's Health Business Elite:** focuses on health care administration and other non-clinical aspects of health care institution management. Topics covered

include hospital management, hospital administration, marketing, human resources, computer technology, facilities management and insurance.

- **MEDLINE:** a leading source for bibliographic and abstract coverage of biomedical literature.
- **PubMed:** a popular alternative to MEDLINE.
- **PsycINFO:** contains citations in the field of psychology and the psychological aspects of related disciplines, such as medicine, psychiatry, nursing, sociology, education, pharmacology, physiology, linguistics, anthropology, business, and law.
- **ERIC:** the Education Resources Information Center contains education research information.

Steps in Developing a Search Strategy for Clinical Research (Fig. 13.1)

Refining your Search Strategy

In the early stages of any research process, the search strategy is an essential aspect to support success. Depending on the number or volume of search results, there are a variety of adjustments that can be made to generate the appropriate results supporting a full exploration of the desired topic. Table 13.1 provides some common adjustment strategies that can be used for any type of search.

Combining Search Concepts

Another way to refine your search strategy is to combine term. When combining search terms or concepts, you may use the terms *AND*, *OR*, and *NOT*. These are called Boolean operators and are used to indicate the relationship between search terms (Table 13.2).

Diagrams of Boolean Operators at Work:

AND (Fig. 13.2)
OR (Fig. 13.3)

The following video tutorials provide additional guidance on the use of Boolean operators:

Western University (2011) Basic Search: Using Boolean operators. Available: http://www.youtube.com/watch?v=1mmdXFOyRDo
Western University (2011) Basic Search: Boolean operators (Advanced). Available: http://www.youtube.com/watch?v=RkCJNdetsmI

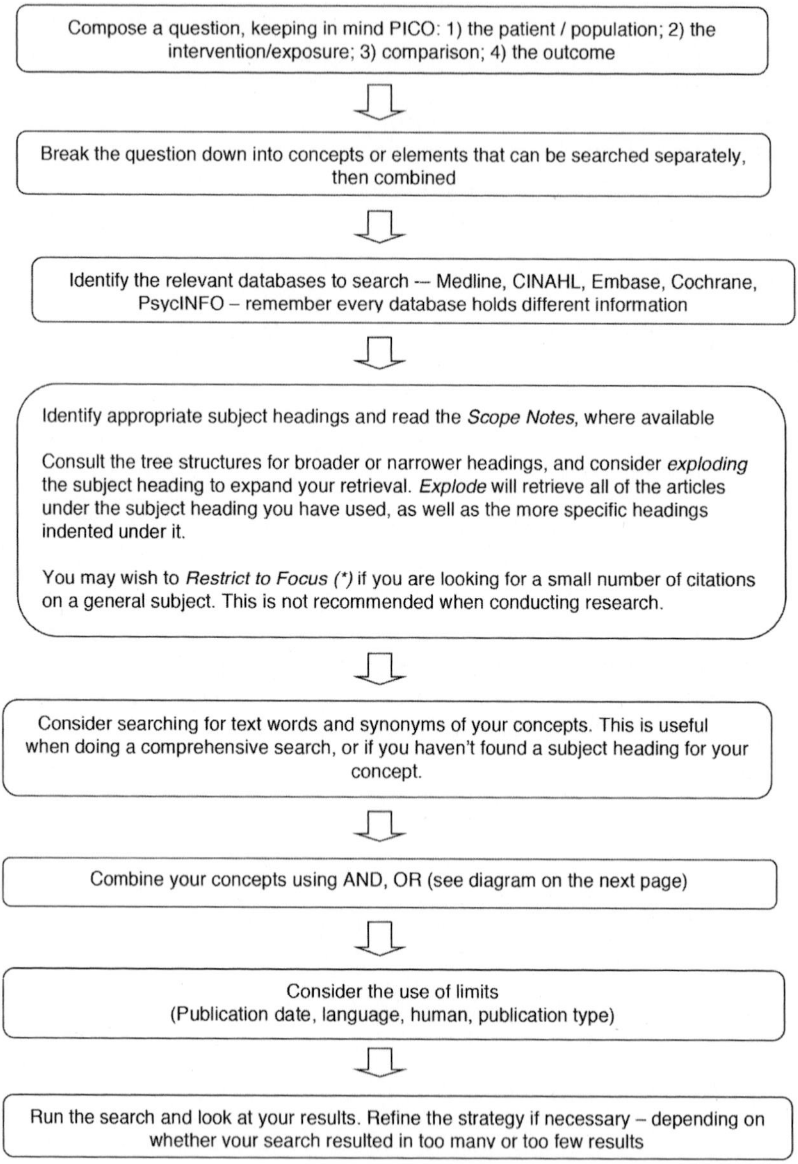

Compose a question, keeping in mind PICO: 1) the patient / population; 2) the intervention/exposure; 3) comparison; 4) the outcome

Break the question down into concepts or elements that can be searched separately, then combined

Identify the relevant databases to search — Medline, CINAHL, Embase, Cochrane, PsycINFO – remember every database holds different information

Identify appropriate subject headings and read the *Scope Notes*, where available

Consult the tree structures for broader or narrower headings, and consider *exploding* the subject heading to expand your retrieval. *Explode* will retrieve all of the articles under the subject heading you have used, as well as the more specific headings indented under it.

You may wish to *Restrict to Focus (*)* if you are looking for a small number of citations on a general subject. This is not recommended when conducting research.

Consider searching for text words and synonyms of your concepts. This is useful when doing a comprehensive search, or if you haven't found a subject heading for your concept.

Combine your concepts using AND, OR (see diagram on the next page)

Consider the use of limits (Publication date, language, human, publication type)

Run the search and look at your results. Refine the strategy if necessary – depending on whether your search resulted in too many or too few results

Fig. 13.1 Steps in developing a search strategy for clinical research

Table 13.1 Strategies for adjusting search results

Too many results
Add in another concept
Use more limits
Use subheadings
Apply Focus to subject heading
Too few results
Remove some limits
Remove Focus on any subject headings
Use more text words
Choose all subheadings
Use broader subject headings
Use the Related articles feature

Table 13.2 Boolean search operators and outcomes

Boolean search operators			
TERM	**AND**	**OR**	**NOT**
ACTION	Narrows search	Broadens search	Narrows search
EXAMPLE	Myocardial infarction AND urokinase	Streptokinase OR urokinase	Streptokinase NOT urokinase
OUTCOME	Retrieves citations containing both terms	Retrieves citations containing one term or the other, or both	Retrieves citations on streptokinase excluding urokinase citations

Choosing a Database for Your Search

The appearance or interface for each database varies from one to the next. All databases can be searched by using keywords while many also allow searches using subject headings. Learning how to use subject headings can improve the results of your literature search. One of the most commonly used subject heading systems is MeSH, the U.S. National Library of Medicine's thesaurus used by the MEDLINE/PubMED databases.

MeSH Terms

Skillful use of subject headings can improve the results of a literature search. MeSH (Medical Subject Headings) is one of the most commonly used subject heading systems controlled by the U.S. National Library of Medicine. It is a vocabulary thesaurus used for indexing articles in PubMed [9]. When it comes to inter-disciplinary

Fig. 13.2 Diagrams of boolean operators at work: AND

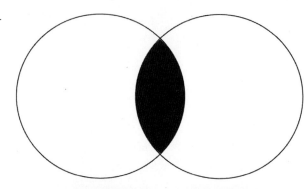

Fig. 13.3 Diagrams of boolean operators at work: OR

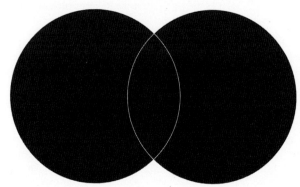

research, knowing what MeSH terms correspond to terms you would normally search by is important. For instance, 'human factors' is not a MeSH term but 'human engineering' is.

All databases should provide the user with the ability to search and save or print their search results. Databases usually contain a section entitled *Search Help*, *Help Topics*, *FAQs (Frequently Asked Questions)* or *Tutorials* to enable the user to learn how to use the database. In addition, many libraries have developed help sheets, online information or YouTube videos on how to search or use specific databases. YouTube video tutorials for using PubMed are linked to the MeSH website (http://www.ncbi.nlm.nih.gov/mesh).

In addition to MEDLINE citations, PubMed also contains in-process citations that provide a record for an article before it is indexed with MeSH and added to MEDLINE as well as citations for books and book chapters available on the NCBI Bookshelf (http://www.ncbi.nlm.nih.gov/books).

Libraries buy access to databases such as MEDLINE and CINAHL and PsycINFO from different vendors such as Ovid and EBSCOhost. Different databases as well as different vendors for database access have different user interfaces and navigation strategies. PubMed now has various sidebar features such as an editable window with the search details so that you can edit the search strategy in the window and re-run the search. PubMed is available not only to scholars but also to the public.

Open Access

Open access journals are gaining popularity with the intent of making journal articles more freely available to readers. Some journals are subsidized and some require payment from the author to publish. Open access journal publishers include PLOS (Public Library of Science) and BMC (BioMed Central).

Open access journals are likely to continue to gain popularity for various reasons: (1) authors are usually in a position to pay the open access fee, (2) students are usually not able to pay for articles, and (3) they sometimes save libraries the cost of a journal subscription. If journal articles are obtained through a university or hospital, whether or not a journal article is an open access article or not, will not be apparent. From outside an academic institution, open access journal articles can be obtained through public access to databases such as PubMed.

Literature Review

Learning to review articles critically and efficiently is an important skill for a researcher. A good guide to the steps for performing a critical appraisal of the literature is 'Reading Research, 5th Edition: A User-Friendly Guide for Health Professionals' by Davies and Logan [10]. The authors of this introductory book take a step-by-step approach to reading research and assessing its quality.

When reviewing literature it is important to (a) have a method of summarizing the information and (b) share the work of reading and summarizing the literature amongst the research group members. Table 13.3 shows an example of a template used by a nursing research team working on a trauma research project. This research team uses Microsoft Word documents to share their review but there are other methods of archiving research summaries and sharing the summaries amongst research team members. By typing in 'online research collaboration tools' into Google, you can find a variety of useful sites, including one at the University of Queensland, Australia. Westlake [11] also provides some practical tips for literature synthesis.

Reference Management Software

The great advantage of using reference management software such as Reference Manager, RefWorks, EndNote, EndNoteWeb, Zotero, Mendeley, and recently Papers 2, is that it provides not only bibliographic storage for citations but it also automatically changes the style of the references depending on what style you need your references to be in for publication or for other types of papers. Choosing the right reference management software for you can be simple if your university, hospital or other organization has a license for reference management software or you have colleagues that already use a particular one. If you are starting from scratch,

Table 13.3 Example of a template used by a nursing research team working on a trauma research project to summarize an article by Duff [15]

Type of research (qual/quan)	Tools used	Sample
Grounded theory research method: constant comparative analysis 16 months for data collection and analysis	1–3 interviews per patient + 12 h clinical observation	11 severe TBI Pts and 25 family members, in PCU/MR from 2 acute neuro centers (Canada). Families followed until patient woke up from coma or died. Length of study was from 7 weeks to 1 year, depending on patients' progress. Ethnic population (TO, the world's most culturally diverse city)

Purpose: To discover the most salient concerns of families who had a close relative with a severe TBI, and how they dealt with the experience during the uncertain trajectory of illness that followed coma

Major Findings: Identified the family's basic social process of "Negotiating Uncertainty", which consisted of 4 phases: Willing Survival, Attending Snow White, Reconstructing the Person and Making it Better

Uncertainty related to both the trajectory of the illness and the eventual cognitive, physical and behavioral outcomes that result

Other Findings:

Willing Survival: Spiritual beliefs, medical miracles and the TBI individual's strength; often determined meaning and provided hope. Families reported that doctors were often pessimistic about outcome, contributing to the family's need to stay close to the patient and be an advocate for care. Virtually all families turned to friends and relatives for support

Snow White: "Waiting for patient to wake up". Family first to notice very detailed improvements in pt's behavior. Family involvement in care very important. Family belief that essential person intact, needs only correct stimuli to awaken from coma/post coma unawareness and return to previous life and personality

If TBI prolonged, family expand efforts to understand brain injury, recovery and rehab, became more adept at negotiating

Transfers both within and outside the hospital were breaking points for family: "very, very traumatic – difficult to overcome fear that he is not ready – not going to be looked after"

If unconsciousness prolonged, dampened hopes and belief in potential for positive outcome. Variable family response: some openly express concerns, some hide fears, afraid that acknowledging/voicing them will negatively affect recovery. Protracted and unpredictable course is very distressing for families. If slow recovery, families often feel forgotten, ignored or patronized

Reconstructing the person: Family constantly engages in process of re-evaluation and reconciliation of pre and post person. Growing realization of long term or permanent effects, resulting in a changed person, and relationships/responsibilities of the family. Degree of recognition and acceptance of families vary widely

With ongoing improvement, HC team more supportive and optimistic for recovery and increased their involvement in care. For pts with limited progress, the HC team (except nurses and SW) do not "see a role" for their services unless the person was acutely ill

Making it Better: Gradual acceptance (timing varies significantly) that person will not return to pre-injury abilities, personality and memories. Families remain committed to helping individual achieve highest level of recovery possible. Often, other pent-up life demands begin to take precedence ("important for me to have some kind of normality") – gradual return to usual routine. Process of making it better facilitated by trusting relationships with HC team and others contributing to well-being of family. Families unable to access acceptable facilities compelled to remain in attendance, change lives or living arrangements (bringing pt home) or suffer guilt

(continued)

Table 13.3 (continued)

Type of research (qual/quan)	Tools used	Sample
Strengths: Richness of data, clinical relevance, followed patients and family over entire coma period, multicultural population, consistent interviewer,		
Weakness: Small sample size, no demographics available, (other than initial coma) and multi-cultural population. Minimal discussion of method of analysis		
Key Points: negotiating uncertainty underlying process, four stages as identified above. Many relevant recommendations for implications for practice and research		
Comparisons: need for hope (Bond, Johnson), need for involvement with care (Serio, etc.), increased stress with transition (Grossman)		
Commentary:		
The richness of the data collected, the examples of statements of family members and the relevance of the clinical observation make this research an excellent example of qualitative research. Unfortunately, the study is limited by the fact that there is no demographic information on the patients and families, and limited definitions of family and the severity of injury		
One of the strengths of Duff's article is the variety of recommendations that she identifies, both in the clinical and research context. Some of the activities she recommends include the involvement of advanced practice nurses in the delivery of information on an early and frequent basis, the development of protocols for experiences the patient undergoes (ie agitation, tracheostomy weaning), which will decrease uncertainty for families and the presence and involvement of families in the patient's care, beginning in the critical phase. Duff emphasizes that although "there are many areas of uncertainty, such as eventual outcomes, that cannot be determined; there are many other causes of uncertainty that can be addressed"		
Excellent article – very clinically relevant		
From Alanna Keenan, MScN, Advanced Practice Nurse (Trauma), The Ottawa Hospital		

you can find various comparisons of these programs. For instance, from the John Hopkin's University library, or by typing 'online research collaboration tools' into a search engine such as Google.

This Reference Manager demo will give you an idea of why reference management software is popular with researchers.

Qualitative Research, Quantitative Research and Mixed Methods Research

The broad choice of research designs can be classified as quantitative, qualitative or mixed methods. Qualitative research investigates a phenomenon in a variety of ways in order to develop a deep understanding or narrative of a phenomenon. The narrative is generated through a variety of research strategies such as ethnography, grounded theory, and other approaches [2, 12]. Quantitative research is often associated with randomized control trials where there are defined independent variables and defined dependent variables. However, there are other types of quantitative designs, often referred to as 'quasi-experimental designs' where it is not possible to randomize [13]. Mixed methods research uses a mixture of quantitative and qualitative methods [14, 16].

Qualitative Research

Qualitative research defined by Polit and Beck [2] is "The investigation of phenomena, typically in an in-depth and holistic fashion, through the collection of rich narrative materials using a flexible research design" (p. 739).

Data Collection

There are many methods of gathering data for qualitative research including interviews and focus groups. Data collection can be done by hand, by computer, or by audiotaping and later transcribing the data into text. MacLean et al. [17] discuss how to improve the accuracy of transcripts. Areas discussed include the following issues:

- Use of voice recognition systems
- Notation choices
- Processing and active listening versus touch typing
- Transcriptionist effect
- Emotionally loaded audiotaped material
- Class and/or cultural differences among interviewee, interviewer, and transcriptionist
- Errors that arise when working in a second language

It is worth noting that voice recognition systems, although used in interactive voice response systems and medical dictation (e.g. Dragon), are more problematic for research use. The challenge for using such technology for interviews is the necessity of voice-training the system. Focus groups pose additional challenges for this type of technology because of the many different speakers. As an alternative method of data collection, Scott et al. [18] discuss the use of court reporters to improve the accuracy of focus group data.

Data Analysis

Thematic analysis of qualitative data can be done without qualitative analysis software if the data set is small. However, for large data sets, a software package that performs thematic analysis is recommended. Qualitative analysis software can select and code data based on the researchers' choice of words and phrases, group the codes, and produce graphical relationships based on the findings. However, the software does not determine the theme, define the codes or interpret the data. The software is a tool to help organize data but is no substitute for keen observation, careful data collection, and analytic interpretation on the part of the researcher.

The University of Surrey in the UK has had a program running for many years called the 'CAQDAS networking project'. CAQDAS stands for 'Computer Assisted Qualitative Data AnalysiS'. This project team has developed many useful resources, including a comparison of qualitative analysis packages such as NVivo and ATLAS.ti as well as many others. Manual methods for organizing qualitative data is reviewed by Polit and Beck [2]. The logic is the same with manual methods as it is with software: both include careful transcription of the data that is captured (usually with audiotapes) and identification of themes. The difference is that you tag pieces of transcribed data when a software package is used and you use a manual method such as colour-coding when not using a software package. This can be done by using a highlighter pen, coloured file cards, paper-clips, or Post-it Notes. Manual methods become unwieldy when the data set is large.

Examples of articles in which qualitative data analysis software was used include an article by Varpio et al. [19] These authors used NVivo to code observations and interview data in a study investigating nurses' responses to patient monitor alarms in a hospital in-patient unit. Another example is an article by Lawton et al. [20]. These researchers conducted interviews with twelve nurses and eight managers on three different hospital medical wards in order to identify latent failures that are perceived to underpin medication errors. Using Braun and Clarke's [21] five stages of thematic content analysis (familiarization with the data, generating initial codes, searching for themes, reviewing themes, and defining and naming themes), Lawton et al. discovered ten themes which were outlined in their article. The authors include a thematic map of the theme 'ward climate' with theme descendents. Bergin [22] describes in detail the process of using NVivo 8 for data analysis of a study he conducted of providers and users of mental health services in Ireland. Polit and Beck [2] describe software such as NVivo and ATLAS.ti as theory-building software.

Concept maps, visually similar to thematic maps, can be used to graphically represent concepts related to nursing theories [23, 24] as an example. The use of concept maps to teach nurses and nursing student critical thinking skills is a lively area of nursing research [25–27].

Quantitative Research

Quantitative research defined by Polit and Beck [2] is "The investigation of phenomena that lend themselves to precise measurement and quantification, often involving a rigorous and controlled design" (p. 739). Examples of study designs that can be classified as quantitative research include randomized control trials (RCTs), experiments, and quasi-experiments (experiments where randomization is not possible). The types of statistical analysis employed in quantitative research include inferential statistics such as analysis of variance (ANOVA) and regression analysis, where the investigator is looking for variables that can predict the values of a dependent variable based on one or more independent variables.

Data Collection

Data collection for quantitative research has changed dramatically over the years due to technology. Paper-based data collection tools such as questionnaires are largely being replaced by online surveys, depending on the population being surveyed. Interactive voice response systems produce data that can be mined for research, as can the variety of databases available for research (see the section on Data Mining in this chapter). The internet itself as well as social media platforms have opened up a whole new area of research. As an example, there are several recent articles related to the quality of YouTube videos for nursing education [28] and medical education [29], as well as analyses of YouTube content for patient education and public health [30].

Clinical data capture for use in nursing research has been revolutionized based on the increase in electronic health record systems in place, mobility devices such as smartphones and tablets, and other wireless technology devices that directly input data into the electronic health record such as vital sign integration devices, infusion pumps, and point-of-care testing devices. Although not flawless, these devices eliminate much of the human error related to manual data entry into the electronic or paper-based chart. Bellomo et al. [31] studied patient outcomes associated with the deployment of electronic automated advisory vital signs monitors on general wards in three different countries, with a sample size of 18,305 patients. The researchers found that use of the electronic automated advisory vital signs monitors were associated with (1) an improvement in the proportion of rapid response team-calls triggered by respiratory criteria, (2) increased survival of patients receiving rapid response team calls, and (3) decreased time required for vital signs measurement and recording.

Data Analysis

Before data analysis begins, it is important to verify the accuracy of the data to be analyzed. Historically, data was entered onto paper either by the research participant or by the researcher. More direct data entry methods have emerged such as internet-mediated research using online questionnaires or by having participants enter data directly into a computer or a smartphone. When data is not entered directly into a computer device by the participant but rather by the research team from paper, Atkinson [32] and Barchard and Pace [33] recommend double data entry to improve accuracy.

There are many statistical software packages for quantitative data analysis. Two of the more common packages include:

- SPSS (Statistical Packages for the Social Sciences), now called IBM SPSS since the IBM purchase of SPSS Inc in 2009
- SAS (Statistical Analysis System) by SAS Institute Inc.

This author's experience is that SPSS is most often used by researchers in nursing and the behavioural sciences while SAS is more often used by epidemiologists and biostatistians who often deal with much larger datasets. Choosing which statistical analysis software to use can be straightforward if your institution only has a site license for one or the other. Who you will be interacting with on the research project may be another consideration (for instance if your thesis advisor uses a particular statistical package). Sometimes, for small datasets where the statistical analysis will not be complex, a spreadsheet program such as Microsoft Excel may suffice.

Mixed Methods

Mixed methods research is research where both quantitative and qualitative methods are used in a study. Although it has its detractors who think that qualitative and quantitative research is separate, mixed methods is gaining popularity in health science research. The U.S. Department of Health and Human Services has an excellent page on 'Best Practices for Mixed Methods Research in the Health Sciences' [14]. This initiative was led by John Creswell, whose excellent book on mixed methods research is now in its 3rd edition [16].

Collecting Data from the Patient Medical Record

Data collection from the patient medical record is often performed by nurses conducting research. Gregory and Radovinsky [34] outline the various strategies for reliable data collection from both paper and electronic patient records, including:

- The development and testing of a data collection tool
- Organization and structure of the data collection tool
- Detailed nature of the data to be collected
- The use of a coding manual guiding data collection
- The selection, training, and management of a research team of data abstractors
- Ensuring and reporting inter-rater reliability

The C-HOBIC project is a good example of a project intended to promote standardized extraction of data from medical records to track patient outcomes [35, 36]. C-HOBIC stands for the Canadian Health Outcomes for Better Information and Care.

Data Mining

Clinical, administrative, and demographic databases at the institutional, network, and governmental level continue to grow in number and scope. Hospitals and other healthcare organizations with integrated electronic health records have a significant research advantage. Consider the time it would take to review data elements in fifty patient charts in a hospital compared to accessing the same data from an electronic health record database. Data mining involves the semi-automatic exploration of large data sets, looking for meaning through patterns in the data.

The researcher's ability to data mine for research purposes is dependent on a number of factors, including accessibility of the data, the completeness of the data in the database and if more than one database is being mined, the compatibility of the data elements in the various databases. Doran et al. [37] used data mining of a college of nurses' database to determine if the demographics of the sample of nurses in their study matched the demographics of nurses in the province as a whole. Lee et al. [38] data mined a hospital incident reporting system and used logistic regression analysis to determine the main predictors of the most common form of pressure ulcer (sacral) in the hospital. These factors were hemoglobin, weight, sex, height, and [lack of] use of an assistive device/re-positioning sheet.

Data Visualization and Graphics

Data visualization is a way of looking at data, usually in some pictorial representation, in order to gain a better understanding of data and the relationships that might exist. Scatterplots are a common data visualization tool. The ease with which data can be visualized with modern computers is very helpful to researchers in exploring their data with the use of such visualization tools within software packages. When reporting research results, use of pictures and graphs can enhance the understanding of the study and study results. David McCandless has done a very interesting TED talk on data visualization. http://www.ted.com/talks/david_mccandless_the_beauty_of_data_visualization

Although data visualization is usually associated with the graphing of quantitative data, the reporting of qualitative data can be enhanced by the presentation of concept maps. A flowchart of the study design is also often presented in publications as well as in research ethics applications.

New and Emerging Research Ethics Concerns

Research Ethics Boards have to change their practices to accommodate new and emerging technology. This includes the security of electronic data, the electronic sharing of data between various organizations involved in a research study, and the use of audiotaping and video-taping of participants. Principles of research ethics are similar in different parts of the world, but they are often based on the same principles, such as the Declaration of Helsinki – Ethical Principles for Medical Research Involving Human Subjects. Contracts or data sharing agreements are often required between organizations if more than one organization is involved in a research study. Cloud computing also poses some risk to human participants and if there is a risk to the participant, this needs to be articulated in the consent form. Cloud computing has implications not only for patient privacy and security but also for data sharing agreements.

Knowledge Translation

Knowledge translation (KT) is the synthesis, dissemination and exchange of knowledge by researchers to the targeted knowledge users [39]. Many grant applications now require the researcher to include a KT/dissemination plan. The following is a diagram on the Canadian Institutes of Health Research (CIHR) depicting the knowledge to action cycle (Fig. 13.4).

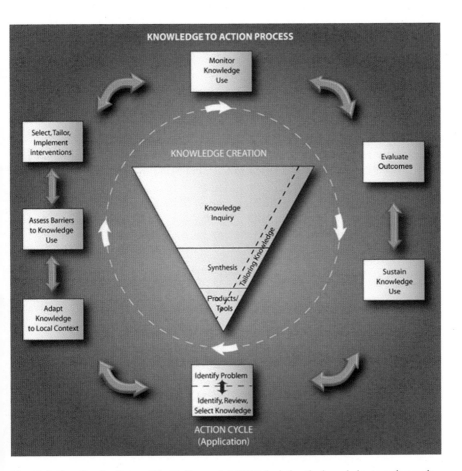

Fig. 13.4 Canadian Institutes of Health Research (CIHR) depicting the knowledge to action cycle

Patient education falls into the KT category and it is often nurses who are the knowledge translators for patients. Research related to health education for patients and harnessing technology to produce and deliver education is a lively area of research. For instance, Gupta et al. [40] report on an online collaborative process to design the content and format of an asthma self-management tool for patients. Participants in the study included pulmonologists, primary care physicians, certified asthma educators, and patients.

The Impact of Technology Innovations on Research

More than ever before, technology innovations are having an impact on how research is conducted and interpreted. For instance, Doran et al's 2012 [37] study of the use of point-of-care devices for accessing evidence by nurses found that PDA users used their devices more frequently than tablet users. However, this study was done before the introduction of more user-friendly tablets such as the iPad (launched in April 2010) and the more user-friendly and smaller iPad mini (launched November, 2012).

Birnbaum's [41] review of human research and data collection via the internet was written before the Facebook launch in February 2004. Since then, collection of data online and online recruitment of research participants has increased greatly. Chu and Snider [42] report on a study where participants were successfully recruited via a Facebook advertisement. Research principles that can threaten the validity of a study remain the same even though the tools for data collection and participant recruitment have changed. These principles include sampling bias, response bias, and experimenter bias. Methodological issues in internet-mediated research (e.g. do you get the same results if questionnaires are completed online versus on paper?) continue to be debated and explored [43].

Nursing Informatics Research

Nursing informatics research covers a variety of topics including studies on how technology affects situation awareness, critical thinking, and decision-making by nurses, how technology affects the nursing care process and tasks related to that process, effects of electronic nursing documentation on patient outcomes and patient safety, and technology usability. Below, two research areas, both related to understanding the work that nurses do and how technology impacts them are discussed.

The Nature of Nursing Work

Time-motion Studies

Time-motion studies were pioneered by Frank and Lillian Gilbreth in the early 1900s. They studied skilled performance in bricklaying, surgical procedures, and design for the handicapped. Frank Gilbreth was a student of Frederick Taylor, who developed the scientific study of work in order to improve efficiency. Taylor was interested in the management of work and workflow whereas the Gilbreths mainly focused on the efficiency of physical movement. The movie 'Cheaper by the Dozen' is based on the life stories of Frank and Lillian Gilbreth. A description of the origin of time-motion studies can be found in David Meister's book, 'The History of Human Factors and Ergonomics' [44].

Time-motion studies of nursing work is performed in order to understand where nurses are spending their time (direct patient care, documentation, etc.), and/or to re-design the way that nurses work prior to or in conjunction with technology implementations. There is active discussion in the literature about the best way to measure clinical work processes and workflow [45]. Time-motion studies may vary in methodology but, in general, involve continuous and independent observations of clinician's work. Hendrich et al. [46] performed a time-motion study in 36 hospitals, partly in order to collect baseline data for an EHR implementation. Other methods that are used to understand the nature of nursing work include work sampling and self-report methods [47].

Technology to Improve Nurses' Situation Awareness

Situation awareness (sometimes referred to as situational awareness) is a construct developed by Mica Endsley in the 1980s [48] to understand the human operator's cognition and performance in complex environments in order to design systems and equipment to improve it. Situation awareness (SA) is described by Endsley as an internalized mental model of the environment. Factors that affect SA include information from a variety of sources, technological and human. In a healthcare environment, on the technology side, this could include the electronic health record, patient whiteboards, infusion pumps, etc. On the human side, this could include interaction with team members, the patient and their family, etc. Situation awareness is arrived at by a synthesis of all this information by the human operator such as the nurse. There are three levels of situation awareness:

- Level 1 is perceiving the elements in the environment
- Level 2 is the comprehension of the current situation
- Level 3 is the projection of the future status

In a healthcare environment, an example of level 1 would be a nurse who has received report on their patient at the start of their shift, conducted a patient assessment, read the pertinent information in the patient's electronic health record, and taken the patient's vital signs. Integrating all this information into a mental model of the patient and their current problems and treatments, would be an example of level 2 situation awareness. Level 3 situation awareness would involve having a good understanding of current state but also being able to project what needs to be done to take care of the patient this shift and in the days coming.

Koch et al. [49] investigated whether or not an integrated ICU display would improve the situational awareness and task completion time of ICU nurses compared to the traditional display. They found that situation awareness accuracy was 85.3 % with the integrated display compared to 61.8 % with the traditional displays and that task completion times were nearly half with the integrated display.

Ashoori et al. [50] looked at the elements of team situation awareness in the birthing unit using a team cognitive work analysis approach. Parush et al. [51] used a communication framework to look at team situation awareness in the operating room and to propose a team situation awareness display.

A tragic example of lack of situation awareness and teamwork is the case of Emily Bromiley, a young mother who lost her life as a result of an elective surgery where a medical emergency combined with lack of situation awareness and poor teamwork led to her death [52].

Downloads

Available from extras.springer.com:

Educational Template (PDF 102 kb)
Educational Template (PPTX 116 kb)

Acknowledgements The author wishes to thank the Library Services staff at The Ottawa Hospital for their help in reviewing the literature search section, supplying the list of common databases, the steps in developing a search strategy, and the description of MeSH terms.

References

1. Hannah KJ, Ball MJ, Edwards MJA. Introduction to nursing informatics. 3rd ed. New York: Springer; 2006.
2. Polit DF, Beck TB. Nursing research: generating and assessing evidence for nursing practice. 9th ed. Philadelphia: Wolters Kluwer Health/Lippincott Williams & Wilkins; 2012.
3. Wink DM. Digital books. Nurse Educ. 2011;36(6):233–5.
4. Wink DM, Killingsworth EK. Optimizing use of library technology. Nurse Educ. 2011; 36(2):48–51.
5. Wink DM. Cloud computing. Nurse Educ. 2012;37(1):3–5.

6. Wink DM, Killingsworth EK. Beyond Google docs. Nurse Educ. 2012;37(2):45–7.
7. Wood MJ, Ross-Kerr JC. Basic steps in planning nursing research. 7th ed. Sudbury: Jones and Bartlett; 2011.
8. Urquhart C, Currell R, Grant MJ, Hardiker NR. Nursing record systems: effects on nursing practice and healthcare outcomes. Cochrane Database Syst Rev. 2009;(1):CD002099. doi: 10.1002/14651858.CD002099.pub2.
9. Using MeSH. National Center for Biotechnology Information, U S National Library of Medicine 2013. Available from URL: http://www.ncbi.nlm.nih.gov/mesh.
10. Davies B, Logan J. Reading research: a user-friendly guide for health professionals. 5th ed. Toronto: Elsevier; 2011.
11. Westlake C. Practical tips for literature synthesis. Clin Nurse Spec. 2012;26(5):244–9.
12. Denzin NK, Lincoln YS. The Sage handbook of qualitative research. 3rd ed. Thousand Oaks: Sage; 2005.
13. Shadish WR, Cook TD, Campbell DT. Experimental and quasi-experimental designs for generalized causal inference. Boston: Houghton Mifflin Company; 2002.
14. Creswell JW, Klassen AC, Plano Clark VL, Smith KC for the Office of Behavioral and Social Sciences Research. Best practices for mixed methods research in the health sciences. August 2011. National Institutes of Health, Bethesda, MD. Retrieved Jan 25 2012. http://obssr.od.nih.gov/mixed_methods_research.
15. Duff, D. Family concerns and responses following a severe traumatic brain injury: a grounded theory study: Codman Award paper. Axone. 2002; 24(2):14–22.
16. Creswell JW. Research design: qualitative, quantitative, and mixed methods approaches. 3rd ed. Thousand Oaks: Sage; 2008.
17. MacLean LM, Meyer M, Estable A. Improving accuracy of transcripts in qualitative research. Qual Health Res. 2004;14:113–23.
18. Scott SD, Sharpe H, O'Leary K, Dehaeck U, Hindmarsh K, Moore JG, et al. Court reporters: a viable solution for the challenges of focus group data collection? Qual Health Res. 2009;19(1):140–6.
19. Varpio LP, Kuziemsky CP, MacDonald CM, King WJM. The helpful or hindering effects of in-hospital patient monitor alarms on nurses: a qualitative analysis. Comput Inform Nurs. 2012;30(4):210–7.
20. Lawton R, Carruthers S, Gardner P, Wright J, McEachan RR. Identifying the latent failures underpinning medication administration errors: an exploratory study. Health Serv Res. 2012; 47(4):1437–59.
21. Braun V, Clarke V. Using thematic analysis in psychology. Qual Res Psychol. 2006;3(2):77–101.
22. Bergin M. NVivo 8 and consistency in data analysis: reflecting on the use of a qualitative data analysis program. Nurse Res. 2011;18(3):6–12.
23. Veo PMRN-B. Concept mapping for applying theory to nursing practice. J Nurses Staff Dev. 2010;26(1):17–22.
24. Hunter Revell SMP. Concept maps and nursing theory: a pedagogical approach. Nurse Educ. 2012;37(3):131–5.
25. Maneval RE, Filburn MJ, Deringer SO, Lum GD. Concept mapping. Does it improve critical thinking ability in practical nursing students? Nurs Educ Perspect. 2011;32(4):229–33.
26. Huang YC, Chen HH, Yeh ML, Chung YC. Case studies combined with or without concept maps improve critical thinking in hospital-based nurses: A randomized-controlled trial. Int J Nurs Stud. 2012;49(6):747–54.
27. Atay S, Karabacak U. Care plans using concept maps and their effects on the critical thinking dispositions of nursing students. Int J Nurs Pract. 2012;18(3):233–9.
28. Duncan I, Yarwood-Ross L, Haigh C. YouTube as a source of clinical skills education. Nurse Educ Today. 2013;33(12):1576–80.
29. Topps D, Helmer J, Ellaway R. YouTube as a platform for publishing clinical skills training videos. Acad Med. 2013;88(2):192–7.
30. Butler DP, Perry F, Shah Z, Leon-Villapalos J. The quality of video information on burn first aid available on YouTube. Burns. 2013;39:856–9.

31. Bellomo R, Ackerman M, Bailey M, Beale R, Clancy G, Danesh V, et al. A controlled trial of electronic automated advisory vital signs monitoring in general hospital wards. Crit Care Med. 2012;40(8):2349–61.
32. Atkinson I. Accuracy of data transfer: double data entry and estimating levels of error. J Clin Nurs. 2012;21(19–20):2730–5.
33. Barchard KA, Pace LA. Preventing human error: the impact of data entry methods on data accuracy and statistical results. Comput Hum Behav. 2011;27(5):1834–9.
34. Gregory KE, Radovinsky L. Research strategies that result in optimal data collection from the patient medical record. Appl Nurs Res. 2012;25(2):108–16.
35. Hannah K, White PA. C-HOBIC: standardized clinical outcomes to support evidence-informed nursing care. Nurs Leadersh (Tor Ont). 2012;25(1):43–6.
36. Jeffs L, Wilson G, Ferris E, Cardiff B, Ng S, Lanceta M, et al. Exploring nurses' perceptions of collecting and using HOBIC measures to guide clinical practice and improve care. Nurs Leadersh (Tor Ont). 2012;25(1):14–28.
37. Doran D, Haynes BR, Estabrooks CA, Kushniruk A, Dubrowski A, Bajnok I, et al. The role of organizational context and individual nurse characteristics in explaining variation in use of information technologies in evidence based practice. Implement Sci. 2012;7:122.
38. Lee TT, Lin KC, Mills ME, Kuo YH. Factors related to the prevention and management of pressure ulcers. Comput Inform Nurs. 2012;30(9):489–95.
39. Canadian Institutes of Health Research. Knowledge translation and commercialization. Available from http://www.cihr-irsc.gc.ca/e/29418.html.
40. Gupta S, Wan FT, Newton D, Bhattacharyya OK, Chignell MH, Straus SE. WikiBuild: a new online collaboration process for multistakeholder tool development and consensus building. J Med Internet Res. 2011;13(4):e108.
41. Birnbaum MH. Human research and data collection via the internet. Annu Rev Psychol. 2004;55:803–32.
42. Chu JL, Snider CE. Use of a social networking web site for recruiting Canadian youth for medical research. J Adolesc Health. 2013;52(6):792–4.
43. Whitehead L. Methodological issues in Internet-mediated research: a randomized comparison of internet versus mailed questionnaires. J Med Internet Res. 2011;13(4):e109.
44. Meister D. The history of human factors and ergonomics. Mahwah: Lawrence Erlbaum; 1999.
45. Zheng K, Guo MH, Hanauer DA. Using the time and motion method to study clinical work processes and workflow: methodological inconsistencies and a call for standardized research. J Am Med Inform Assoc. 2011;18(5):704–10.
46. Hendrich A, Chow MP, Skierczynski BA, Lu Z. A 36-hospital time and motion study: how do medical-surgical nurses spend their time? Perm J. 2008;12(3):25–34.
47. Ampt A, Westbrook J, Creswick N, Mallock N. A comparison of self-reported and observational work sampling techniques for measuring time in nursing tasks. J Health Serv Res Policy. 2007;12(1):18–24.
48. Endsley M. Design and evaluation for situation awareness enhancement. Thousand OaKs: Sage; 1988. p. 97–101.
49. Koch SH, Weir C, Westenskow D, Gondan M, Agutter J, Haar M, et al. Evaluation of the effect of information integration in displays for ICU nurses on situation awareness and task completion time: a prospective randomized controlled study. Int J Med Inform. 2013;82(8):665–75.
50. Ashoori M, Burns C, Momtahan K, d'Entremont B. Control task analysis in action: collaboration in the operating room. Thousand Oaks: Sage; 2011. p. 272–6.
51. Parush A, Kramer C, Foster-Hunt T, Momtahan K, Hunter A, Sohmer B. Communication and team situation awareness in the OR: implications for augmentative information display. J Biomed Inform. 2011;44(3):477–85.
52. Bromiley M, Mitchell L. Would you speak up if the consultant got it wrong? …and would you listen if someone said you'd got it wrong? J Perioper Pract. 2009;19(10):326–9.

Chapter 14
Case Studies Introduction: Transformational Research

Pamela Hussey and Fintan Sheerin

Abstract Chapter 14 reports on nursing informatics in relation to change management. It introduces the proceeding chapters which are presented as case studies on the various perspectives and differing approaches from authors working in the sphere of nursing informatics. The cross cutting theme evident in the case studies is that health care systems and nursing informatics are in various stages of transition. Authors report within the case studies how ICT is shaping nursing while highlighting the importance of implementing in parallel effective change management strategies to maximize effectiveness. Chapter 14 offers a summary overview of change management principles and how they can be applied in practice. It also includes a summary report on the ACENDIO Conference on eHealth and Nursing Innovations for the Future.

Keywords Change management • Nursing informatics • Health care delivery • International strategic planning

Key Concepts

Change Management
Nursing Informatics
Health Care Delivery
International Strategic Planning

The online version of this chapter (doi:10.1007/978-1-4471-2999-8_14) contains supplementary material, which is available to authorized users.

P. Hussey, RN, RCN, MEd, MSc, PhD (✉)
School of Nursing and Human Sciences, Dublin City University, Dublin, Ireland
e-mail: pamela.hussey@dcu.ie

F. Sheerin, BNS, MA, PhD, RNID, FEANS
School of Nursing and Midwifery, Trinity College Dublin, Dublin, Ireland

© Springer-Verlag London 2015
K.J. Hannah et al. (eds.), *Introduction to Nursing Informatics*,
Health Informatics, DOI 10.1007/978-1-4471-2999-8_14

Introduction

Nursing Informatics, health and healthcare are globally in various stages of transition and change. IMIA-NI the International Medical Informatics Association Special Interest Groups Strategic Plan 2007–2015 calls on the *nursing informatics community to encourage global knowledge leaders to come together to effectively and efficiently create, assemble, integrate, synthesise or assimilate intellectual knowledge that is required worldwide to advance nursing/health informatics in its role of improving health and healthcare* [1, p. 3]. Key objectives identified for 2015 include exploration of the scope of nursing informatics, and its development across the continuum of health. Promotion of linkages by the establishment of collaborative activities and the development/publishing of guidelines tools and courses relating to nursing informatics which are likely to maximise visibility are particularly important [1, p. 6]. Such activities offer the potential to facilitate a smooth transition process that supports sustainable change. Managing this transition presents nursing with a number of challenges which requires careful change management implementation practices. In the proceeding chapters, we present case studies which offer insight on how such activities are in process within practice, additionally Dr Fintan Sheerin offers a summary overview of the 2013 ACENDIO [2] conference (Association of European Nursing Diagnosis Interventions and Outcomes organisation) and the existing papers contributed by the international informatics community on nursing language and terminology. The case studies presented Chaps. 15, 16, 17, 18 and 19 depict the current state of practice and present examples of nurses actively seeking clarity while offering solutions on how ambiguous processes relating to eHealth can be delivered. This approach ensures that opportunities which can deliver better patient care are not wasted but optimised. As a preamble to the cases presented in the proceeding chapters, a short introduction on change management theory follows. The case studies are also introduced as follows.

In Chap. 15, **Case Study 1: Nursing Informatics and eHealth in Australia** is written by Joanne Foster who offers a summary of the eHealth and Nursing Informatics landscape in Australia. In this chapter, the recently launched PCEHR [3] is introduced and key challenges for nursing informatics in Australia are discussed. A call for nursing informatics to be integrated into all nursing undergraduate and postgraduate programmes in Australia is proposed, and a stronger focus on taking control of the nursing role in future health care is suggested. Strategies to achieve greater control and actively engage with eHealth developments include participating in active debate on policy decisions and management of eHealth developments.

Chapter 16, **Case Study 2,** presents the TIGER Virtual Learning Environment (VLE) [4] introduced by Sally Schlak. The TIGER Initiative initially introduced in this edition in Chap. 1 is an international collaboration entitled Technology Informatics Guiding Educational Reform. The recently launched virtual learning environment is described in this case study and an associated WebEx is also provided offering a tour of key VLE screens and functionality. For ease of reading, this chapter also includes key screen shots from the TIGER VLE resource.

In Chap. 17 **Case Study 3,** Beverley Thomas provides a summary overview of past and current ICT strategy in Wales. Describing how the nursing community in Wales is actively translating policy agendas into practice, this case study offers a comprehensive timeline with insight on how the change management and transition process has evolved in the past and is currently being managed in Wales. Examples of innovations completed in Wales include collaborative workshops with tactical outputs such as an agreed set of guiding principles for community nurses and creation of a new role within Wales of clinical nursing informaticist.

The last case study in Chap. 18, **Case Study 4,** is provided by Polun Chang, Shaio-Jyue Lu, Ming-Chuan and Jessie Kuo who report on the uptake and use of mobile technologies in Taiwan. The authors present two examples, firstly a chemotherapy medication administration solution which includes evidence-based guidelines and documentation process administration; the second example focuses on the deployment of a mobile device within an Intensive Care Unit for nursing to assess and document pressure sore management.

As a preamble to the proceeding chapters, a summary report from the 2013 ACENDIO Conference is also included at the end of this chapter, demonstrating the active contribution the nursing community is making to the eHealth policy debate.

Change Management and Transition

Recent reports indicate that health care professionals are increasingly dissatisfied with Electronic Health Records (EHR) implemented in healthcare, and particularly on the impact that the transition to electronic records is having on their routine working practices. Presented in March 2013 at the Health Information and Management Systems Society (HIMSS), the American EHR data collection report completed on over 4,239 physicians, noted a 12 % decrease in EHR user satisfaction from 2010 to 2012, with 39 % of clinicians not recommending their EHR to a colleague. Specifically they reported on issues with impact on productivity as the primary reason [5].

So why is this the case? Change management theory suggests that altering practice involves two key concepts, firstly *change processes* and secondly *transition processes* [6]. Both of these concepts can be distinguished as follows; change can be described as observable things that happen or are done differently usually involving alteration of structural processes on work practice routines. On the other hand, transition processes relate more to the emotional aspects around what people feel, experience, or consider important in their practice. Early recognition that both concepts are required for successful implementation of national eHealth programs is important [7].

The costs of national programmes relating to ICT are prohibitive, and underestimating the importance of an effective change management program can be a costly business. Recent investment in the United States on health transition and change management offers one example of how on a global scale, governments are progressively recognizing change management programs as a priority. The Health Information Technology for Economic and Clinical Health (HITECH) Act has allocated 27 billion dollars for meaningful use of electronic health records by physicians and hospitals between 2011 and 2015 [8]. In the past decade, early adopters such as United Kingdom have invested significant funds in their national programmes for IT. In England between 2003 and 2010, the National program for IT (NPfIT) was estimated to cost 20.6 Billion dollars and its overall success was declared to be limited throughout the literature [9, 10]. In light of the perception of limited value for investment, healthcare leaders must ask what models of change theory exist and what guiding principles of change management practice can be used within the nursing informatics community? The literature on this topic is extensive; here we offer a summary of some of the concepts and theories relating to the topic.

Change management principles relating to electronic health records and information technology implementation have been well documented over the years [11, 12]. Recent publications emphasise the importance of establishing both frameworks and models to facilitate sharing and collaborating on the transition process in order to ensure a smooth translation from paper based records to electronic records is achieved. Bridging the gap between *what we know* and *what we do* in order to maximise the translation of evidence into practice requires effective communication [13, p. 20]. The importance and complexity of communication within the change management/transition process is well illustrated in the following quote:

> eHealth program is best conceptualised not as a blue print and implementation plan for a state of the art technical system but as a series of overlapping, conflicting, and mutually misunderstood language games that combine to produce a situation of ambiguity, paradox, incompleteness and confusion. [10, p. 534].

Identifying the need for change with practitioners and devising strong leadership with clear aims and objectives are critical components of the change management process [7]. Other key requisites for change realisation include creating and communicating a vision [14, 15]. From the informatics perspective, it is important to consider key roles and linkages to identified expertise within organisations for specific change innovations to succeed. Change management programmes need to be rooted in practitioner's wisdom [10, p. 7]. Information systems implementation in healthcare practice (as opposed to other change implementations in healthcare practice) is recognised as particularly difficult and there is much written on the topic [16–19]. Advancing eHealth agendas therefore requires change management programmes, not only to succeed in single organisations structures, but also increasingly to cross institutional boundaries, thus adding an additional layer of complexity to an already tense and challenging process [20, 21]. The consequences of such innovations affect health care professionals' working practices in a number of ways. For example, healthcare professionals may need to invest significant effort on acquiring new skills on security measures, training on routine documenting and referral practices while concurrently managing patient care to avoid adverse outcomes. Clarity on realisable benefits or incentives, not just for the organisation but for the individual practitioners involved, by identifying why they should make such a time investment needs to clearly articulated [12].

For those individuals most impacted upon by the change in their working practice, it is important that they feel comfortable using new information systems and decide that the time investment is a worthwhile and worthy venture [6]. Generally, the nursing community are open to embracing change, established nurse practice development units are often seen for this reason as a vehicle for change management programmes within health care institutions [22]. Previous individual experiences, whether negative or positive, may have a direct influence on the degree of future engagement [7].

The initial approach from the outset of how organisations approach and resource change programmes is a critical factor. Careful planning on whether to use a top down, bottom up or a combined approach to deployment are all important aspects for consideration. Key adopted and adapted tools/models for planning change include the SMART model, as devised by Doran in the 1980s [23]. The acronym SMART identifies the various components for setting realistic targets in project planning. Doran advocates that core objectives need to be Specific, Measurable, Achievable, Realistic, and Time Specific. In the health and social science domain, top down approaches with early focused collaboration and engagement with health care professionals is increasingly seen as the preferred option. Reflection on cycles of existing and past implementation programmes to inform the next stages of development specifically on large scale implementations is increasingly noted as an informative and cost effective exercise [10]. Pawson maintains that due consideration of core components and structures within the health care setting are useful to identify the complex footprints of programme implementation programmes. Often labelled as the context mechanism and outcomes of the planned or existing implementation programme they can be summarised by asking a set of questions which broadly summarise such activities as *what is it about this programme that works for whom, in what circumstances, in what respects, in which duration, and why?* [16, p. 15].

Other early business models that are used in the informatics domain and which have been found effective in planning change management processes include benefit realisation management by Joseph Peppard et al. [12]. As is the case with other change management models, this tool also advocates early engagement of staff impacted upon by any change programme. Benefit Management Analysis stresses the need for comprehensive stakeholder consultation, and identification of the benefits and disbenefits of each of the core stakeholder groups identified.

The role of culture and collective team engagement in promoting innovation and supporting behavioural change is consistently referenced in the literature and recent publications on studies exploring nurses' uptake and use of ICT in Canada is one such example [24]. One theory as to why team members individually respond to change differently at various times over the lifecycle of a project can be explained by classifying individuals by both behaviour and type. Rodger classified individuals in teams into different groups who he considered to behave differently over time. He maintained that groups who engage with change programmes broadly fall into categories; Innovators, Early Adopters, and Laggards, thus informing the basis of his theory *Rodgers Diffusion Theory* [25]. Rodgers described Laggards as those individuals who only choose to engage in change management innovations toward the end of any change process. Therefore advocating changing management facilitators that early identification of staff into group formations can be a worthy exercise in successfully managing the change environment. The majority of individuals Rodgers suggests have a tendency to be classified into Early or Late Majority Adopters, with only a small number of the population classified as Innovators. It is however the innovators who are seen as key champions of change within organisational group theory. A similar notion is also presented by Gladwell in his bestselling book on change management *The Tipping Point*. Three agents of change are presented by Gladwell: (1) The Law of the Few, (2) The Stickiness Factor and (3) The Power of Context. Gladwell advocates the 80/20 rule when he considers organisational theory which suggests that 80 % of work is done by 20 % of the participants in innovations. He also classifies individuals into group types although he offers different titles to the group types such as Connectors and Mavens [19, 25, 26].

Staying with organisational group theory, additional popular terms used within the literature on change management includes the term *Readiness for Change*. Shute et al. [22] identifies and offers a succinct summary of change management theory relevant to nursing underpinned by a study completed in 2008 by Weiner et al. [27], which describes over 40 different instruments relating to readiness for change [22].

This short introductory section on change management will conclude with a perhaps the most widely acknowledged change theorist Karl Lewin. Known as the father of action research who in 1940s introduced the notion of force field analysis. Lewin describes how certain forces affect change, Lewin's theories have been extensively adopted, adapted and modified in change management programmes over a number of years including the work by Rodgers in 2003 [18, 25, 28] Briefly Lewin's theory involves three key elements:

1. Unfreezing existing processes when change is needed
2. Moving when change is initiated
3. Refreezing when equilibrium has been established.

In summary, this section offers a brief overview of some of the critical factors that can influence change management within the domain of nursing informatics. The topic is a vast one to explore and this section has offered only a brief introduction to the topic from an informatics perspective.

European Perspectives Summary Reports on ACENDIO

ACENDIO 2013. eHealth and Nursing: Innovating for the Future

The Association for Common European Nursing Diagnoses, Interventions and Outcomes (ACENDIO) held its 9th Biennial European Conference in the Radisson Blu Royal Hotel, Dublin from 22 to 23 March 2013. The association, which has been in existence since 1995, promotes the use standardised languages to support nurses and midwives to communicate the contribution that they make to health care. This allows us to describe nursing – its practice, its focus and its expert decisions – so that this contribution can be properly quantified, resourced and researched, ensuring quality health care for patients. In recent years, ACENDIO has been exploring the importance of eHealth in the changing health care environment. This has included the development of a coherent nursing input to the European eHealth Strategy, work which was undertaken at a working group in Dublin in 2012. The ACENDIO conference was an opportunity for Irish nurses to come together in the company of 130 international experts from more than 20 countries. The conference was opened by Dr. Michael Shannon, Chief Nursing Executive, Health Service Executive and Ms. Elizabeth Adams, Head of Professional Development, Irish Nurses and Midwives Organisation who set a national and European National Nurses Association perspective on informatics and eHealth. Keynote speakers included Prof. Anne-Marie Rafferty from Kings College London, Prof. Jane Grimson of the Irish Healthcare Informatics and Quality Authority, Dr. Liam MacGabhann of Dublin City University and Prof. Bonnie Westra from University of Minnesota.

While focused on eHealth, the 45 parallel papers, 39 posters and 6 workshops addressed many topics related to nursing informatics including: nursing diagnoses, interventions and outcomes; standardisation of nursing language; datasets and terminologies; the electronic patient record; patient safety and population health; self-care in the community; nursing decision-making and decision support. Work was progressed on two of ACENDIO's most exciting projects. The first of these is the development of a nursing contribution to the European eHealth Strategy. This work was commenced at the 2011 ACENDIO conference, in Madeira, which led to the formation of an eHealth Working Group. The work was progressed through a 'bottom-up' process involving sequential online surveys and Working Group meetings in Dublin, Reykjavik and Turin. This project is ongoing and the draft report will be made available via the ACENDIO website. The second initiative, which was discussed over the past 2 years, is the European Observatory on Nursing Standards. This project is being developed through a partnership between ACENDIO and the Spanish nursing informatics group, AENTDE, and is in an advanced planning stage. Healthcare informatics is evolving at an accelerated rate and often nurses and midwives are not central to the key decisions that will impact on their practice and, consequently, on their patients. This is a subject which is relevant to all areas of nursing and it is imperative that nurses become actively involved in its development.

Downloads

Available from extras.springer.com:

Educational Template (PDF 7160 kb)
Educational Template (PPTX 3625 kb)

References

1. International Medical Informatics Association Nursing Informatics Special Interest Group IMIA NI Strategic Plan Toward IMIA-NI −2015. Geneva; 2007.
2. ACENDIO Association of European Nursing Diagnosis Interventions and Outcomes. Available from: http://www.acendio.net/. Accessed 2 July 2013.
3. Australian Government. Bringing the PCEHR to Life. 2011. Available at: http://www.youtube.com/watch?v=3IOoUMwSGMI. Accessed 2 July 2013.
4. Tiger website. Available from: http://www.thetigerinitiative.org. Accessed 24 Apr 2013.
5. Brookstone A EHR dissatisfaction diminishing American EHR blog. Available from: http://www.americanehr.com/blog/2013/03/himss13-ehr-satisfaction-diminishing/. Accessed 7 July 2013.
6. McLean C. Change and transition: what is the difference? Br J Sch Nurs. 2011;6(2):78–81.
7. Hewitt-Taylor J. Planning successful change incorporating processes and people. Nurs Stand [serial on the Internet]. 2013 May 22 [cited 2013 July 2];27(38):35–40. Available from: CINAHL Plus with Full Text.
8. Blumenthal D, Tavenner M. The "meaningful use" regulation for electronic health records. N Engl J Med. 2010;363(6):501–4.
9. National Audit Office. The national programme for IT in the NHS: an update on the delivery of detailed record systems. London:HMSO; 2011
10. Greenhalgh T, Russell J, Ashcroft RE, Parsons W. Why national eHealth programs need dead philosophers: wittgensteinian reflections on Policymakers' reluctance to learn. Millbank Q. 2011;89(4):533–63.
11. Coiera E. Putting the technical back into socio-technical systems research. Int J Med Inform. 2007;76 Suppl 1:S98–103.
12. Peppard J, Ward JM, Daniel E. Managing the realisation of business benefits from IT investments. MIS Q Exec. 2007;6:1–11.
13. Thomson L, Schneider J, Wright N. Developing communities of practice to support the implementation of research into clinical practice. Leadersh Health Serv. 2013;26(1):20–33.
14. Kotter J. Leading change: why transformation efforts fail. Harvard Business Review 1995. Available from: http://lighthouseconsultants.co.uk/wp-content/uploads/2010/08/Kotter-Leading-Change-Why-transformation-efforts-fail.pdf. Accessed 7 July 2013.
15. Alonso I. Navigating triage to meet targets for waiting times. Emerg Nurse [serial on the Internet]. 2013, June [cited 2013 July 2];21(3):20–26. Available from: CINAHL Plus with Full Text.
16. Pawson R. The science of evaluation a realist manifesto. London: Sage; 2013.
17. Greenhalgh T, Potts HW, Wong G, Bark P, Swinglehurst D. Tensions and paradoxes in electronic patient record research: a systematic literature review using the meta-narrative method. Milbank Q. 2009;87(4):729–88.
18. Mitchell G. Selecting the best theory to implement planned change. Nurs Manag UK [serial on the Internet]. 2013 Apr [cited 2013 July 2];20(1):32–37. Available from: CINAHL Plus with Full Text.
19. Gladwell M. The tipping point how little things can make a big difference. Boston: Little Brown; 2000.
20. Milne P, Coyne A, Pilgrim D. Improving the quality of primary care. Qual Prim Care [serial on the Internet]. 2012 Nov [cited 2013 July 2];20(6):435–442. Available from: CINAHL Plus with Full Text.
21. Golden R, Shier G. What does 'care transitions' really mean? Generations [serial on the Internet]. 2012 Dec [cited 2013 July 2];36(4):6–12. Available from: CINAHL Plus with Full Text.
22. Shute R, Harrison K, Forsyth K, Melton J, Thompson S, Fear C. Supporting implementation of health service change. Br J Healthc Manag [serial on the Internet]. 2012 Dec [cited 2013 July 2];18(12):638–643. Available from: CINAHL Plus with Full Text.

23. Doran GT. There's a SMART way to write management's goals and objectives. Manage Rev. 1981;70(11):35–6.
24. Doran D, Haynes BR, Estabrooks CA, Kushniruk A, Dubrowski A, Bajnok I, Hall LM, Mingyang L, Carryer J, Jedras D, Bai YQ. The role of organisational context and individual characteristics in explaining variation in use of information technologies in evidence based practice. Implement Sci. 2012;7:122.
25. Rogers EM. Diffusion of innovations. 4th ed. New York: Free Press; 1995.
26. Hall GE, Hord SM. Implementing change: patterns, principles and potholes. 3rd ed. London: Pearson; 2011.
27. Weiner BJ, Amick H, Shoou-Yih DL. Conceptualisation and measurement of organisational readiness for change. A review of the literature in health services research and other fields. Med Care Res Rev. 2008;64(4):379–436.
28. Lewin K. Field theory in social science. London: Tavistock Publications; 1951.

Chapter 15
Case Study 1: Nursing Informatics and eHealth in Australia

Joanne Foster

Abstract There are currently many changes happening in nursing and healthcare in Australia. Healthcare reform has been high on the national government agenda and has created many changes in healthcare including eHealth. Healthcare information technologies and informatics are providing many challenges and excitement for the future of healthcare in Australia. The challenge for professional nursing organisations and nursing leaders of Australia is to be proactive in developments and initiatives for nursing to remain visible and viable in health care systems to safeguard the profession for the future as health care reform is implemented.

Keywords Nursing informatics • eHealth • Australia • Case study • Health Workforce Reform

Key Concepts

Healthcare reform
Australian Healthcare System
Australian Personally Controlled Electronic Health Record (PCEHR)
Health Workforce Reform
Nursing informatics education
Nursing informatics challenges

Introduction

There are currently many changes happening in nursing and healthcare in Australia. Healthcare reform has been high on the national government agenda and has created many changes in healthcare including eHealth. This chapter will highlight some of these changes from a national and nursing focus, reflecting key initiatives and priorities, workforce capacity and future directions for nursing and healthcare in Australia.

J. Foster, RN, DipAppSc-NsgEdn, BN, GradDipClEdn, MEdnTech
School of Nursing, Queensland University of Technology, Kelvin Grove, QLD, Australia
e-mail: j.foster@qut.edu.au

© Springer-Verlag London 2015
K.J. Hannah et al. (eds.), *Introduction to Nursing Informatics*,
Health Informatics, DOI 10.1007/978-1-4471-2999-8_15

National Developments

Informatics and Australian Health Care System

All States and Territories in Australia have their own governments that are under the auspices of the Australian government, which has led to many disparate systems over the years. The Australian government has introduced healthcare reform and major funding to develop and implement national eHealth projects over the past 3–5 years in particular to address these inefficiencies. The development of the Personally Controlled Electronic Health Record (PCEHR) [1] has been the focus over the last 3 years as a major first step in involving the health consumer and professionals in managing health data and information for improved health care outcomes. Even though this has mainly had a medical and chronic illness focus during the implementation the outcome has benefits for all health professionals. The project for a national broadband network is also part of the infrastructure to enable all Australians to access health information 'anytime – anywhere' and provide effective and safe health care to all. The overarching national plan for using health data and information more efficiently and effectively for improved health care for all Australians is good however, it takes all health professionals, politicians, vendors and consumers to work together to achieve a high level health outcome for all involved.

Australian nurses need to be involved in all these developments to ensure that relevant nursing data is collected for expert nursing practice in primary, secondary and tertiary levels of health care. Currently there is limited input by nurses into any developments in this country and many systems are not end user friendly which promotes the negativity towards the use of health information technologies in practice. Nurses are the only health professionals with patients 24 h a day and collect the majority of health data but have little input into developments. It is logical therefore to suggest that systems will not work if nurses are not included. Is this going to change? Not from what has been and is occurring nationally with developments in Australia in this area.

There are many individual Health Informatics (HI) and Nursing Informatics (NI) projects that are undertaken in specific clinical areas but many of these are either not shared or not taken up by others. This can be because of jurisdictional boundaries and requirements, copyright or IP issues. This is another issue of how do we deal with this? This adds another layer of complexity that needs to be included in attempting to provide solutions.

Key Organizations in Informatics in Australia?

Australian Government: Department of Health and Aging (DOHA) [2]

The Department of Health and Ageing has responsibility of "better health and active ageing for all Australians" of which eHealth is one of the major programs within current health reform. It is the department that controls all of health care for Australia and all States and Territories report to this department.

Australian Government: National eHealth Transition Authority (NeHTA) [3]

NeHTA was established by the Australian, State and Territory governments to develop better ways of electronically collecting and securely exchanging health information. They have been responsible for development of the infrastructure of the PCEHR and other eHealth initiatives and is a major player in Australian informatics.

Australian Government: Department of Human Services (DHS) [4]

The Department of Human Services is responsible for the development of service delivery policy and provides access to social, health and other payments and services. Medicare [5] is one area of this department which looks after the health of Australians through the efficient delivery of programs such as the Pharmaceutical Benefits Scheme, the Australian Childhood Immunisation Register and the Australian Organ Donor Register. It also manages the Individual Health Identifier Service, which is central to eHealth.

Australian Government: Health Workforce Australia (HWA) [6]

HWA delivers change collaboration and innovation to build a sustainable health workforce that meets the healthcare needs of all Australians and is an initiative of the Australian Government. Australian health informatics workforce issues are part of the work of the HWA.

Australasian College of Health Informatics (ACHI) [7]

ACHI is the professional body for Health Informatics in the Asia-Pacific Region. The credentialed Fellows and Members of the College are national and international experts, thought leaders and trusted advisers in Health Informatics. ACHI sets standards for education and professional practice in Health Informatics, supports initiatives, facilitates collaboration and mentors the community.

Health Informatics Society of Australia (HISA) [8]

HISA is a not-for-profit membership organisation for health informaticians and those with an interest in health informatics. HISA members are leaders in the field and are actively involved in national and international leadership positions in e-health and health informatics.

Nursing Informatics Australia (NIA) [9]

Nursing Informatics Australia (NIA) is the pre-eminent group of nursing informaticians in Australia. This HISA Special Interest Group (SIG) is the reference point to learn about the developments in Nursing Informatics both nationally and internationally. NIA aims to promote nursing informatics priorities such as appropriate language, education and ongoing research and to engender nursing to embrace information and communication technologies, and establish strong foundations for taking these developments forward.

Health Reform

Australia's healthcare system is among the best in the world. However, an ageing population, increasing rates of chronic and preventable disease, new technological advances, changes to consumer health demands, increasing use of social media in health, and continuing rising health care costs have all placed huge demands on the current systems. Therefore critical solutions need to be introduced by the federal and state governments to take on these challenges [10].

The overarching solution was for national health reform, which resulted in the National Health Reform Agreement being negotiated in late 2011 between the federal and state governments to deliver better healthcare for all Australians and to secure a sustainable national health system for the future. The major reforms included in the Agreement included organisation, funding and delivery of health and aged care [10, 11]. These reforms aim to deliver better access to services, improved local accountability and transparency, greater responsiveness to local communities and provide a stronger financial basis for our health system into the future [12].

eHealth Reform and the Electronic Health Record

eHealth reform has been conducted in Australia in a very fragmented and uncoordinated way for many years. This lack of coordination came to national prominence in the late 2000s with calls to ensure the provision of a coordinated, accountable, affordable, and sustainable twenty-first century system providing quality and safety at the core to enhance healthcare delivery for all [13, 14].

Nationally the first step was to develop and implement the Personally Controlled Electronic Health Record (PCEHR) System (Fig. 15.1) [15]. The PCEHR System enables secure sharing of health information between individual's healthcare providers, while enabling the individual to control who can access their PCEHR (Fig. 15.2) [13, 14]. The PCEHR was launched nationally on July 1 2012. The

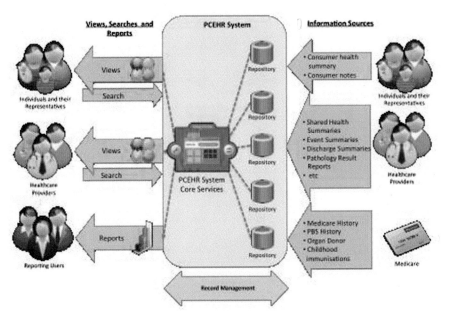

Fig. 15.1 The personally controlled electronic health record (PCEHR) system [15]

PCEHR is an ongoing developing dynamic system with increasing services and functionality being added over time. This also aligns with the government's commitment to self-management of health – as the PCEHR provides an electronic solution for individuals to control their health information. Australia has taken an "opt-in" approach to the PCEHR – meaning that individuals need to actively subscribe to this service. Healthcare organisations can register to participate in the PCEHR record system and authorise doctors, nurses and other appropriate users within their organisation to view patient records through the secure online provider portal [16].

The core components of the PCEHR are centred around health and event summaries as can be seen in Fig. 15.3 [17]. These particular areas were seen to be the most important aspects to include in the initial version of the PCEHR with the focus on specific groups in the community such as aged care and chronic illness. The system has been developed to enable functionalities to be added as they are developed. The PCEHR is not a replacement for organisational clinical records and the clinical component contains copies, not originals and the "source of truth" remains where it is today – in local clinical records.

Consumers and health professionals have access to a Learning Portal (Fig. 15.4) [17] which covers the major aspects of the PCEHR such as why it is needed, how to access and how to use it. There are a number of modules which are easily accessible and easy to use from the website and as this is a national development there are no variations between Australian states and territories. Currently only Medical Practitioners, Registered Nurses and Aboriginal Health workers are the authorised

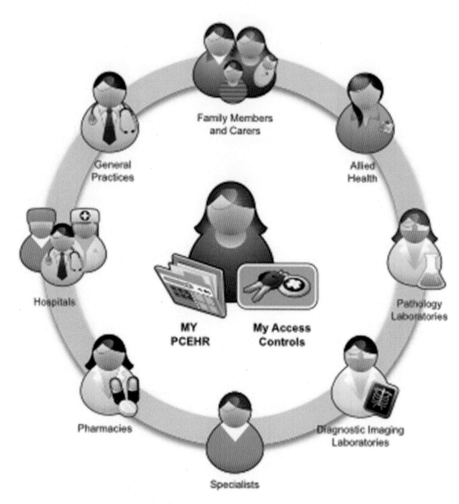

Fig. 15.2 The PCEHR concept [14]

health professionals who can upload and commence the original shared health summary in the PCEHR. Every Australian can register a PCEHR but it is only after they consent to having the PCEHR used can the above mentioned health professionals upload the health summary. Event summaries can be added by any registered health professional following the initialisation of the PCEHR and with the individuals consent. Individuals have control of the PCEHR and access to the majority of information and who can access it. They also have the ability to hide specific health information of a personal nature that they do not want shared.

As the PCEHR is a health record and not a medical or clinical record has resulted in some confusion but hopefully this will resolve over time as everyone becomes more confident and comfortable using the system. There is some conjecture that eventually the PCEHR will become the only electronic health record in the future in

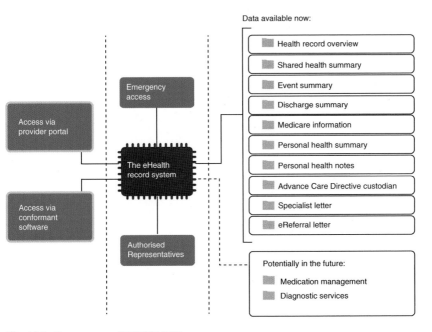

Fig. 15.3 Components of PCEHR [17]

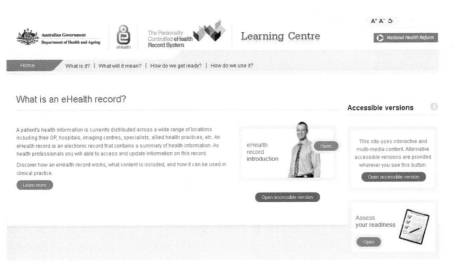

Fig. 15.4 PCEHR learning centre [17]

Australia. However, as this is still new in Australia with only being available since July 1 2012 it is still in its infancy and has more development needed over the next few years as it starts to mature and Australians become increasingly engaged in the use of eHealth.

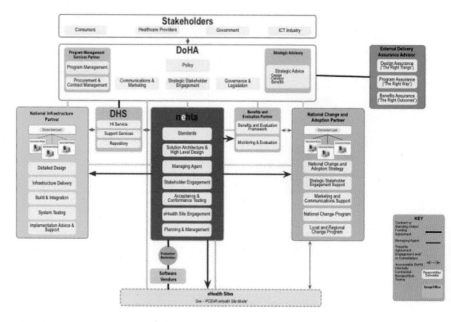

Fig. 15.5 PCEHR source model [18]

Governance of the PCEHR is with the Australian Government. New federal leg-islation was enacted for the PCEHR and Individual Health Identifiers (IHI) in 2012 and 2010 respectively. Standards for these developments have been undertaken within Standards Australia and the National eHealth Transition Authority (NeHTA), which has developed the major infrastructure of the PCEHR and the IHI's. National Privacy guidelines have also been incorporated into all developments however, some State and Territory laws must still be accommodated where appropriate. A number of other organisations are also involved in the PCEHR and the complex-ity of this type of development is shown in Fig. 15.5 [18].

The PCEHR has been rolled out in phases or managed stages. Individual informa-tion from Medicare, including Medicare Benefits Schedule (MBS), Pharmaceutical Benefits Schedule (PBS), Australian Organ Donor Register and Australian Childhood Immunisation Register data, will be incorporated into the PCEHR system for indi-viduals who request this information to be part of their record.

Significant advertising and promotion is underway nationally for individuals to sign up to the PCEHR. There is a dedicated web site [19] for anyone to access for further information on the PCEHR.

Healthcare Identifiers Service

Prior to 2010, Australia had no national system of individual identification and patients/clients were identified by their Medicare Number and each individual health care agency filing system. These are not individual identifiers for national use

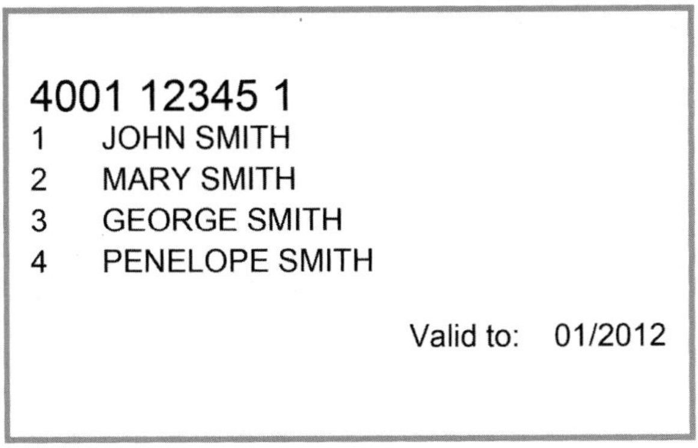

Fig. 15.6 Diagrammatic
example of an Australian
Medicare Card

```
4001 12345 1
1    JOHN SMITH
2    MARY SMITH
3    GEORGE SMITH
4    PENELOPE SMITH

                              Valid to:    01/2012
```

as Medicare numbers may have more than one individual person on each card with the same number however, each person will have a different list number For example see Fig. 15.6.

An urgent need was identified to develop a system to ensure security, privacy and confidentiality of eHealth information. The Healthcare Identifiers Service (HI Service) was established in 2010–2011 as a foundation service for e-health initiatives in Australia. A healthcare identifier is a unique number that has been be assigned to healthcare consumers, and to healthcare providers and organisations that provide health services [20].

The identifiers are assigned, administered and operated by Medicare Australia. A key aim of healthcare identifiers is to ensure that individuals and providers can have confidence that individuals are identified uniquely and unambiguously, and that the correct health information is associated with the correct individual at the point of care. This service is supported by a strong and effective legislative framework that includes governance arrangements, permitted uses, and privacy safeguards. The legislation and regulations to support the HI Service are available and can be viewed at ComLaw [20].

Health Workforce Australia Reform

For national health reform to succeed, the health workforce must have capacity to respond to future health system challenges and changes. Government priorities are concerned with improved access and health services for all Australians. Therefore, expansion of the health and aged care workforce and providing education, knowledge and skill opportunities for all health professionals is paramount to prepare for the future [21].

HWA is a national body and operates across the health and education sectors addressing Australia's critical health workforce planning, training and reform priorities.

Health Information Workforce

Health Workforce Australia received requests from the National eHealth Transition Authority (NeHTA) and the Australasian College of Health Informatics (ACHI) to undertake a study of the Australian health information workforce. A discussion paper was released in 2011 with the proposed methodology for the project and the Final Report published in 2012 [22].

It was identified that the definition of this workforce was not agreed upon and the workforce boundaries were ill-defined. However, this was not seen as uncommon with newer workforces and the factors that impact. This workforce has multiple occupational titles and discipline areas with workers drawn from the main discipline areas of health, information and computer science. The composition of this workforce varied considerably and appeared to be influenced by the adoption levels of electronic health records and processes [22]. Therefore these issues made it difficult to identify, quantify and predict workforce requirements now and for the future.

Much of the discussion and findings are about health information managers and clinical coders as they are the only current identified occupational code in this area in Australia. These areas have well documented workforce shortages [22–25]. However, this signifies that many health professionals working within the area of health and nursing informatics are not included and therefore the project outcomes may be misrepresenting current and future workforce issues. However, the report has identified in the findings that consensus on role descriptions and definitions are required. Education was also highlighted as a finding that requires review of current curricular in both the higher education and vocational education and training (VET) sectors as well as strategies to raise the profile to attract more students to this critical area. Formation of a single advisory council was an identified need for workforce issues in this area, which would act specifically for all health informatics stakeholders. Identification of exemplar EMR/EHR/digital adoption sites to identify implications for workforce issues over time was also seen as a critical development [22].

Australian Health Practitioner Regulation Agency (AHPRA)

The government established a single national registration and accreditation scheme for health professionals which was introduced in 2010. AHPRA's operations are governed by the Health Practitioner Regulation National Law, and is in force in each state and territory (the National Law), which came into effect on 1 July 2010. This law means that for the first time in Australia, 14 health professions are regulated by nationally consistent legislation under the National Registration and Accreditation Scheme. It currently regulates the Health professions as listed in Table 15.1.

Table 15.1 Australian register professions [26, 27]

Nurses and midwives	Medical practitioners
Dental practitioners (including dentists, dental hygienists, dental prosthetists & dental therapists)	Optometrists
Chiropractors	Physiotherapists
Pharmacists	Podiatrists
Psychologists	Osteopaths
Medical radiation practitioners	Aboriginal and Torres Strait Islander health practitioners
Chinese medicine practitioners	Occupational therapists

Australian Nursing Informatics

The discipline of Nursing Informatics (NI) in Australia has been slow in developing as with many other countries. It has mainly been early adopters and passionate advocates that have lead the discipline and developments for the past 21 years. It began with a small group of nurses in Victoria in 1989 who realised that technology was important for nursing practice and patient care. This group became the Nursing Computer Group Victoria (Inc) (NCGV Inc) and were successful in hosting the 1991 Fourth International Nursing Informatics Congress in Melbourne, Victoria in conjunction with International Medical Informatics Association (IMIA) – Working Group 8. This congress was very successful and a number of the early pioneers of NI in Australia emerged from this conference.

From this auspicious start developments in health and nursing informatics started to advance and from the NCGV grew two major groups: Health Informatics Society of Australia (HISA) [8] and Nursing Informatics Australia (NIA) [9]. The great platform originating all those years ago has been the catalyst for where both health and nursing informatics are in this country today.

Nursing Informatics Australia (NIA) celebrated their 21st birthday in 2012 at the annual NIA conference and are the preeminent group of nurse informaticians in the country. This was a great milestone to achieve and the members of this group over the years have added to the national and international nursing informatics knowledge and skill base. A number of current members are actively involved in national and international developments, professional and political organisations in this area. NI members have been resolute in ensuring nursing is on the current health reform and eHealth agendas in all political and professional arenas in Australia. For example; National Board position on HISA; NIA position on Coalition of National Nursing Organisations (CoNNO); selected as Clinical leads and Reference Group Chairs and members for eHealth developments at NeHTA; Australian representation on International Medical Informatics Association – Nursing Informatics (IMIA NI) which includes being a current Vice Chair and member of the Education Sub Committee; invitations to national eHealth workshops and events.

Nursing Informatics Competencies

Nursing Informatics Competencies have been and are still being developed globally. In Australia, a project to develop National Nursing Informatics Competencies for all Registered Nurses was undertaken from 2009 to 2011. This project was funded by the Australian Government Department of Health and Aging and managed through the Australian Nursing Federation (ANF). The ANF contracted Queensland University of Technology, School of Nursing to undertake the research and development of the NI Competencies. The final report and competencies, completed in 2011, are currently still with the ANF for publication. It was recommended that such competence development be a requirement for all higher education and vocational education nursing programs in Australia and for the competency standards to be adopted as one of the standards for registration as a nurse in Australia. However at this time, this has not been adopted.

Studies of Australian nurses and information technology reported that nurses generally are poorly prepared to engage with information technology in their practice. The study reported that almost two thirds of nurses had not received any formal training in basic software applications and of the 90 % of nurses who used computers or other information technology applications, only one third had any formal training [28]. This landmark study revealed a gross deficit in the capacity of the nursing workforce to engage in the digital processing of information.

Another study [29] undertaken which investigated perceptions and attitudes of Australian nursing students regarding eHealth reported that the majority of respondents regularly use computers and the internet but their awareness of eHealth was limited. This study also supported the inclusion of nursing informatics and eHealth into undergraduate nursing curricula. These two Australian studies supported the work undertaken in the development of the Australian NI Competencies. Other earlier studies related to computer and informatics skills and knowledge as well as the need for NI competencies had been undertaken and supported the competency development [30–33].

Nursing Informatics Education

Currently, there are no nursing informatics courses available in Australia. There are a small number of eHealth and health informatics programs available in a small number of universities only. These are usually at the postgraduate level or as Summer Schools. This is a major area for growth in the future for all health disciplines.

There has been a pervasive sense of nursing informatics not being essential in heavy undergraduate curricula and not presenting any real interest for post graduate courses in this speciality. There are very few qualified/experienced academics to teach nursing informatics in the higher education sector or even at the VET sector level. This exacerbates the lack of urgency and need for this area to be included in curricula nationally. However, health/nursing informatics and health technology are now part of the Accreditation Standards for all Australian Schools of Nursing [34], which necessitates inclusion of these specialties into all curricula for any future accreditation. Currently at QLD University of Technology, nursing informatics is being integrated across the 3-year undergraduate curricular in 2013 and a nursing informatics and eHealth elective is planned for 3rd year undergraduate students in 2014. Hopefully other universities around Australia will instigate similar initiatives in the future. Once the undergraduate area initiative is completed, there will be a move to getting a specialty postgraduate course in the future.

There is ample literature available to support the need for nursing informatics to be included in curricular and the issues surrounding this inclusion, however, it still appears that implementation into curricula globally is still inconsistent [35–46].

Many of these authors suggest further research is necessary as to what the critical aspects/concepts are that need to be included. Consensus may never be reached on this issue and as time quickly ticks by the urgency for education for all nurses about nursing informatics and its impact must be included in curricula now. As the rapid pace of development, implementation and use of information technology and eHealth worldwide continues, it is imperative that the nursing profession ensures all Registered Nurses have basic education in this speciality if nursing is to remain visible in current health information systems and in the future. The responsibility of providing nurses with the knowledge and skills needed lies with all professional and educational organisations by ensuring that nursing informatics is high on national and international political, educational and professional agendas.

Australian Informatics Challenges

The lack of interaction and interest in health and nursing informatics by nurses has a number of inherent issues from political apathy to support nurses, medical domination in political arenas, high levels of management and micro management, lack of strong nursing leaders and professional organisations as well as lack of educational opportunities in this specialty area. Current eHealth developments do not have specific nursing data documented in the PCEHR or in many of the clinical information systems. There are some aspects of patient care that are incorporated and could be inclusive of nursing however nursing data and standardised nursing language is mostly not included. The future of the International Classification of Nursing Practice (ICNP) being included in future versions of SNOMED may go some way in rectifying this issue. Australia is progressing toward SNOMED CT AU being the common core for all health information systems in Australia and the inclusion of the ICNP will be the first time real nursing data will be available for use in Australia. The ongoing development of the ICNP by international nurses involvement via collaborations such as the International Health Terminology Standards Development Organisation (IHTSDO) Nursing Group continue to evolve the ICNP to be a true international standardised nursing classification.

Australian professional nursing organisations are very slow in realising the importance of nursing informatics, data standards, nursing language and classifications in health information systems. The invisibility of nursing in these systems has been overt for many years and will continue unless these organisations and Australian nursing leaders take this critical area more seriously and support developments by nursing informatics experts as well as foster relationships with state and federal health departments for nursing informatics and eHealth initiatives.

One argument about this lack of interaction and interest by nurses is based on transactional analysis of 'bystanders' as discussed by Brinkman [47]. She suggests nurses continue along the continuum of becoming involved or interacting with professional issues, which ranges from apathy to integration [47] Each nurse needs to assess their personal self-management and identify where we each sit on this continuum so that we can recognise the variations of other nurses. This should enhance understanding of inaction and enable greater interaction among nurses to promote professional collaboration and involvement politically and professionally. As the largest health care professional group, nurses could influence the political agendas and ensure rigorous debate and feedback on current and future issues and directions for healthcare now and in the future [47].

What can be done to overcome these challenges? This is not easy to answer, as it is a complex issue. Nursing informatics advocates and early adopters continue to engage in debates, discussions, developments, implementations, education and political lobbying, but the change is slow. The definitive solutions are not evident in the literature as it appears this is a global issue and one that all nurses are attempting to solve. Things do change over time and as a profession if all nurses can support the changes needed then change will occur. However, whilst horizontal violence and lack of support amongst the profession itself continues then the changes that are needed will not occur and nurses will become invisible forever in health information systems and nursing's role will become obsolete. Is this what we want to happen?

There needs to be debate and discussion around these issues by all nurses nationally and internationally so that informed decisions and change can occur. Nursing Informatics needs to be recognised as a formal nursing specialist role in Australia and roles such as Clinical Nursing Informatics Officer (CNIO) and Nursing Informatics Specialist need to be introduced with specific role descriptions. Education for Nursing Informatics at postgraduate levels also needs to be introduced into curricular to enable nurses to have the specific knowledge and skills required for these roles. Professional organisations and nurse leaders need to be insistent for more of these roles to be formally built into nursing career structures and be recognised within the wider health informatics and health communities. These need to be nationally recognised and not state specific to prevent fragmentation of the discipline. Development of certification for the specialty and recognition of this within the national registration boards for remuneration aspects to be included in career structures would be vital.

The challenge is there for professional nursing organisations and nursing leaders of Australia to be proactive in these developments and initiatives for nursing to remain visible and viable in health care systems and health care to safeguard the profession for the future as health care reform is implemented.

The Future

What does the digital future hold for healthcare and nursing? Rapidly evolving technologies and abilities outstrip the abilities of large healthcare and professional organisations to keep up or be proactive when one is still dealing with old and disparate systems that cannot be removed as well as funding issues, governance, legalities, etc. Adding to the complexity for healthcare change is the reality that many changes come from other areas of computer and information technology, (for example: gaming, capabilities of new technologies, nanotechnology, robotics, artificial intelligence, genomics, and biomedical aspects).

For nursing, it is critical that nursing informatics education be included in all undergraduate nursing programs. Nurses must become involved in debate, policy decisions, developments and management of where professional nursing practice is headed for the future. As a profession, it is time for nurses to take control of nursing's future in this country. Nurses are moving to claim their role as information managers of patient care. Many changes in how individuals will interact with healthcare in the future necessitate changes to education, practice, development and change within the profession. This will require changes to perceptions and long held beliefs about what nursing was and may lead to a very different nursing in the future. This will not be an easy transition for many within the nursing profession and will require many changes in all aspects of nursing.

Conclusion

Health and nursing informatics in Australia is an international leader in some aspects and slower in others. Overall, it is on par with the majority of countries using health information technology today. It is a significant time of healthcare change based on healthcare information technologies which are providing many challenges and excitement for the future. It is hoped that the nursing profession here in Australia is ready to be involved and to be visible, vibrant and dynamic in this new era of healthcare. The change to facilitation of care and self-management with health consumers in the future is an exciting one and nurses should be at the forefront of these developments and in primary healthcare. These are roles that nurse education, knowledge and skills are tailored for with the broad knowledge base and would adapt very easily to these requirements. However, the nursing profession in Australia would need to support the changes needed in education, management and practice. It is not the technology that is the issue but the change processes to use it appropriately.

If Australia wants to lead these developments, much change would be needed. The healthcare reforms, changes for health education, eHealth developments, national broadband infrastructure, and PCEHR developments are all encouraging signs for a national focus on the use of health information technology to promote a more effective, efficient, safe healthcare system for all Australians.

References

1. Australian Government. Bringing the PCEHR to Life. 2011. Available at: http://www.youtube.com/watch?v=3IOoUMwSGMI.
2. Australian Government. Department of Health and Aging. 2013. Available at: http://www.health.gov.au/.
3. Australian Government. National eHealth Transition Authority. 2013. Available at: http://www.nehta.gov.au/.
4. Australian Government – Department of Human Services. 2013. Available at: http://www.humanservices.gov.au/.
5. Australian Government – Medicare. 2013. Available at: http://www.humanservices.gov.au/customer/dhs/medicare.
6. Australian Government – Health Workforce Australia. 2013. Available at: http://www.hwa.gov.au/.
7. Australasian College of Health Informatics. 2013. Available at: http://www.achi.org.au/.
8. Health Informatics Society of Australia. 2013. Available at: http://www.hisa.org.au/.
9. Nursing Informatics Australia. 2013. Available at: http://www.hisa.org.au/members/group.asp?id=85335.
10. Australian Government. National Health Reform. 2013. Available at: http://www.yourhealth.gov.au/internet/yourhealth/publishing.nsf/Content/home#.UVezsPLhdhI.
11. Australian Government. About National Health. 2012. Available at: http://www.yourhealth.gov.au/internet/yourhealth/publishing.nsf/Content/health-reform-overview#.UVezW_LhdhJ.
12. Australian Government. National Health Reform Agreement.2011. Available at: http://www.yourhealth.gov.au/internet/yourhealth/publishing.nsf/Content/nhra-justreleased#.UVfBj_LhdhI.
13. Australian Government. Concept of operations: relating to the introduction of a personally controlled electronic health record system. 2011. Available at: http://www.yourhealth.gov.au/internet/yourhealth/publishing.nsf/Content/PCEHRS-Intro-toc~ch1#.UVfEufLhdhI.
14. National eHealth Health Transition Authority. Concept of operations: relating to the introduction of a personally controlled electronic health record system. The PCEHR Concept. 2011. Available at: http://www.yourhealth.gov.au/internet/yourhealth/publishing.nsf/Content/PCEHRS-Intro-toc~ch1~1_2#.UXpvSUpuI6g.
15. National eHealth Transition Authority. Concept of operations: relating to the introduction of a personally controlled electronic health record system. The PCEHR System. 2011. Available at: http://www.yourhealth.gov.au/internet/yourhealth/publishing.nsf/Content/PCEHRS-Intro-toc~ch1~1_2#.UXvWcUpuI6g.
16. Australian Government. e-Health. 2013. Available at: http://www.yourhealth.gov.au/internet/yourhealth/publishing.nsf/Content/theme-ehealth#.UVe0GPLhdhI.
17. Australian Government. Learning centre. 2013. Available at: http://publiclearning.ehealth.gov.au/hcp/.
18. Australian Government. Concept of operations: relating to the introduction of a personally controlled electronic health record system. The sourcing model. Available at: http://www.yourhealth.gov.au/internet/yourhealth/publishing.nsf/Content/PCEHRS-Intro-toc~ch8~8_3#.UXpuv0puI6g.

19. Australian Government. Welcome to ehealth.gov.au. 2013. Available at: http://www.ehealth. gov.au/internet/ehealth/publishing.nsf/content/home.
20. Australian Government. Healthcare Identifiers Act 2010 – C2012C00590. 2012. Available at: http://www.comlaw.gov.au/Details/C2012C00590.
21. Australian Government. Health Workforce. 2011. Available at: http://www.yourhealth.gov.au/ internet/yourhealth/publishing.nsf/Content/theme-workforce#.UVfQhfLhdhI.
22. Ridoutt L, Pilbeam V, Bagnulo J. Health information workforce study – volume 1. Health Workforce Australia. 2012. Available at: http://www.humancapitalalliance.com.au/down-loads/DH63%20Final_REPORT_Health%20_Information_workforce.pdf.
23. Australian Institute of Health and Welfare (AIHW). The coding workforce shortfall. 2010. Available at: http://www.aihw.gov.au/WorkArea/DownloadAsset.aspx?id=6442472765.
24. Bennett V. Health information management workforce-when opportunities abound. Health Info Manag J. 2010;39(3):4–6.
25. Shepheard J. Health information management and clinical coding workforce issues. Health Info Manag J. 2010;39(3):37–41.
26. Australian Health Practitioner Regulation Agency. Who we are. 2010–2013. Available at: http://www.ahpra.gov.au/About-AHPRA/Who-We-Are.aspx.
27. Australian Government. National partnership agreement on hospital and health workforce reform. 2011. Available at: http://www.ahwo.gov.au/documents/COAG/National%20 Partnership%20Agreement%20on%20Hospital%20and%20Health%20Workforce%20 Reform.pdf.
28. Hegney D, Buikstra E, Eley R, Fallon T, Gilmore V, Soar J. Nurses and information technology: final report. 2007. Available at: http://anf.org.au/pages/it-project.
29. Edirippulige S, Smith A, Beattie H, Davies E, Wooton R. Pre-registration nurses: an investigation of knowledge, experience and comprehension of e-health. Aust J Adv Nurs. 2008;25(2):78–83.
30. Carter B, Axford R. Assessment of computer learning needs and priorities of registered nurses practicing in hospitals. Comput Nurs. 1993;11(3):122–6.
31. Kenny A. Online learning: enhancing nurse education? J Adv Nurs. 2002;38(2):127–35. doi:10.1046/j.1365-2648.2002.02156.x.
32. Conrick M, Hovenga E, Cook R, Laracuente T, Morgan T. A framework for nursing informatics in Australia: a strategic paper. 2004. Available at: https://www.resource/group/3db28856-9ef5-42f4-8700-5bc9aabfacd4/nursinginformaticsinaustrali.pdf.
33. Garde S, Harrison D, Hovenga E. Skill needs for nurses in their role as health informatics professionals: a survey in the context of global health informatics education. Int J Med Inform. 2005;74(11–12):899–907.
34. Nursing and Midwifery Board of Australia (NMBA). Accreditation. 2010–2013. Available at: http://www.nursingmidwiferyboard.gov.au/Accreditation.aspx.
35. Desjardins KS, Cook SS, Jenkins M, Bakken S. Effect of an informatics for evidence-based practice curriculum on nursing informatics competencies. Int J Med Inform. 2005;74(11–12):1012–20.
36. Thompson B, Skiba D. Informatics in the nursing curriculum: a national survey of nursing informatics requirements in nursing curricula. Nurs Educ Perspect. 2008;29(5):312–7.
37. Fetter MS. Graduating nurses' self-evaluation of information technology competencies. J Nurs Educ. 2009;48(2):86–90.
38. Ericksen AB. Informatics: the future of nursing. RN. 2009;72(7):34–7.
39. Bond C, Procter P. Prescription for nursing informatics in pre-registration nurse education. Health Informatics J. 2009;15(1):55–64. doi:10.1177/1460458208099868.
40. Jetté S, Tribble DS, Gagnon J, Mathieu L. Nursing students' perceptions of their resources toward the development of competencies in nursing informatics. Nurse Educ Today. 2010;30(8):742–6. doi:10.1016/j.nedt.2010.01.016.
41. Flood LS, Gasiewicz N, Delpier T. Integrating information literacy across a BSN curriculum. J Nurs Educ. 2010;49(2):101–4.
42. Chang J, Poynton MR, Gassert CA, Staggers N. Nursing informatics competencies required of nurses in Taiwan. Int J Med Inform. 2011;80(5):332–40.

43. Nguyen DN, Zierler B, Nguyen HQ. A survey of nursing faculty needs for training in use of new technologies for education and practice. J Nurs Educ. 2011;50(4):181–9.
44. Gray K, Dattakumar A, Maeder A, Chenery H. Educating future clinicians about clinical informatics: a review of implementation and evaluation cases. Eur J Biomed Inform. 2011;7(2):48–57.
45. Spencer J. Integrating informatics in undergraduate nursing curricula: using the QSEN framework as a guide. J Nurs Educ. 2012;51(12):697–701. doi:10.3928/01484834-20121011-01.
46. DeGagne J, Bisanar W, Makowski J, Neumann J. Integrating informatics into the BSN curriculum: a review of the literature. Nurse Educ Today. 2012;32(6):675–82.
47. Brinkman A. Getting involved – from apathy to integration. Nurs N Z. 2012;18(6):30.

Chapter 16
Case Study 2: The TIGER Initiative Foundation – Technology Informatics Guiding Education Reform

Sally E. Schlak

Abstract The TIGER Initiative, an acronym for Technology Informatics Guiding Education Reform, was launched in 2004 to bring together nursing stakeholders to develop a shared vision, strategies, and specific actions for improving nursing practice, education, and the delivery of patient care with health IT. In 2011, TIGER became The TIGER Initiative Foundation, incorporated as a 501(c) (Institute of Medicine. The future of nursing: leading change, advancing health. Committee on the Robert Wood Johnson Foundation Initiative on the Future of Nursing, at the Institute of Medicine, The National Academies of Press; 2011.p. 172. HIMSH) organization operating for charitable, educational, and scientific purposes. To educate the workforce to use health IT, TIGER has developed a Virtual Learning Environment, which provides multi-faceted, virtual learning experiences and virtual communities to develop knowledge, skills, and awareness of technology and informatics to contribute to a safer, more effective, efficient, patient-centered, timely and equitable healthcare system.

Keywords TIGER • Technology • Virtual learning environment • Informatics • Nursing informatics • Education reform • health IT • Nursing practice

Key Concepts

TIGER
Technology
Virtual learning environment
Informatics
Nursing informatics
Education reform
health IT
Nursing practice – hope this is enough

S.E. Schlak, BSN, MBA
The TIGER Initiative Foundation, 33 West Monroe St. Suite 1700, Chicago, IL 60603, USA
e-mail: seschlak@gmail.com

© Springer-Verlag London 2015   323
K.J. Hannah et al. (eds.), *Introduction to Nursing Informatics*,
Health Informatics, DOI 10.1007/978-1-4471-2999-8_16

Introduction

In 2004, David J. Brailer, MD, PhD, appointed to the new position of National Coordinator for Health Information technology, held the first national meeting announcing the Federal Strategic Framework for the Decade of Healthcare Technology. Several influential nursing informatics leaders and nursing informatics advocates attended and noticed that nursing was not included on the panels. The potential implications on nursing were recognized as being significant. Nursing informatics advocates realized that the nursing contribution to achieving these national goals and participating in implementing, improving and sustaining the new health technology infrastructure would not be recognized. This realization was worrying as nurses comprise approximately 55 % of the healthcare workforce and are integral to any transformation that would take place in healthcare. Following this meeting, a small group of nursing leaders and advocates came together and determined that action was required to mitigate this situation. Thus Technology Informatics Guiding Education Reform (TIGER) was created, thereby initiating a grass roots movement, which was essential to transforming nursing practice, leadership and education through information technology [1]. Since then, much as been achieved through this grass roots movement. For example there has been success in the educational environment to recognize the importance of informatics and technology and the contribution to the nursing body of knowledge through publications and presentations has been prevalent (www.thetigerinitiative.org) [2]. TIGER has also been incorporated as a nonprofit foundation and has recently launched its long awaited educational platform, the TIGER Virtual Learning Environment (VLE) utilizing the INXPO Virtual Platform [5]. Complementing this chapter is a tour of the TIGER Virtual Learning Environment and an opportunity to view this resource via a demonstration of the VLE via a short WebEx.

Critical Success Factors and TIGER

TIGER's successes have been dependent upon its grass roots origins and the support of many volunteers and organizations. TIGER success in education is evident where the American Association of Colleges of Nursing (AACN) Board unanimously approved the revised *Essentials of Baccalaureate Nursing Education* which recommended that graduates must have basic competence in technical skills, which includes the use of computers, as well as the application of patient care technologies such as monitors, data gathering devices, and other technological supports for patient care interventions. In addition, nursing informatics organizations such as Alliance for Nursing Informatics (ANI), American Medical Informatics Association (AMIA), Healthcare Information Management Systems Society (HIMSS), American Nurses Informatics Association (ANIA), Minnesota Nursing Informatics Group (MINING), New England Informatics Nursing Consortium (NENIC) have embraced the TIGER agenda, providing staff resources and financial support to the initiative. Nursing leadership, including American Nurses Association (ANA), Sigma Theta Tau International (STTI), American Academy of Nursing, American Organization of Nurse Executives, (AONE), (Nursing Organizations Alliance (NOA), and specialty organizations including the Association of periOperative Registered Nurses (AORN), National Association of Clinical Nurse Specialist (NACNS), The Association of Women's Health, Obstetric and Neonatal Nurses (AWHONN) provided critical support for TIGER, enhancing visibility and access to nursing executives. Health care IT vendors were active supporters and participants in the initiative, sponsoring the TIGER Summit Gallery Walk, webinars, seminars and components of the TIGER Virtual Learning Environment.

TIGER has made multiple contributions to the nursing body of knowledge through publications, national and international presentations. TIGER recommendations were included in the 2011 *IOM Future of Nursing Report* [3]. Also instrumental has been the publication of *Nursing Informatics: Where Technology and Caring Meet,* 4th Edition, Ball et al. [1].

TIGER published nine collaborative reports, which cover standards and interoperability, national policy, educational and faculty development, usability and clinical application design, leadership development, virtual learning center, consumer empowerment and personal health records and informatics competencies. The collaborative reports can be accessed and downloaded for free from the TIGER Website at www.tigerinitiative.org [2].

In 2013, the TIGER Initiative Foundation continues to build on its history of transforming nursing and interprofessional colleagues to advance the integration of health informatics and to transform practice, education and consumer engagement. Over the last 18 months, through the assistance of HIMSS [4], TIGER has become a nonprofit foundation, and established a structure to its grass roots initiative. TIGER remains focused on its purpose of preparing nurses and interprofessional colleagues to use informatics and emerging technologies to make healthcare safer, more effective, efficient, patient-centered, timely and equitable. TIGER continues to advance the integration of health informatics through a number of communication vehicles: TIGER Website, TIGER List Serv communications, and publication of a monthly TIGER e-newsletter. TIGER has also jumped into the realm of social media with Facebook and Twitter @ABoutTIGER [2].

Most recently, TIGER has launched its long anticipated Virtual Learning Environment. TIGER utilized a collaborative workgroup approach to advance education on Health Information Technology (HIT) topics. The TIGER Virtual Demonstration Collaborative workgroup studied the benefits and challenges of a virtual learning environment to expedite innovation and adoption of HIT and identified that a dynamic and sustainable platform was needed to continuously showcase the most effective and efficient current technology-enabled and near future-enabling technologies to advance nursing practice, education and research.

With the launch of the TIGER VLE, the goal is to increase understanding and adoption of health informatics by frontline clinicians, to provide faculty and educators with tools and resources to prepare the current and future health professions workforce, and to engage consumers in the future technology-enabled care environments is now a step closer. The TIGER Initiative Foundation's Virtual Learning Environment (VLE) provides an interactive web based learning opportunity, which includes information about HIT and related topics for health professionals and consumers. There are a wide range of topics included in the VLE: electronic health records, usability, clinical decision support, health information exchange, care coordination, meaningful use, standards and interoperability, consumer health information, mobile health, privacy and security, exemplars of how health information technology support nursing practice and others. To facilitate adoption of information technologies, the VLE provides not only an opportunity for educational content buts also provide learners with exposure to new and enabling technologies. TIGER has a collaborative approach to engaging with sponsors to demonstrate the use and utility of technology for improving practice and patient outcomes

Unlimited access to the VLE for 1 year is provided through a registration fee of $25. The VLE currently has a national and international broad healthcare professional audience. Faculty, students, clinical and informatics professionals from healthcare institutions, industry and professional associations along with international participants make up a rich diverse audience of learners.

A virtual tour is available to view from this link composed for this text. For ease of reading we have also included some screen shots, which depict the key screens in the TIGER VLE describing briefly their core purpose and function.

Tiger VLE Key Screens Function and Purpose

We will begin our exploration of the TIGER VLE. The first time you log into the event your profile will be displayed. Your profile contains your personal biography and message. Filling out this information allows others in the environment to network with you (Fig. 16.1).

After logging into the VLE, you will be taken to the TIGER Lobby (Fig. 16.2). From the lobby page you have access to TIGER social media on Facebook and Twitter, find out what new content has been added, see a list of TIGER Sightings, upcoming events and read a brief history of TIGER. The lobby page also provides different navigation options.

Navigating to the TIGER Resource Center (Fig. 16.3) enables learners to browse content by subject and sponsor. Resources cover many topics and include; presentations, webinars, links, e-brochures, documented sources and white papers. Faculty can benefit from the resources to enhance curriculum, provide additional resources for students, or provide content material with assignments for discussion boards or online live chats.

The TIGER Communities page (Fig. 16.4) provides learners the opportunity to browse content by various communities. Communities are groups of like-minded individuals with similar interests or professions. Content placed in communities is focused toward each different community's interests. TIGER currently has seven communities- Faculty Development, Leadership & Management, Patient/Consumer Engagement, Policy, Student, Underserved /Rural, and Workforce Development.

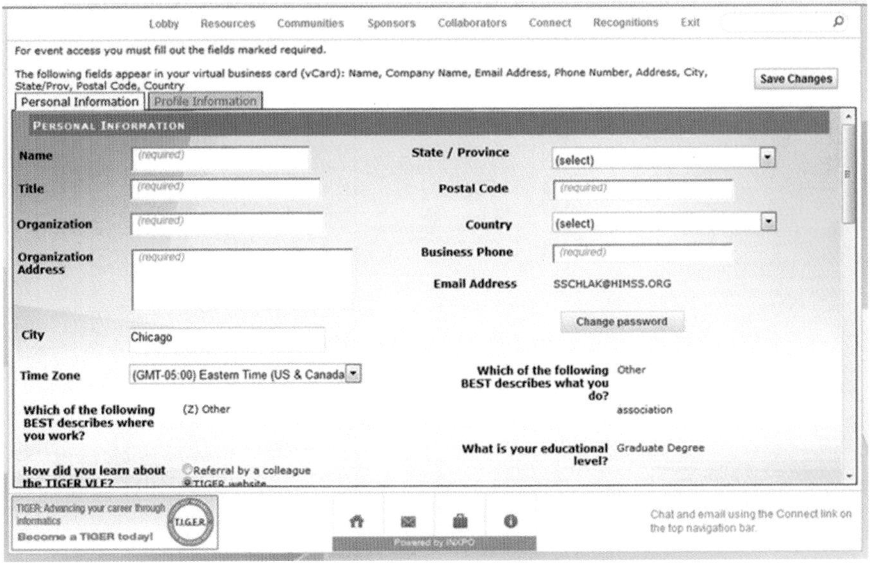

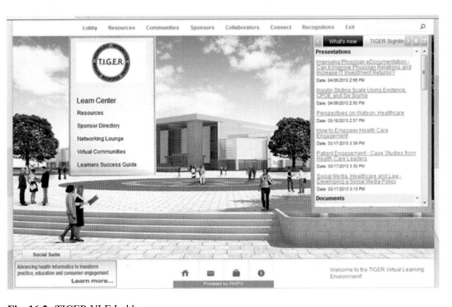

Fig. 16.1 Learner profile

Fig. 16.2 TIGER VLE Lobby

Moving onto the Sponsors page (Fig. 16.5), the Exhibit Floor provides the learner with opportunities to view healthcare informatics technology solutions. The Virtual Demonstration Collaborative identified early on that there was a need to expose nursing and interprofessional colleagues to the broad array of technology available

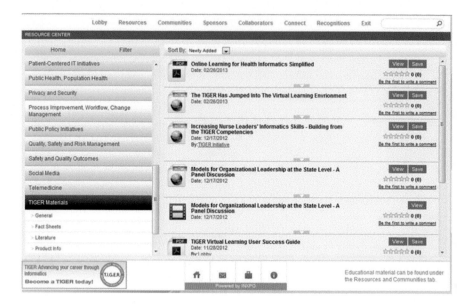

Fig. 16.3 TIGER Resource Center

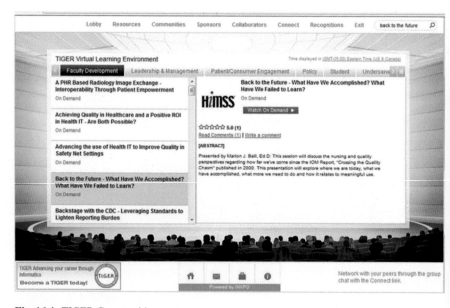

Fig. 16.4 TIGER Communities page

to support healthcare process and outcomes. TIGER's collaborative business model provides opportunities for healthcare information technology solutions companies to gain product visibility and at the same time showcase innovative technology, which supports clinical processes and outcomes. Educational institutions have

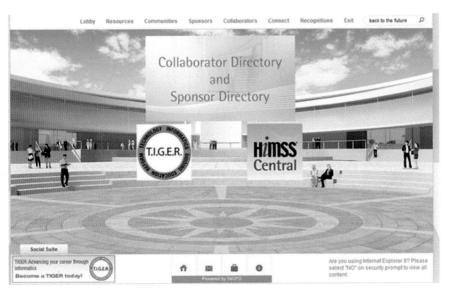

Fig. 16.5 TIGER Sponsor page

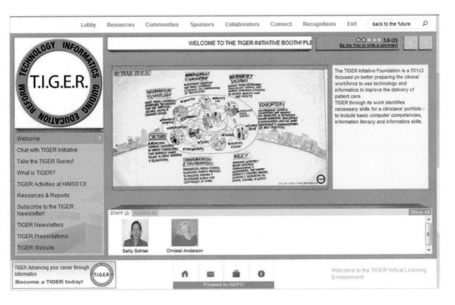

Fig. 16.6 Sponsor booth

expressed interest in sharing their programs, so potential students can see the many educational nursing and informatics programs. Entering a booth exposes the learner to healthcare technology products, education and information. The booth (Fig. 16.6) provides various tools/mediums for showcasing and exploring technology.

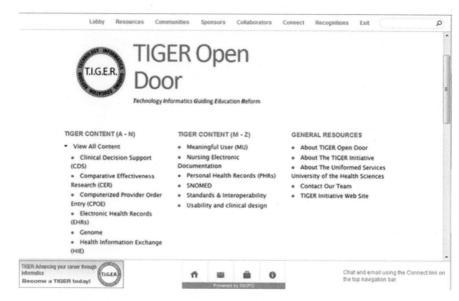

Fig. 16.7 TIGER Open Door

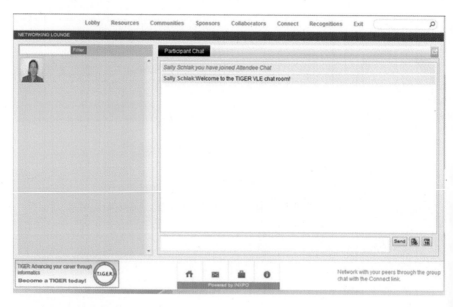

Fig. 16.8 TIGER Connect!

The Collaborator Page (Fig. 16.7) provides an ability to view collaborators and see the recently completed TIGER Open Door Project, sponsored by the National Library of Medicine and hosted on the James A. Zimble Learning Resource Center, Uniformed Services University of the Health Sciences. The TIGER Open Door

Project is a clearinghouse of publically available content organized by health IT topics. This can also be accessed from the TIGER Website.

TIGER Connect (Fig. 16.8) provides an opportunity to chat with others in the environment.

The TIGER VLE also has capabilities to internally privately chat, send emails, play games and earn TIGER recognitions. Virtual business cards may be sent within the environment. Finally, items may be downloaded into your tote bag and saved to your computer.

In summary, coordination and collaboration with industry leaders and experts, nursing and interdisciplinary professional organizations, educational institutions and government agencies at the state, regional and national level will enhance the variety of offerings, and facilitate outreach to a diverse and expansive learning audience. The TIGER VLE and other TIGER efforts will enable The TIGER Initiative Foundation to make a significant contribution to the national HIT agenda to advance nursing and other clinical professions to meet the challenge of transforming healthcare.

References

1. Ball MJ, Douglas JV, Walker PH. Nursing informatics where caring and technology meet. London: Springer; 2011.
2. Tiger website online resource available from: http://www.thetigerinitiative.org. Accessed 24 Apr 2013.
3. Institute of Medicine. The future of nursing: leading change, advancing health. Committee on the Robert Wood Johnson Foundation Initiative on the Future of Nursing, at the Institute of Medicine, Washington D.C.: The National Academies of Press; 2011.p. 172. HIMSH.
4. HIMSS Healthcare Information and Management System Society. www.himss.org.
5. INXPO. The Power to Reach: Next Generation Webcasting. 2014. Available: http://www.inxpo.com/aboutus/company-overview/.

Chapter 17
Case Study 3: Nursing Informatics – Highlights from Wales

Beverley Thomas

Abstract Chapter 17 describes the importance of effectively engaging nurses from an NHS Wales perspective, to support the Welsh Governments strategic approach to utilizing Information Communication Technology for care planning and delivery.

An outline of the Welsh NHS and the history of Welsh nursing informatics between 2007 and 2013 is provided. The eight principles that underpin the approach to nursing informatics in Wales are discussed.

Keywords Information Communication Technology • Enabling improved health care delivery • Welsh nursing informatics

Key Concepts

Information Communication Technology
Enabling improved health care delivery
Welsh nursing informatics

Introduction

Change in the way health services will be delivered in Wales is intended to ensure patients are the central concern of the NHS in Wales. Improvements in patient/client/citizen care will include: addressing the needs of an aging population and those with chronic conditions, tackling public health issues, and delivery of care closer to a person's home. In addition, service delivery will require simplification of the management structures, consideration of a whole system approach to care delivery, and a focus on value for money.

Enabling this vision will require effective use of information communication technologies, engagement of the clinical workforce, and a framework to measure success.

B. Thomas, RN, Cert Ed (FE). MPH. Dip HSM
NHS Wales Informatics Service, Cardiff, Wales, UK
e-mail: bev.thomas@wales.nhs.uk

© Springer-Verlag London 2015   333
K.J. Hannah et al. (eds.), *Introduction to Nursing Informatics*,
Health Informatics, DOI 10.1007/978-1-4471-2999-8_17

An outline of the Welsh NHS is provided in the box below. This is followed by a summary overview of changes in the utilization of information technology and an historical overview of Welsh nursing informatics between 2007 and 2013. The overview is presented within the context of the Welsh Government strategy for informatics.

Welsh National Health Services in Context

Wales has a population of approximately three million; it is one of the four constituent countries of the United Kingdom. Wales has devolved political powers, which means that the central Government of the United Kingdom has granted the Welsh Government statutory powers *at a sub national level*. Twenty areas of responsibility, known as 'subjects' have been granted and one of these is health. Healthcare is provided by the Welsh public health service, National Health Service (NHS) Wales.

The NHS in Wales employs close to 72,000 staff which makes it Wales' biggest employer. NHS Staff are drawn from many professions and occupational groups. In addition to staff employed directly by the NHS, there are contractor professions including dentists, opticians, pharmacists and nearly 2,000 General Practitioners (GPs) who predominantly work in primary care settings.

The NHS Wales health services were reconfigured in 2009, in order to deliver better healthcare to the population of Wales. The changes associated with the reconfiguration of services came into effect on the 1st October 2009; seven Health Boards and three Trusts were created, replacing 22 Local Health Boards and 7 Trusts. Figure 17.1 illustrates the geographical areas covered by the Health Boards. The three Trusts; the Welsh Ambulance Services NHS Trust, Public Health Wales and the Velindre NHS Trust offer specialist services and have an all Wales focus.

The Welsh Government's Departments are headed by senior civil servants; the Director General for Health and Social Services is also Chief Executive of NHS Wales. As Chief Executive, NHS Wales, the Director is accountable to the Minister for Health and Social Services, and is responsible for providing policy advice and exercising strategic leadership and management of the NHS.

The Director General receives professional nursing advice from the Chief Nursing Officer (CNO) for Wales, who is the head of the Nursing and Midwifery Professions in NHS Wales (the largest single group of health professionals within the NHS in Wales) and is responsible for the professional performance and development of Nurse Directors and the nursing profession. The CNO provides expert professional advice on nursing, midwifery and specialist community public health matters to Welsh Government.

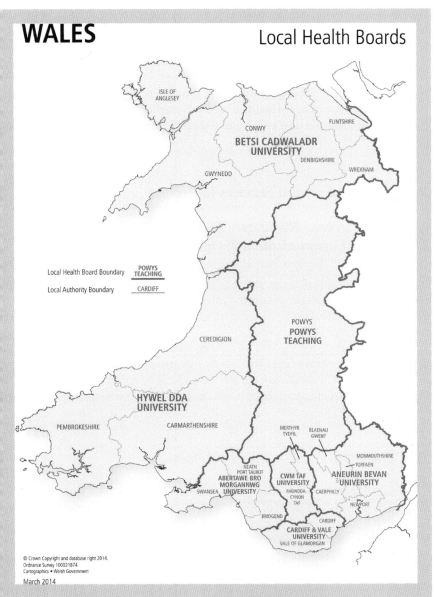

Fig. 17.1 NHS Wales Local Health Boards. Contains Ordnance Survey data © Crown copyright and database right 2014 (Reproduced with permission)

The description of some of the key nursing informatics strategic decision within Wales is intended to illustrate the importance of professional collabora tion at national and international levels in order to reduce duplication of effor and to efficiently share good practice. It is hoped that the lessons from Wale: will signpost readers to other local Welsh informatics initiatives that have no been explicitly described in this chapter, a number of which are sponsored by Welsh Universities, Local Health Boards, Welsh Trusts, the Royal College o Nursing[1] and local nursing and Allied Health Professional informatics interes groups.

Welsh National Health Services in Context

Enabling Improved Healthcare Delivery in Wales – Utilizing Information Communication Technology (ICT)

In order to improve health care delivery supported by ICT, the Welsh Governmen sponsored a key strategic document titled Informing Healthcare a National IT Programme for Wales [1] in 2004. The Informing Healthcare Programme (IHC) was established to progress this agenda.

The remit of IHC, subsequently the NHS Wales Informatics Service (NWIS), is to enable service improvement. Welsh policy directives have underpinned the direc- tion of all Wales ICT developments, the most recent being Together for Health [2]. The content of this chapter considers the impact of health informatics in Wales on Welsh Nurses.

The Use of ICT to Enable Improved Care Delivery

The strategic objectives of the Welsh Government in relation to healthcare services are to position patients and citizens at the centre of modern, efficient and high quality services [1, 2] and to ensure that individuals have greater access to information about their health and the ability to provide feedback on the quality of services they receive. One of the organizations committed to enabling this approach is NHS Wales Informatics Service (NWIS), the national IT programme for Wales, formed in April 2010, which was previously known as Informing Healthcare [1]. NWIS is concerned with the development of new methods, tools and technologies to transform NHS Wales for the benefit of the people of Wales. Modernizing eHealth service delivery and promoting new ways of working through better access to information and

---

[1] The **Royal College of Nursing (RCN)** is a union membership organization with over 395,000 members in the United Kingdom. It was founded in 1916, receiving its Royal Charter in 1928.

knowledge is a key aim of the national IT Programme. Recognition within the current health and social care environment regarding the range of constraints to the effective use of information communication technology supporting the delivery of care has been a critical step in the transformational process. Constraints identified include:

- Poor preparation of users of ICT;
- Poor access to information technology systems;
- A limited range of systems to address the effective management of patient/client information;
- Variability in staff skills and experience in the use of technology; and
- Inadequate education and training of system users.

Involving nurses in developments utilizing ICT to deliver improved clinical care in Wales is fully supported by the country's senior nurses. Some of the prerequisites of effective delivery of technology supported by nurses have been identified as understanding;

- the clinical and business requirements, including the design of the planned service,
- the process for the delivery of the service,
- utilization and/ or defining technical and information standards; and
- the preparation of the users of the new technologies.

The importance of involving nurses in ICT developments has been described by Thomas and Warm [3]. Survey reports by the Royal College of Nursing [4] indicated that nurses have clear opinions on the ways in which information technology can help to deliver care to patients. Early studies undertaken by the Nomina Group [5] highlighted developments in nursing, health informatics, and the management and use of nursing information. The recommendations contained in this report are still relevant; in particular the recommendation that the nursing profession should be actively involved in all programs leading to the development of electronic health records.

Oroviogoicoechea et al. [6] suggests that for effective implementation of information and communication technology (ICT) systems, that are to be used by nurses, critical issues such as attitude and culture as well as broader technological solutions need to be addressed. This notion is supported by Hannah et al. [7] and Clark [8] who suggest that nurses need to be at the forefront of informatics development, to achieve this aspiration; nurses should be actively included in informatics developments and have opportunities to develop their understanding of the benefits of clinical informatics. Nurses competent in change management can lead transformation in the use of ICT [9].

Surveys from several countries, show that front line nurses are not necessarily confident or have the necessary skills to use ICT effectively [10, 11]. The DKIW Framework, discussed in chapter one emphasizes the importance of nursing informatics education and the importance of good data to create a strong knowledge framework for the profession.

Table 17.1 The key principles underpinning the Informing Healthcare framework in Wales

Listening – The view of nurses and midwives about the potential benefits and application of information communication technology (ICT) to enhance the provision of care by defining the most appropriate way of capturing the clinical expertise of nurses from all disciplines and at all levels within organizations, formed a key component of the implementation of the framework

Influencing – Ensuring that the nursing and midwifery profession in Wales has the opportunity to shape the design and testing of new technological methods early in the process. This requires engagement at both a national and local level

Evaluation – Measuring the effectiveness of the engagement process and subsequently applying the lessons learned from the process

Overview of Welsh Nursing Informatics 2007–2013

The Welsh national IT Programme, Informing Healthcare (subsequently NHS Wales Informatics Service) supported the introduction of new processes through incremental service improvement projects. These projects ensured that new ICT and information services, based on sound evidence, delivered real benefits to patients and the public. The organization's founding principle was continuous consultation and engagement with clinicians and key stakeholders to drive service development.

In 2007, the Informing Healthcare programme appointed a National Nurse Lead to support the development of clinical informatics and to establish effective engagement with the nursing profession in Wales. During 2007/2008 senior nurses in Wales were consulted about a framework (the framework) for engaging nurses, midwives and specialist public health nurses in the Informing Healthcare change management agenda.

The aim of the framework was to work in partnership with nurses and other healthcare professionals in Wales to identify, develop, test and evaluate the benefits of potential electronic solutions to assist and improve the outcomes of care for patients, carers and service users.

The objectives of the framework included:

- Creating a useful and manageable method of two way communication and dissemination of information within and between key stakeholder groups;
- Contributing to testing new technological methods from a nursing and clinical perspective; and
- Evaluating the contribution of the framework in relation to influencing the ICT agenda in Wales.

The key principles underpinning the framework were listening, influencing and evaluating. Table 17.1 provides more detail.

To enact the aims and objectives, as agreed by senior nurses in Wales, a National Nursing and Midwifery Advisory Group (the advisory group) was established. Outputs from the advisory group included; contributing to the development of IHC products and services including associated clinical risk management/ patient safety

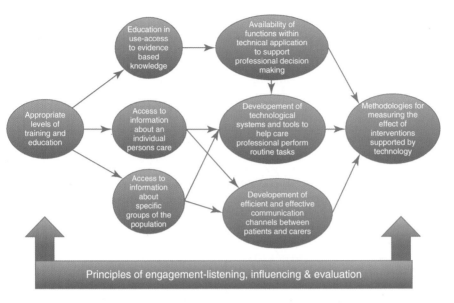

Fig. 17.2 Conceptual overview of the eight Principles in Community Nursing Strategy in support of emerging nursing eHealth agenda in Wales

activities, and influencing the e-health agenda associated with the Welsh Government initiatives in particular the Community Nursing Strategy for Wales (2009) [12].

   To provide a context for the advisory group, a draft set of eight principles were developed in order to guide the group's activities. These principles were subsequently endorsed by senior nurses in Wales and included in the Community Nursing Strategy for Wales. Figure 17.2 offers a conceptual overview of the eight principles and a summary Table 17.2, which provides an illustration of the eight principles.

Eight Principles to Support the Emerging Nursing E-Health Agenda In Wales

Welsh Nurses opinions about ICT supporting community nursing services informed a Community Nursing Strategy which was launched in September 2009 by the Welsh Government. The strategy contains a range of chapters that cover the areas of particular relevance to community nurses. Chapter eight of the strategy discusses the impact of the e-health agenda on the nursing profession in Wales. The development of the e-health chapter was led by Informing Healthcares National Nurse Lead with input from the advisory group and others, for example the Royal College of Nursing in Wales.

   The core set of principles relating to Information Communication Technology enabled healthcare delivery in this eHealth chapter are of particular importance, as

Table 17.2 Principles eHealth Agenda

Access to up to date, evidence based knowledge to support the delivery of modern health and social care services:
The efficient and effective collection, retrieval, analysis and communication of information enables informed decisions to support treatment and care planning options that can provide the data necessary to support service planning and resource management. Knowledge management and the subsequent development of knowledge management tools will provide: the evidence upon which the provision of health care can be informed; support for clinical audit; the evidence to support service planning and resource management, and assistance with research and development activities
Access to information about an individual persons care (*contained in an individual's health record*):
Supporting staff to undertake their day to day activities through the capture of real time standardized patient/ client information, should be the ultimate goal. Clinical staff need to be able to receive and record information at the point of care using appropriate devices such as laptops, mobile computers with touch screens/graphic tablet screens, or Personal Digital Assistants (PDAs)
Access to information about specific groups of the population:
The ability to access accurate information about specific groups within the population and subsequently to introduce a more community focused service for patients/ clients is a challenge for health and social care service providers. The ability to identify people at risk of, either unplanned admission to hospital services or those in need of additional packages of care, has the potential to inform proactive care management
The development of efficient and effective communication channels between patients/ clients and care givers and between professional groups that provide care:
New and emerging plans for the redesign of services need to consider the linkages and impact of information technology to these services. Managing the information available within and between health, social care, independent and voluntary sector organizations and other public sector organizations is fundamental to the creation of improved service design. Digital communications, use of e –mail, conference call facilities and call centers as communications as a means of communication have become an essential part of working practice for many employed in the NHS in Wales
The provision of technological systems and tools that help the health professional perform routine tasks:
There are a number of system options that could be used to support the delivery of health care, as a minimum the system should provide functionality that allows effective and efficient recoding of information to support; the record of assessment of care need, development of care plans and monitoring of care delivered
The availability of functions within technical applications to support professional decision making:
Supporting professional decision making with technical applications has been proven to be efficient and effective. Functions that are available to improve safety include; alerts and warnings for example, relating to administration of medications. As more complex care is delivered in community settings, including people's homes this functionality will be extremely important
Appropriate levels of training and education:
The training and education of clinical staff is critically important, preparation for clinical practice in an electronic world is should be embedded in all clinical education learning programs. The challenge is to embed within all educational learning programs an understanding of information management, information governance requirements and the underlying principles upon which information systems and the proper use of IT in healthcare depend
Methodologies for measuring the effect of interventions supported by technology:
Audit packages, scheduling systems and the development of intelligent performance indicators are potential methods for measuring the effectiveness of interventions supported by technology

Table 17.3 ICT supporting community nursing services

There must be appropriate financial investment in the system and associated technical equipment (for example mobile devices);
The design of ICT systems must be informed by nurses;
Information systems need to satisfy clinical and managerial requirements;
ICT solutions must enable seamless sharing of essential information to support service delivery; and
All nurses should receive appropriate training and support in the use of technology solutions

set out in Table 17.2. These principles continue to be relevant for nurses in Wales as the e-health agenda progresses.

Following the launch of the Community Nursing Strategy, during 2009, a survey that utilized the principles outlined in the strategy, was undertaken by IHCs Clinical Informaticist (Nursing). The survey involved 144 district nurses and health visitors; the themes identified by those responding to the survey questionnaire, with respect to the vision for a community nursing service supported by ICT, have been included in Table 17.3.

The results of the survey have been instrumental in informing the requirements of the emerging approach to the procurement of a community system for Wales and are equally relevant to acute and specialist care settings.

The National IT Programme – NHS Wales Informatics Service

On 1 October 2009, NHS Wales Informatics Service (NWIS) reaffirmed its commitment to developing clinical informatics skills to support the NHS in Wales. Large-scale NHS reforms took place in Wales, 22 Local Health Boards (LHBs) and seven NHS Trusts were replaced with seven integrated Local Health Boards, responsible for all health care services. In addition, three new Trusts were formed: Public Health Wales NHS Trust, Velindre NHS Trust, the specialist cancer Trust and Welsh Ambulance Services NHS Trust.

As part of the Welsh healthcare reform programme 2009, the NHS Wales Informatics Service (NWIS) was established on April, 1, 2010, replacing the Informing Healthcare programme. The new arrangements will allow ICT resources to work together more closely to support a consistent approach to health informatics and the implementation of common national systems. The new organization was formed by merging Informing Healthcare, Health Solutions Wales, the Business Services Centre (Information Management and Technology section), the Corporate Health Information Programme and the Primary Care informatics Programme. The new organization has a national remit to support the transformation of NHS Wales making better use of ICT skills and resources.

New technologies affect many aspects of care delivery, from patient administration and clinical documentation systems to decision support aids. Hersh [13] highlights the importance of involving the expertise and knowledge of healthcare professionals to ensure emerging technologies are appropriate for clinical use.

Ensuring clinicians are skilled in the use of new technologies is essential, particularly if they are to describe the clinical requirements to system developers, and help implement these new technologies. Huryk in 2010 [14] reported that nurses are more likely to be satisfied with a system if they have been involved in its design. Stevens in 2010 [15] suggested that nurse involvement in system design can yield positive results because they understand the context in which the system will be used and can link it with issues such as patient safety and user acceptance.

Warm and Thomas [16] reviewed the effectiveness of the clinical informaticist role and findings supported earlier studies [17–20] demonstrating that excluding healthcare professionals from the development of IM&T systems is likely to be detrimental to their design. Helping clinicians to understand the importance and benefit of technology, and including their input in the design process, can help ensure that patients receive the best possible care [21, 22].

Hersh [13] reviewed the literature and established that the role of an informatician includes involving a local expert who is representing the user community, providing a link between IM&T and clinical staff. Likewise studies completed in the United States [23, 24] indicated that developing clinical informatics as a subspecialty of medicine and health care is an important role. They pointed to work undertaken by the American Medical Informatics Association to identify the key tasks performed by clinical informatics staff, categorizing these tasks into four knowledge and skills areas: fundamentals of care and technology use; clinical decision making and care process improvement; health information systems; and leadership and management of change.

To explore the potential influence that clinicians with an interest in informatics could make in the Welsh context, there are a range of part and full time clinical posts within the Clinical Directorate of the NHS Wales Informatics Service. In 2009, Informing Healthcare created two new Clinical Informaticist posts as secondment opportunities (subsequently permanent appointments); one nursing and one Allied Health Professional post. The aim was to create a learning environment for the post holders to be able to build upon their existing skills and interests in informatics. The purpose of these roles is to provide professional expertise to NWIS, to influence policy and (in respect of the nursing post) to promote nursing and nurse engagement in informatics development.

Many e-health developments need to be led by clinical professionals with appropriate skills to ensure that they are suitable for use in a clinical setting and provide enhanced delivery of care to patients and citizens. Warm and Thomas [16] describe the impact of the appointment of new Clinical Informaticist roles within the NHS Informatics Service (NWIS) and the intention of the posts to support the delivery of ICT initiatives.

An evaluation of the impact of the NWIS Clinical Informaticists roles was undertaken in 2010–2011. While the evaluation was based on a small sample size of interviewees, the findings suggest that the post holders have a positive impact on; the strategic development and delivery of ICT in NHS Wales; contribution to NWIS business activities, provide support for all Wales e-health initiatives and in the provision of subject matter expertise both within NWIS and broader NHS Wales.

In the first instance, the areas of responsibility identified for the Clinical Informaticists, employed initially within IHC and subsequently NWIS included:

Providing clinical leadership and advice to NWIS programme and project managers on the key clinical aspects of project development;
Ensuring adherence to professional standards;
Enabling nurses and allied health professional engagement in programmer and project development; and
Developing and agreeing on new policies, protocols and procedures to ensure sufficient local guidance, with the aim to promote safe and efficient delivery of care.

Some of the post holders main activities are; reviewing NWIS Clinical risk management process, engaging with professional groups, peer-to-peer contact, testing products, reviewing standards and guidance documentation, and attending meetings and conferences.

Evaluation Responses

Post holder responses to the evaluation questions indicate that from their perspective they: actively support NWIS Programmes and projects, including product testing, they make an important contribution to the design of products and services and are instrumental in identifying potential patient safety risks, and importantly have improved engagement activities with NHS colleagues.

Although engagement with the post holders is good, some interviewees said there is scope for the role to be more clearly defined, particularly in relation to knowing in which activities the post holders could be asked to become involved.

The interviewees reported that clinical experience and understanding were the most important attributes of the Clinical Informaticist role. Particular reference was made to professional integrity and the commitment to safeguarding the interests of the patient and wider public. Interviewees also highlighted the importance of clinical knowledge and experience and the ability to work with non-clinicians to translate the clinical requirement in support of ICT developments.

Since commencing employment the nursing, post holder has been involved in:

Undertaking a national survey to elicit the information requirements for community nurses and facilitating workshops to validate these requirements;
Representing Welsh nursing informatics at UK wide meetings;
Influencing the inclusion of informatics learning outcomes in the pre-registration nursing curriculum;
Supporting the development of information standards for national nursing care quality indicators;
Supporting the NHS Wales Informatics Service clinical risk management process, by encouraging nurses to become actively involved in clinical risk management workshops;

- Steering the development of a 'National Complex Care Database[2]' through the governance and quality assurance process;
- Influencing the design of the Welsh Clinical Portal[3];
- Undertaking technical testing of the Individual Health Record (IHR[4]);

Similar activities have been undertaken by other members of the Clinical Directorate under the leadership of the NWIS Nurse Director.

In addition to the work undertaken to support national ICT initiatives, nurses across Wales are actively involved in local ICT developments. Many of these activities are supporting national developments, though senior nurses in Wales recognize the requirement to share and develop local initiatives more widely.

Senior Nurses in Wales Reaffirm the Direction for Nursing and eHealth Agenda

During 2012 senior nurses in Wales recognized the need to reaffirm the direction for nursing in relation to the e-health agenda both within and outside Wales. The modernization agenda requires a nursing workforce confident in using information and communication technology to underpin practice and improve care delivery.

To enable the effective use of ICT, a Welsh e-Health nursing action plan has been approved by the Chief Nursing Officer and Nurse Directors in Wales. The four areas that have been identified for development in nursing informatics are developing clinical leadership, ensuring fitness for practice, encouraging collaborative working, and supporting patient focused activities.

Developing Clinical Leadership is achieved by:

- Ensuring nurses are at the fore-front of the design, implementation and quality assurance (particularly clinical risk management) of information communication technology;
- Involving nurses in requirements gathering and requirements assurance to influence system and service design and development; and
- Proactively managing the potential "data burden" as nurses collect and interpret data and information associated with quality improvement and performance management.

---

[2] Continuing NHS Healthcare (CHC) involves a package of ongoing care arranged and funded by the NHS. Determination of eligibility for adults is undertaken via a nationally defined process, and based upon multi-disciplinary and multi-agency assessment. Such assessments, and the subsequent decision process, can be complex and are undertaken within the context of an evolving legal position. A requirement for all Health Boards in Wales to have access to National Complex Care Database has been achieved.

[3] The Welsh Clinical Portal (WCP) is a secure health space, where key elements of information, from a range of computer systems and databases used in NHS Wales is brought together. It provides clinical staff with a single immediate view of information needed to support clinical decisions. Existing functionality includes; patient lists, electronic pathology test requesting and results viewing and radiology reported and image viewing.

[4] NHS Wales Informatics Service is working with a major General Practitioner system supplier to deliver a national Individual Health Record (IHR) solution. The IHR enables health staff working in 'Out of Hours' services to view important elements of the patients general practice record.

Ensuring Fitness for Practice

- Preparing nurses, both pre- and post-registration, to utilise Information Communication Technology as part of their everyday activities by ensuring they are able to acquire appropriate skill levels supported by professional standards;
- Supporting nurses through the change management process associated with the transition from traditional forms of nursing practice to those that utilise the benefits of ICT; and
- Ensuring nurses have the skills to critique and interpret information and use it to improve care delivery.

Encouraging Collaborative Working

- Sharing all Wales Nursing skills, resource and best practice in nursing informatics; and
- Creating links with nursing informatics groups across the UK and beyond.

Supporting Patient Focused Activities

- Involvement of nurses in activities associated with ensuring ICT systems are clinically safe;
- Enabling nurses to harness ICT to maximise time spent on direct clinical care;
- Ensuring the appropriate Information Governance[5] arrangements are in place to protect patient privacy; and
- Empowering patients to be involved in their own care planning including assisting them with the use of new technologies for example social media and assistive technologies.

To take forward this exciting agenda, the Nurse Directors in Wales have sponsored a Welsh e-health Nursing Forum (the Forum) and have nominated representatives from their respective organizations to provide the expertise necessary to take forward the work of the Forum on their behalf. The work plan of the Forum will reflect the changing emphasis of the use of informatics within the profession.

The actions and suggested tasks to deliver the actions, as discussed by the Chief Nursing Officer for Wales and Nurse Directors in Wales, have been included below. They are not presented in order of priority, though all will be drivers for the Welsh e-Health Nursing Forum terms of reference (Table 17.4).

---

[5] **Information governance**, or **IG**, is an emerging term used to encompass the set of multidisciplinary structures, policies, procedures, processes and controls implemented to manage information at an enterprise level, supporting an organization's immediate and future regulatory, legal, risk, environmental and operational requirements.

Table 17.4 e-health Forum action plan 2013

Action:

Develop a competent Welsh nursing workforce capable of applying nursing informatics skills to improve patient/ client care

Delivery task(s)

Work with Health Boards, academic institutes and other relevant organisations to create learning opportunities for nurses to develop competencies in nursing informatics

Encourage the publication of research and interest articles on nursing informatics

Action:

Utilise the informatics nursing skills and experience that has been developed by the national programme (NWIS) to support the implementation of national projects and to provide expert advice for the development of local projects

Delivery task(s):

Explore the potential opportunities and benefits of developing Clinical Informaticist roles as part of mainstream service development

Undertake a baseline review of the numbers of nurses working in local organisations who, as part of their current role, undertake/lead on nurse informatics activities for their organisation. Identify priorities and gaps in nursing informatics and make recommendations for future developments

Action:

Create collaborative partnerships with influential nursing organisations and nursing colleagues within and outwith the UK

Delivery Task(s):

Develop a communication strategy to ensure nurses and other care givers are fully engaged with the work of the Welsh e-Health Nursing Forum

Continue the important work currently being undertaken by the 4 UK Home Countries e-Health Leads Partnership, which is sponsored by the UK Chief Nursing Officers

Action:

Support Patient Focused ICT Activities

Delivery task(s)

Consider ways to effectively empowering patients to be involved in their own care planning including assisting them with the use of new technologies for example social media and assistive technologies

In order to demonstrate the effectiveness of the Welsh e-Health Nursing Forum, an evaluation framework will consider the four key areas of development in nursing informatics (i.e. clinical leadership, fitness for practice, collaborative working and support for patient focused activities) This framework is likely to include the following measurement criteria:

Levels of engagement with the e-health Forum by front line nurses including requests for support with local projects;

Number of specific Clinical Informaticist roles within clinical areas

Evidence that informatics skills are becoming mandatory as part of nurse education training and development; and

The number of nurse led initiatives associated with social media and assistive technologies

---

Use of Information to Support and Monitor Improvements Relating to Care

The use of information to support and monitor health care improvements involving nurses in Wales is ongoing. In this section, four core examples are used for illustrative purposes: first, nursing quality metrics, secondly the electronic recording of nursing assessments, thirdly the use of social media, and finally telehealth services.

Nursing Quality Metrics

The use of nursing quality metrics as a tool to measure the nursing contribution to care delivery is increasingly being used in the United Kingdom. The concept of nursing metrics should show how successful nursing care is in a specific area and should focus on the outcomes for which nurses can realistically be held accountable [25].

The Fundamentals of Care Guidance for Health and Social Care Staff (2003) [26] underpins part of a Welsh Government initiative, Free to Lead Free to Care (2008) [27] the intention, to improve the quality aspects of health and social care for adults. The Fundamentals of Care guidance lists 12 aspects of care that have been identified by patients and caregivers as being the most important, when they or a loved one, is in receipt of health or social care. The aspects of care are:

- Communication and information;
- Respecting people;
- Ensuring safety;
- Promoting independence;
- Relationships;
- Rest, sleep and activity;
- Ensuring comfort alleviating pain;
- Personal hygiene and appearance and foot care;
- Eating and drinking;
- Oral health and hygiene;
- Toilet needs; and
- Preventing pressure sores.

All Local Health Boards and Trusts in Wales are required to report progress on an annual basis against these areas of activity. Ensuring that the collection of meaningful data occurs, a Welsh electronic data collection system is used. This system, the design of which has been driven by frontline nursing staff, is currently being upgraded in response to new requirements that have emerged since its initial implementation. In addition to being the system to support the annual audit requirement, it also supports the collection of local quality care metrics; this information feeds the emerging national quality indicators.

Electronic Recording of Nursing Assessments

An emergent area of development in support of improved nursing care delivery is the electronic recording of nursing assessments. The principles and professional standards associated with good record keeping will inform and influence the approach to electronic recording of patient information in Wales [5, 28].

As electronic health records develop and the move towards integrated care records evolves, it is essential that information is consistent and transferrable across health and social care settings. Extensive work to develop clinical and technical information standards has been undertaken by a number of international groups, though enforcing standards has not been particularly effective in the United Kingdom. As record keeping practices and record structures change, relevant and appropriate informatics standards will inform the approach that will be taken in Wales.

Use of Social Media

Nurses as knowledgeable professionals communicate and collaborate with patients to assist with person/ patient centered care planning, and are well placed to utilize social media as a tool to assist with this process. Demystifying social media tools is essential if nurses are to embrace the opportunities social media can provide in supporting modern healthcare delivery.

There are undoubtedly benefits to using social media in healthcare. For example, fostering professional connections, educating and informing healthcare professionals, promoting timely communication with patients and their family, such opportunities for nurses are both exciting and necessary, although keeping abreast of good practice developments and constraints and emerging problems is essential.

Social media tools can improve the quality and access to education resources, offering nurse learners the opportunity to share knowledge, offer each other peer to peer support, including the creation of communities of learning/forums.

Communication technologies are available to help manage treatment-related symptoms, particularly in the community and remote and rural settings, and nurses are well placed to develop patient-driven models of care that will challenge traditional care giving models by actively encouraging patient engagement.

Social media can and should be used by nurses as a vehicle for communicating public health messages. Citizens are getting organized; they are collaborating and using social media sites like PatientsLikeMe [29], and building their own self-help sites. This suggests that patients are taking greater control of their health and that in the near future, online interaction with nurses will be an expectation. Technology will not replace the expert nurse; the challenge for nurses is to embrace technology as a key enabler to transform the delivery of health services.

Nurse leaders and managers of healthcare organizations have a duty to capitalize on the opportunities presented, encouraging nurse's use of the internet and social media tools to support healthcare delivery and patient involvement in care planning. Nurse leaders must provide guidance to nurses on the effective use of electronic media in a way that maintains the correct level of patient privacy and confidentiality.

Telecare, Telehealth and Assistive Technologies

Telecare, telehealth and assistive technology[6] developments are emerging across the UK; they have been used to support intermediate care, rehabilitation services and to reduce the use of unscheduled care services.

Nurses have an opportunity to actively encourage and empower people to be involved in their care. This empowerment happens through information sharing and inclusion in care planning and the application of technology to support the care plan. The trend in the use of smart phones and mobile applications in healthcare, particularly amongst individuals with chronic conditions is increasing.

These new technologies have the potential to improve quality of life, reduce unnecessary hospital and care home admissions, and support care integration by providing care and disease management from multi-disciplinary care teams linked remotely to users.

Next Steps for Nursing Informatics In Wales......

Organizations in NHS Wales adhere to national policies and procedures and develop local policies and procedures to protect individuals who receive care and those that provide it. Respecting dignity and privacy is integral to this approach.

In June 2010, the UK Government Secretary of State for Health launched a full public inquiry chaired by Robert Francis, Queens Council Barrister (QC) into the standard of care delivered at the Mid Staffordshire Foundation NHS Trust. The remit of the public inquiry was "*to examine the operation of the commissioning, supervisory and regulatory organizations and other agencies, including the culture and systems of those organizations in relation to their monitoring role at Mid Staffordshire NHS Foundation Trust between January 2005 and March 2009 and to examine why problems at the Trust were not identified sooner, and appropriate action taken*" [30, p.xx]

In February 2012, Robert Francis QC published the findings of the independent report into the concerns about the poor quality of care at Mid Staffordshire Foundation NHS Trust. The full report of the public inquiry was published in February 2013.

---

[6] **Assistive Technology** is a term that includes assistive, adaptive, and rehabilitative devices that interact with technology for people with disabilities.

The headline of the inquiry identified, "*a story of terrible and unnecessary suffering of hundreds of people who were failed by a system which ignored the warning signs of poor care and put corporate self interest and cost control ahead of patients and their safety.*"

While the remit of the report focuses on England, there are significant implications for Wales and Welsh nurses, including the requirement to develop strategies to ensure a situation similar to the one that occurred in Mid Staffordshire Foundation NHS Trust does not occur in Wales.

The recommendations contained in the Francis Report [30] are targeted at changes required by; Central Government, Regulatory Bodies (including the General Medical Council, the Nursing and Midwifery Council and the Royal College of Nursing), Commissioners and Providers of services. Of particular note is the concept of criminal liability for failures in care. The implication of this decision is that data and information relating to service quality and performance must be timely, accurate, reliable and easily available.

The main emphasis within the Francis Report is the requirement to improve the culture of the NHS, in particular to raise concerns about the delivery of unacceptable patient care, unacceptable clinical practice and unacceptable risk. Clearly the recommendations have implications for frontline clinical and nursing care and in the context of e-health there are links to the importance of:

- The creation of a usable electronic record, with appropriate safeguards to ensure safe communication of patient information;
- Patient access to their records, including the ability to enter information into the record; and
- Transparent publication of data and information.

Senior nurses in Wales are committed to ensuring effective collaboration with all appropriate nursing groups in Wales and beyond, in order to deliver agreed development activities that will address the implications of the Mid Staffordshire NHS Trust inquiry and aim to answer the following questions:

- What activities are required to determine the most efficient and effective nursing service models that can be supported by ICT?
- What are the relevant outcome measures that can/ should be introduced to demonstrate the effectiveness, or otherwise, of agreed nursing interventions and the outcomes of the interventions?
- What is the most appropriate and efficient methodology for creating information standards to enable accurate comparison of nursing performance locally, nationally, internationally?

The approach to answering these questions will be informed by the newly formed e Health Forum. Members of the Forum have been tasked with ensuring that the nursing profession influences the change associated with the use of technology to improve patient care and support the protection of the public.

It is anticipated that some of the mechanisms to improve the effective use of technology in support of improved healthcare delivery will include:

- partnerships with appropriate organisations/ehealth Forums;
- effective management of healthcare data;
- identification of information requirements to support service improvement;
- influencing the development of clinical and technical standards;
- supporting the assurance processes in particular the clinical safety of ICT products;
- identification of the benefits of new technologies;
- effective sharing good practice, by creating e-links with established networks;
- a reference group for nursing initiatives in Wales, that involves the use of information and communication technologies; and
- evaluation and publication of the Forums activities.

Conclusion

There can be little doubt that as countries across the globe grapple with austerity, the need for new healthcare service models that can be enabled by information and communications technologies will materialize. The rapid development of technology coupled with greater availability and ease of access by citizens and health care professionals, particularly access to demographic and personal information is changing the fabric of societies.

The principles adopted by senior nurses in Wales are listed below:

- Access to up-to-date, evidence-based knowledge to support the delivery of modern health and social care services;
- Access to information about an individual person's care (contained in an individual's health record);
- Access to information about specific groups of the population;
- The development of efficient and effective communication channels between patients/clients and care givers and between professional groups that provide care;
- The provision of technological systems and tools that help the health professional perform routine tasks;
- The availability of functions within technical applications to support professional decision making;
- Appropriate levels of training and education; and
- Methodologies for measuring the effect of interventions supported by technology continue to be the focus of nursing informatics developments.

The goal for Welsh nurse leaders is to pursue opportunities for collaboration with nurses and clinical professionals with an interest in clinical informatics, both within and out with Wales and the United Kingdom.

Acknowledgements My grateful thanks are extended to many dedicated Welsh nurses who have contributed to the exciting nursing informatics journey in Wales, the nursing informatics highlights describing the past 6 years of development would not have been possible without their commitment and determination. I would like to acknowledge in particular; Dr Daniel Warm and Mrs. Anne Owen colleagues I have worked closely with, as the content of this chapter has been produced.

References

1. Informing Healthcare – National IT Programme for Wales set up in 2003 by the Welsh Assembly Government. Available from http://www.wales.nhs.uk/sitesplus/documents/956/ihc_a5-e.pdf. Accessed 5 June 2013.
2. Welsh Government 2012 Together for Health Public Information Delivery Plan Welsh Government. Available from http://wales.gov.uk/docs/dhss/publications/111101togetheren.pdf. Accessed 5 June 2013.
3. Thomas B, Warm D. Providing support for the informing healthcare programme. Nurs Stand. 2009;26:35–41.
4. Royal College of Nursing. Speaking up; nurses and NHS IT developments: qualitative analysis results of an online survey by Nursix.com on behalf of the Royal College of Nursing http://tinyurl.com/3j5lagc. (Last accessed 17 June 2011), 2004.
5. Nomina Group. The Nursing Information Research Project: final report for the project board NHS Centre for coding and classification. http://tinyurl.com/3qifxqt (Last accessed 17 June 2011), 1988.
6. Oroviogoicoechea C, Elliott B, Watson R. Review evaluating information systems in nursing. J Clin Nurs. 2007;17:567–75.
7. Hannah KJ, Ball MJ, Edwards MJA. Introduction to nursing informatics. 3rd ed. New York: Springer; 2006.
8. Clarke J. Embrace new technology or others will decide how we end up using it (letter). Nurs Stand. 2008;22:17–32.
9. Courtney K, Alexander G, Demiris G. Information technology from novice to expert implementation implications. J Nurs Manag. 2008;16:692–9.
10. Cole IJ, Kelsy A. Computer and information literacy in post qualifying education. Nurse Educ Pract. 2004;4:190–9.
11. Eley R, Fallon T, Soar J, Bulkstra E, Hegney D. Nurses' confidence and experience in using information technology. Aust J Adv Nurs. 2008;25:23–35.
12. Welsh Assembly Government. Community nursing strategy Welsh Assembly Government; 2009.
13. Hersh W. Who are the informaticians? What we know and should know. J Am Med Inform Assoc. 2006;13:166–70.
14. Huryk L. Factors influencing nurses' attitudes towards healthcare information technology. J Nurs Manag. 2009;18:606–12.
15. Stevens M. Nurses as power users: the role of nursing informatics in health IT is growing http://tinyurl.com/43oev9y (Last accessed 17 June 2011), 2010.
16. Warm D, Thomas B. A review of the effectiveness of the clinical informaticist role. Nurs Stand. 2011;24:35–8.
17. McManus B. A move to electronic patient records in the community: a qualitative case study of a clinical data collection system, problems caused by inattention to users and human error. Top Health Inf Manage. 2000;20:23–37.
18. Harrop S, Wood-Harper A, Gilles A. Neglected user perspectives in the design of an online hospital bed-state system: implications for the National Programme for IT in the NHS. Health Informatics J. 2006;12:293–303.
19. Saleem N, Jones D, Van Tran H, Moses B. Forming design teams to develop healthcare information systems. Hosp Top. 2006;84:22–30.
20. Hannan T. Physicians need to understand the importance information technology in the 21st century (editorial). Int Med J. 2009;39:633–5.
21. Chaudry B, Wang J, Wu S, et al. Systematic review: impact of health information technology on quality, efficiency and costs of medical care. Ann Intern Med. 2006;144:742–52.
22. Black AD, Car J, Pagilari C, et al. The impact of eHealth on the quality and safety of healthcare: a systematic overview. PLoS Med. 2011;8(1):e1000387.

23. Detmer D, Lumpkin J, Williamson J. Defining the medical subspeciality of clinical informatics. J Am Med Inform Assoc. 2009;16:167–8.
24. Gardner R, Overhage M, Steen E, et al. Core content of the subspeciality of clinical informatics. J Am Med Inform Assoc. 2009;16:153–7.
25. Foulkes M. Nursing metrics: measuring quality in patient care. Nurs Stand. 2011;25:40–5.
26. Fundamentals for Health and Social Care 2003 http://www.wales.nhs.uk/document/acf1153.pdf.
27. Free to lead free to care. http://www.wales.nhs.uk/documents/cleanliness-report.pdf.
28. Patients like me. http://www.patientslikeme.com/.
29. Nursing and Midwifery Council. Nursing and Midwifery Council Record keeping: guidance for nurses and midwives; 2009.
30. Report of the mid Staffordshire NHS Foundation Trust Public Inquiry; 2013, London Stationery Office. ISBN 9780102981476.

Chapter 18
Case Study 4: Mobile Nursing in Health Information Systems

Polun Chang, Ming-Chuan Jessie Kuo, and Shaio-Jyue Lu

Abstract Mobile nursing has been a well-noticed but still emerging and exciting care delivery model for nursing. Nursing using mobile information technology such as notebooks, handheld devices, and mobile carts has been naturally designed and well documented due to the features of point of care provided by nurses (Lu et al., Int J Med Inform 74:409–422, 2005). Many design issues for useful mobile nursing have also been studied and reported (Chang et al., Comput Inform Nurs 29(3):174–183, 2011). Quality issues such as patient safety and medication administration also stimulate the use of mobile technology such as barcode readers. Various kinds of mobile nursing products and solutions can also be easily found on websites. It will not be a surprise that mobile nursing has and should become a very important care delivery model for nurses at practice today and the future.

Keywords Case study • Mobile Nursing • Handheld • Health Information Systems

Key Concepts

Case study
Mobile Nursing
Handheld
Health Information Systems

P. Chang, PhD (✉)
Institute of Biomedical Informatics, National Yang-Ming University, Taipei, Taiwan, ROC
e-mail: polunchang@gmail.com

M.-C.J. Kuo, RN, MS
Nursing Department, Cathay General Hospital, Taipei, Taiwan, ROC
e-mail: jessiemkuo@gmail.com

S.-J. Lu, RN, MS
Nursing Department, Taichung Veterans General Hospital, VACRS, Taichung, Taiwan, ROC
e-mail: sjlu@vghtc.gov.tw

© Springer-Verlag London 2015
K.J. Hannah et al. (eds.), *Introduction to Nursing Informatics*,
Health Informatics, DOI 10.1007/978-1-4471-2999-8_18

Mobile Nursing

Mobile nursing has been a well-noticed but still emerging and exciting care delivery model for nursing. Nursing using mobile information technology such as notebooks, handheld devices, and mobile carts has been naturally designed and well documented due to the features of point of care provided by nurses [1]. Many design issues for useful mobile nursing have also been studied and reported [2]. Quality issues such as patient safety and medication administration also stimulate the use of mobile technology such as barcode readers. Various kinds of mobile nursing products and solutions can also be easily found on websites. It will not be a surprise that mobile nursing has and should become a very important care delivery model for nurses at practice today and the future.

Mobile Nursing is not only dynamic in concept but also evolving in content, which makes it an exciting and unique nursing informatics topic. Though mobile devices have been used by nurses before 2007, the power of mobile nursing was recognized in 2007 when Apple launched the first iPhone. This introduction inspired clinical professionals, who have long complained the low usability of healthcare information systems, that the medical informatics applications could actually be easy to use, fun to use, and cause disruptive changes of caring models with creative imagination. Handheld mobile devices used in healthcare were no longer only for documentation, reference searching or communication. Integrated with cloud network and decision support modules, mobile devices could be used to design intelligent, cost-effective and evidence-based clinical information systems. The systems could support accurate and safe care to be efficiently delivered to patients at the point of care. Furthermore, from patient's perspective, with the right accessories and applications, smartphones could become convenient tools for people to automatically record their vital signs, such as blood pressure and heart rate, and transmit the data to nurse for care management and planning. This new environment of Mobile Health, integrated with mobile nursing, will no doubt bring up an exciting revolutionized healthcare opportunity [3].

The rapid advancement of ICT also makes Mobile Nursing more practical, affordable and acceptable. For example, handheld PDA has made nurses' documentation more simple barcode reader has made patient identification checking and prevention of medication administration errors easier; and mobile carts have brought the hospital information system closer to bedsides and made caring documentation more immediate. The integration of these features into a new product today makes the mobile nursing more feasible. Handheld devices integrated with barcode readers have been no more new toy and could be easily found from websites [4, 5]. To integrate with larger Pad-size display, these handheld devices will further enhance the usability of mobile solutions [6]. More mobile devices specifically designed for healthcare professionals for use at the point of care will be developed and launched to the market. When these mobile devices are installed with creative apps and cloud services, mobile nursing will become a new stimulating model and possibility for nursing.

However, the development of mobile nursing application is distinct and more conceptually complex than just putting a web-based system into mobile devices for viewing. Mobile devices are unique in its many features such as small display size, to be handheld, to be carried anytime, and being used in a mobile context. Usability issues like interface design, workflow reengineering, as well as creativity and involvement of nurses are highly important to create effective and useful mobile nursing applications. The following two examples will demonstrate the development process of effective mobile applications and how these applications are changing the way nurses provide better and safer care. Encouragingly, these two mobile solutions, led by nurses, were not only highly accepted by clinical nurses but also widely endorsed and supported by physicians.

The first case is about how a complex, heavy loading, and time consuming chemotherapy medication administration was improved by a mobile solution which simultaneously considered the factors of work reengineering, evidence-based guideline, decision support, identification and double checking into traditional medication administration and documentation process [7]. The second case is about how a NI team, which is mainly composed of nurses, designed a handheld pressure sore assessment support system for ICU nurses to improve assessment, documentation and coordinated care quality.

Case #1: Mobile Chemotherapy Medication Administration

The chemotherapy medication administration (CMA) process has been a very time-consuming nursing task with great safety responsibility [8]. There are a total of four safety double-checking points in the original manual process, as shown in Fig. 18.1, to assure the patient safety. The nurse needs to be very careful checking the medication and calculating the right IV drop rate. A 722-bed teaching, tertiary care medical center in Taipei serves more than 5,000 chemotherapy patients every year, has adopted a mobile cart solution with an electronic medication administration system, as shown in Fig. 18.2. Despite this technology to support practice, there continues to be complex, time consuming and difficult to manage as the cart cannot be easily mobilized to bedside, a standalone barcode reader is not well integrated into the workflow, and important caring guidelines are not readily available. The nursing leaders decided to develop the mobile CMA (mCMA) to simplify and streamline the work process while assuring the patient safety at the same time. In 2010, a task force, composed of one nursing informatics specialist and three IT engineers, was set up to work with the 10-staffed 59-bed Hematology & Oncology Ward.

Workflow Reengineering

The business process reengineering was used to design the mCMA. This process started with analyzing the current work process and its difficulty shown in Fig. 18.1. Eight work items were identified and determined after close discussion with the head nurse and staffs as the core functions of the new solution: patient identification, medication administration reminding, medication checking, physician order checking,

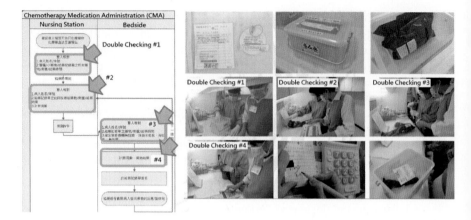

Fig. 18.1 Chemotherapy Medication Administration Process. There are four double-checking steps to assure the correctness of medication before administration (Courtesy of Cathay General Hospital, Taipei, Taiwan)

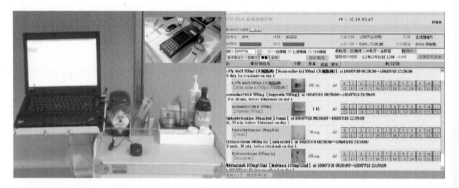

Fig. 18.2 Mobile car solution with first generation of barcode readers, left, and home-made electronic medication administration system, right

SOP guidelines, dosage automatic calculation, observation documentation and accident response. A prototype approach was used to design the interface so nurses could understand what the application would look like and how it would be used during their medication administration. IT engineers started to design the database and to code the application after the mCMA prototype model was approved by the NI specialist.

Developing Mobile Solution

A handheld 6″ sterilizable Wifi Android Pad with barcode reader was chosen as the hardware [6]. A non-web-based Android native application was developed using the open source Eclipse development toolset by IT engineers. Medication barcodes were placed on all medication containers and used for identification checking compared to the ordered medication list shown on the screen of Pad after patient's wristband barcode was scanned. An alert is issued whenever there is a mismatch between the data read by the barcode reader and the data read from hospital information system. Hospital care pathway guidelines for the accident prevention and response were included. All ten nurses from the unit were invited to evaluate the mCMA system. A 4-point Likert scale, in which 1 and 4 means completely disagree and completely agree respectively, questionnaire designed by the Technology Acceptance Model for Mobile Service model was used to evaluate nurses' acceptance of the system.

System and Nurse's Acceptance

Representative screen shots of the mCMA are shown in Figs. 18.3, 18.4, 18.5, 18.6, 18.7, 18.8 and 18.9. Nurse will see their patient list, Fig. 18.3, after log in. The application was designed based on nurses' workflow, Fig. 18.4, starting from medication preparation (Fig. 18.5), administration preparation (Fig. 18.6) to bedside administration (Fig. 18.7). During preparation, application could assist nurse on drip rate calculation, Fig. 18.8, or check the guidelines, Fig. 18.9. Nurse could check physician's order, Fig. 18.10. Nurse could documentation all necessary tasks such as biohazard waste disposal, Fig. 18.11. All tasks could be done in this single mobile solution.

The evaluation results confirmed nurses' high acceptance of the mobile system. Nurses showed high recognition of the system in all five measures, as shown in Fig. 18.12. Out of score of 4 ("strongly agree") on each measure, the results were Usefulness 3.95, Ease of Use 3.78, Ease to Learn 3.8, Acceptance 3.95 and Satisfaction 3.7. The Overall acceptance score is 3.83. Nurses commented that their work was simplified, guidelines were handy and it was helpful to train new members. The attending physicians showed positive support for this solution as they believed this could better assure patient's safety. There are currently more expectations on this mCMA, as nurses recommended the font could be larger so the system is easier to read and physicians wanted to join to enhance the documentation of patient's response to the medication. Consequently, this project is under modification to make it easier to use and to support the care team to better control and manage the outcomes of medication treatment.

Case #2: Mobile Support System of Prevention and Management of Pressure Sore

Prevention and management of pressure ulcers for patients in hospitals has been an important quality indicator for nursing. This issue is important in ICUs because it is one of most common problems in ICUs [9]. Due to the unique layout, limited space

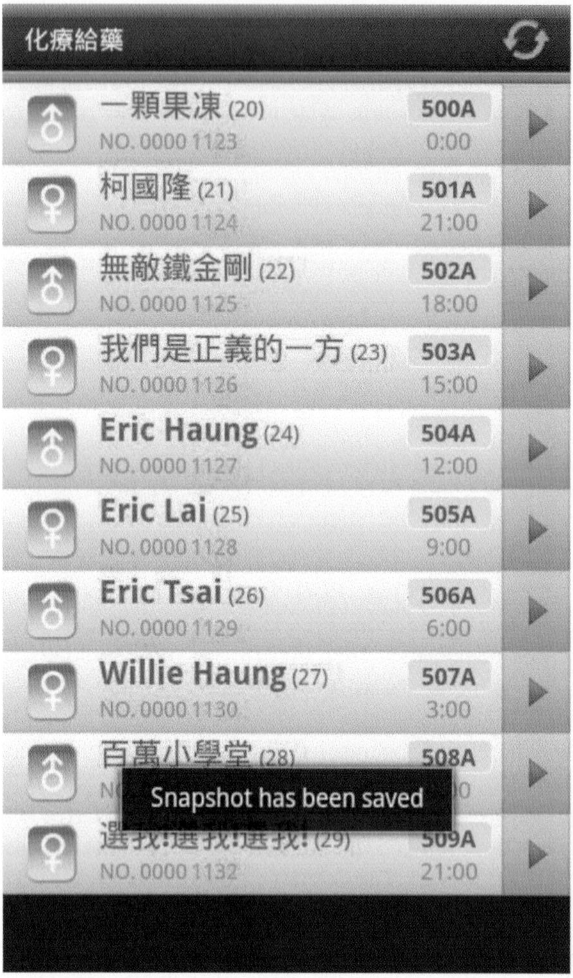

Fig. 18.3 Patient list after log in the application

and requirements of sterilization, there has been lack of appropriate information system support for ICU nurses in a 1,500-bed tertiary, teaching medical center in central Taiwan though this hospital has been well known for its nursing information system. In mid 2011, the internal study showed that there was as high as 25 % of error rate for pressure ulcer grading in ICUs. The nursing leaders decided to design a mobile support system for ICU nurses to improve their grading capability. A team, composed of one deputy nursing director, 4 ICU head nurses, as well as one NI specialist, was established to look for the mobile solution. The project was led, managed, and coded by nurses.

Fig. 18.4 CMA workflow

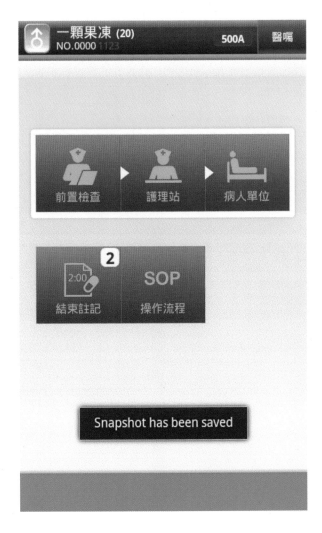

Designing Mobile Solution

The basic objective of this project was to support the documentation of patients' pressure ulcers by ICU nurses using the information system. In terms of hardware, due to the environment constraints and variety of devices, no cart solution was possible and only an Android handheld mobile solution was considered. Android development tools, such as Android SDKs and open source Eclipse tool kits were used for coding the Android native application. The application was designed to interact with the HIS. The application server was IBM WebsSphere

Fig. 18.5 Medication preparation

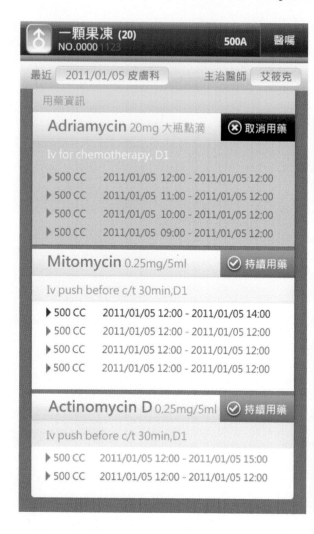

6.1 with Oracle 10G database. Two smartphones and three pad models for front line documentation were evaluated. Battery hours, barcode scanning response time and picture quality were the three key variables in evaluating the performance of solutions. The advanced objectives of this project were to better assure patient safety and to improve care coordination among care teams, especially between nurses and physicians. Contents of the mobile application were determined based on the consensus among care team. All care team members, including both nurses and physicians, were invited for evaluation. Nurses expressed their preferences from workflow, operating and caring process perspectives. Physicians mainly judged the quality of pictures taken and the facilitation of improving their treatment decisions.

Fig. 18.6 Administration
preparation

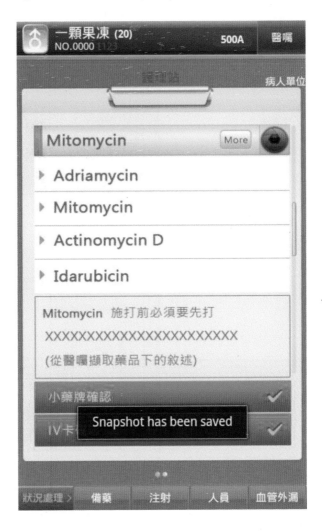

System and Nurses' Acceptance

A 6″ Pad with barcode reader was finally chosen due to its short barcode response time, large display size and clinical-setting specifications like sterilizability, waterproof and rug resistance. The mobile solution started with identifying patient's name with barcode reader, as shown in Fig. 18.13, after nurse logs into the system. The nurse then selects the pressure ulcer grading assessment and takes pictures, as shown in Fig. 18.14, for assessment and documentation. Both assessment results and pictures were saved to the hospital information system, as shown in Fig. 18.15, so all stakeholders including the attending physician and quality management nurse could read and respond immediately.

Fig. 18.7 Bedside administration

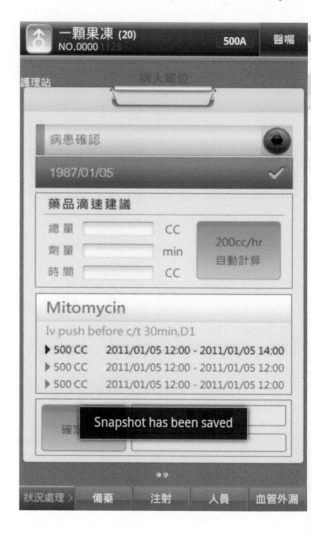

Though no complete evaluation of the mobile solution was done, this handheld mobile solution was put into practice right after it was designed because it was well accepted by ICU nurses with great satisfaction. By April 2013, 3,476 real cases were supported using this solution. It was found that the average of total operating time from scanning patient's wrist bands, assessing the pressure sore, documenting, taking pictures and uploading to system was only 2.6 min. This was very acceptable by ICU nurses. Nurses were satisfied with this new process because they could complete the entire process with one single mobile device. More importantly, the error

Fig. 18.8 Calculation of
drip rate

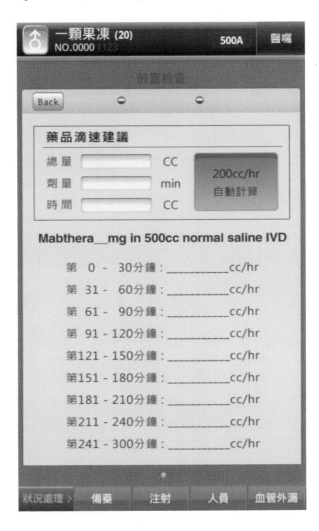

rate of grading pressure ulcers was decreased by 20 % so far. Better documentation
with more quality pictures also improved the shift report effectiveness and satisfaction among care team members. They found this system was also useful to train ICU
nurses in pressure ulcer assessment. Encouragingly, the physicians in the care team
expressed great support for this solution because they were very satisfied with the
pictures taken which highly improved their decisions in treating patient's pressure
ulcer. Currently, the nursing department has decided to extend the application of this
handheld mobile solution into wound caring and bundle care.

Fig. 18.9 Guidelines of CMA workflow

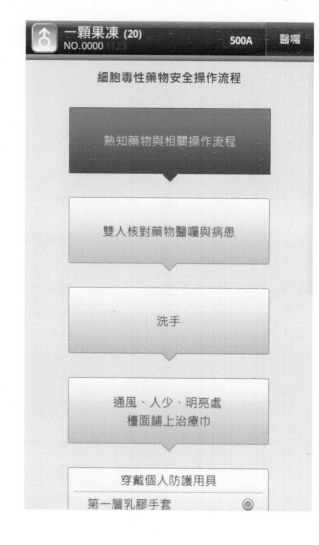

Fig. 18.10 Physician's order

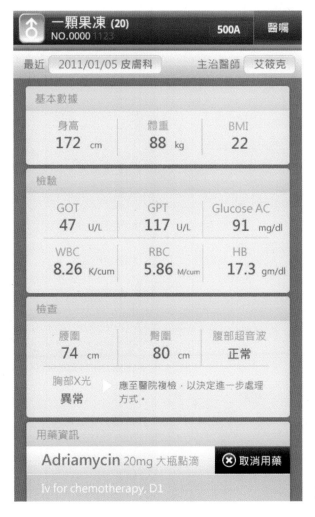

Fig. 18.11 Documentation for biohazard waste disposal

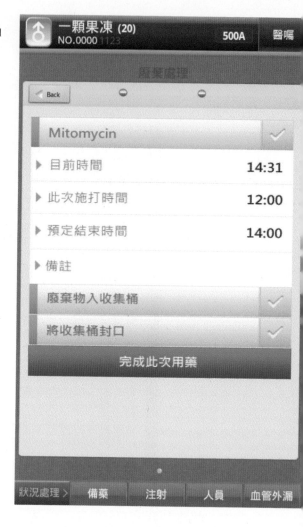

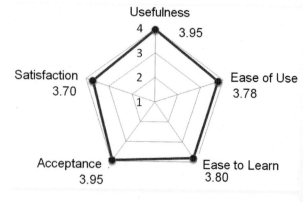

Fig. 18.12 Spider diagram of evaluation results of nurses' perceived acceptance of mobile chemotherapy medical administration solution. From a 4-point Likert scale, in which 4 means strongly agree, the results show nurses' high acceptance of solution

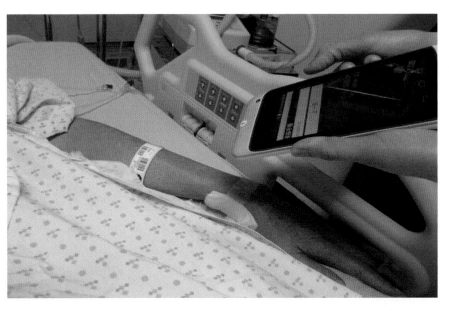

Fig. 18.13 ICU nurse assure patient's identity using handheld device with barcode reader

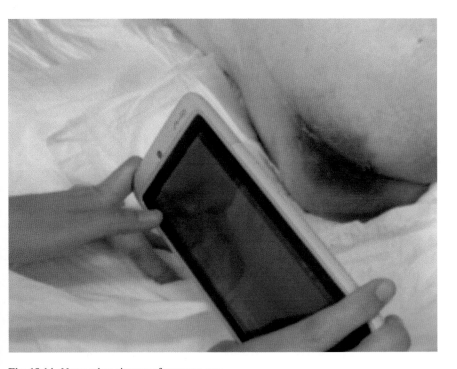

Fig. 18.14 Nurse takes pictures of pressure sore

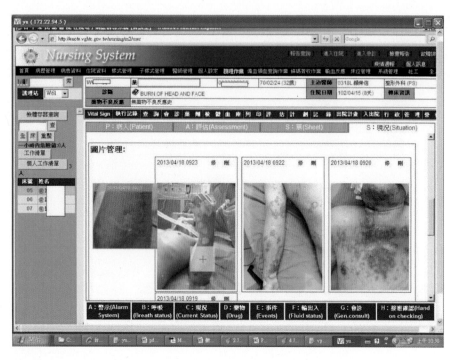

Fig. 18.15 Assessment results and pictures are saved into the hospital information system

References

1. Lu YC, Xiao Y, Sears A, et al. A review and a framework of handheld computer adoption in healthcare. Int J Med Inform. 2005;74:409–22.
2. Chang P, Hsu CL, Liou YM, Kuo YY, Lan CF. Design and development of interface design principles for complex documentation using PDAs. Comput Inform Nurs. 2011;29(3):174–83.
3. Kumar S, Nilsen W, Pavel M, Srivastava M. Mobile health: revolutionizing healthcare through trans-disciplinary research. Computer. 2013;46(1):28–35.
4. Mobility in Nursing. Available on http://www.motorola.com/web/Business/Products/Mobile%20Computers/Handheld%20Computers/MC75A0-HC/Documents/_staticfiles/Mobile-Nurse_SB_0910.pdf. Accessed on 4 May 2013.
5. Bedside Medication Administration. Available on http://codecorp.com/medicationadministration.php. Access on 4 May 2014.
6. Pocket-sized table computer designed for healthcare. Available on http://miocare.mio.com/index_enGBR.asp. Accessed on 4 May 2013.
7. Kuo MC, Chang P. Developing a Chemotherapy mMAR Support System. Poster presented at the American Medical Informatics Association 2012 Symposium, 2012, Chicago, IL, USA.
8. Jacobson JO, Polovich M, McNiff KK, LeFebvre KB, Cummings C, Galioto M, Bonelli KR, McCorkle MR. American Society of Clinical Oncology/Oncology Nursing Society chemotherapy administration safety standards. J Clin Oncol. 2009;27:5469–75.
9. Reilly EF, Karakousis GC, Schrag SP, Stawicki SP. Pressure ulcers in the intensive care unit: the "forgotten" enemy. OPUS 12 Scientist. 2007;1(2):17–30.

Chapter 19
The Future Is a Sharp 90° Turn

Stephen P. Murray

"Is Health Informatics the panacea of an ailing Health Sector: rising costs, limited resources, higher patient acuity, fractured organizations, conflicting priorities?" "Are you and nursing informatics part of the solution or part of the challenge?" You decide.

Abstract The future of health informatics has no bounds; the areas of consideration encompass technologies, both hardware and software, processes, knowledge creation, delivering services, and surviving the relentless march of time and change. Technologies of all kinds will continue to evolve, and healthcare, like other industries and domains of society will continue to encounter evolution in terms determining how to interact with new technologies and manage the impact of new technologies. This chapter will focus on the future context of nursing informatics, present scenarios for reflection and propose a "survival kit" providing nurses entering the work force with choices and which contributes in a meaningful way to shaping the elusive interim state which was yesterday's future. Without being too philosophical, the future can only be realized in the present.

Keywords Future • Healthcare • Mind mapping • Consumerism • Transformation • Digital workspace • Intrapreneurship • Five elements of business • Change dynamic Disruptive technologies • Performance metric • Service management • Social networking • Dialectic learning • Cloud computing • Visualization

Key Concepts

Mind mapping knowledge is a spatial reality
Consumerism and Transformation
1st Generation Digital Workspace
Intra-preneurship
Five Elements of Business

The online version of this chapter (doi:10.1007/978-1-4471-2999-8_19) contains supplementary material, which is available to authorized users.

S.P. Murray, BSc, EBU, MBA, PMP, ISP, CPHIMS
Whiteshadow Inc., Charlottetown, PE, Canada
e-mail: smurray@islandtelecom.com

© Springer-Verlag London 2015
K.J. Hannah et al. (eds.), *Introduction to Nursing Informatics*,
Health Informatics, DOI 10.1007/978-1-4471-2999-8_19

371

Disruptive Technologies
Change Dynamic
Service Management
Performance Metric
Social Networking and Dialectic Learning
Cloud Computing
Visualization
Autonomic Database and "Big Data"

Introduction

The future of health informatics has no bounds; the areas of consideration encompass technologies, both hardware and software, processes, knowledge creation, delivering services, and surviving the relentless march of time and change. Technologies of all kinds will continue to evolve, and healthcare, like other industries and domains of society will continue to encounter evolution in terms determining how to interact with new technologies and manage the impact of new technologies. This chapter will focus on the future context of nursing informatics, provide scenarios for reflection and propose a "survival kit" providing nurses entering the work force with choices and which contributes in a meaningful way to shaping the elusive interim state which was yesterday's future. Without being too philosophical, the future can only be realized in the present.

The importance of postulating the future is to be prepared for probably, or even potential, events and issues, and based on reason, predictability, and critical thinking, be able to anticipate the next steps, the next technologies, and the rate upon which these visions come into view. A good way to illustrate this phenomenon is by providing a practical example.

> You drive your car through a park at 10 km an hour. You can anticipate children crossing the road, see the wild life, and visually and mentally take snapshots of the experience. At 100 km an hour, you cannot anticipate a child running into the traffic and the wild life becomes a blur. You will, in both cases, reach your destination but did you experience or take into consideration all the things you need to realize your goal?

There are three key characteristics that manifest the future: it is not predictable, it is always changing, and you don't know when you get there. This chapter will challenge what you understand to be the present versus the future and provoke your thinking about how to survive in a changing information technology and communications (ICT) world by anticipating change and putting tools in place to alert you to the change dynamic. The goal is not simply to be reactive to change, but to anticipate it and be proactive. The change dynamic depicts the rate of change and the influencing factors that move a product, processes or technology along the adoption s-curve. There is no crystal ball but there are ways to monitor and assess trends and formulate scenarios, which could, in part or in whole, represent a future-state. While considering the future state, the top eight questions that will be addressed in this chapter are:

1. Will technologies replace the need for critical thinking?
2. What role does nursing have in facilitating change in a system that is increasingly impacted by health informatics?
3. Is it possible for health informatics to inform and enforce consistent clinical practice thus increasing both the quality of care and patient safety?
4. By using mind mapping is it possible to better understand work processes, the change dynamic and identify gaps? The world is not flat so does thinking large, looking at the big picture, using mind mapping without boundaries tend to reveal the future?
5. Healthcare is a very large business. Is it possible to institute service management to improve outcomes?
6. Does the future have a place for informatics and does it foster mediocrity or excellence in structures and work processes?
7. Can an individual's life-plan impact their effective use of technology in the delivery of care or improving patient outcomes?
8. "*Intra-preneurs*", enterprising entrepreneurial employees internal to your organization, accelerate the research, design, development and implementation of innovations and transformative technologies. How can social networking facilitate this dynamic?

Scenario One

A graduate nurse has been hired and was taught that clinical nursing at the bedside is the most important type of practice. Part of the nurse's education included the practice that everything needs to be documented in case of an adverse event, such as a patient death or a lawsuit against the hospital. The shift nurse is a strong union representative and has been trained that "if it is not on paper, it doesn't exist". What is now the graduate nurse's focus?

Foundation Lenses

Building a baseline of thought, knowledge, and clinical practice lays the foundation upon which the future can be considered. The first step is to consider the scope of the issue or problem statement. Is the problem statement considering mobile technologies and security or is it something more fundamental – such as ordering of materials such as pens to prepare nursing progress notes in the event of power outages that require staff to go to disaster recovery procedures and revert to documenting care on paper.

The second step in the process is to understand the baseline dynamics upon which the mind map of nursing practice can apply critical, reflective and active thinking. Is the future predictable? No! Can a nurse influence factors that determine the future? Yes! If an event or a change in a contributing factor should occur that changes the predictability of the future, can Change Management be instituted to restore the predictability? Yes! Is it anticipated that the future state will remain the same? The answer is typically, yes but is that a reasonable expectation? No!

Where does a change intervention leave a critical thinking nurse? It introduces a dilemma for the nurse. Should the nurse influence the situational factors to maintain the initial expected outcome because the framework is scripted – or actively think through the context, seek advice, and initiate a new future state with predictable outcomes that are logical and relevant and are the results of a collaborative experience?

Louis and Sutton [1; p56] argue that,

> An individual or group needs to be adept at (1) functioning in an automatic cognitive mode, (2) sensing when reliance on habits of mind or automatic processing is inappropriate, (3) switching from automatic to conscious cognitive processing, (4) functioning in a conscious cognitive mode, (5) sensing when active thinking is no longer necessary, and (6) switching from the conscious to automatic cognitive mode.

Louis and Sutton [1; p22, 58] characterize active thinking or conscious cognitive processing where an individual possesses awareness, attention, reflection, by noticing oneself, one's tasks, one's context. This suggests that clinical pathways and prescriptive workflow does foster consistent work but the individual especially in the clinical setting needs to be able to switch from automatic processing to active thinking.

What role does the nurse provide? Is the role the agent of change, the provider of care, the mentor of knowledge, the delivery manager, social media moderator, the business manager or the innovator/*intrapreneur*? In the future, nursing practise will involve all these roles in varying degrees, especially as an informatics nurse. Chap. 12, *The Role of the Informatics Nurse*, speaks to the current roles of nursing. The key aspects to the foundation lenses for the future are: (1) the continual refresh of the knowledge state and a commitment to life-long learning, (2) understanding the change dynamic, (3) be intuitively aware of one's self-conscious cognitive processing mode, and (4) know the emerging future roles. The pathway to the future is not a straight line and it is part of a continual state of flux and new mindsets. Embracing the future, active thinking, and mind mapping one's context gives an individual the lenses to see the world wide open. Have the courage to take action!

> Rather, ten times, die in the surf, heralding the way to a new world, than stand idly on the shore. —— Florence Nightingale

Scenario Two

Significant effort has been applied to the definition and the implementation of electronic pathways for patient care. A patient presents to the Emergency Department and the graduate nurse logs into the e-Heath system that has been implemented for several years. The clinical pathway prescribes the steps for the nursing staff to provide optimal care to a patient. The patient presents with chest pain. All the tests in the clinical pathway are ordered and the labels affixed to the container. The patient is given medication ordered by the attending physician. There is an adverse reaction. Would the nurse rely on the electronic clinical pathway or revert to sound critical thinking informed by data, knowledge, and experience?

Back to the Future

Florence Nightingale got it right in that she dared in an era when women had no stature to record her observations. Nightingale recorded not just her actions but the outcomes and then discerned from her journal what was working and what was not. This vision and critical thinking would come to make nursing the catalyst for better outcomes regardless of discipline or area of practice. However, nursing in the rush to serve the volume of patients became technicians, housekeepers, administrators, and clerks in addition to their clinical roles.

Health informatics encompasses information, knowledge products and raw data on the coal face of healthcare regardless of location or discipline. The missing elements are the tools: the journal and pencil or quill of the Crimean War front and the cognitive lens that allow the nursing profession to enable, collect, assimilate, research, discern, formulate, establish a plan of care, and communicate both actions and outcomes. This high-level workflow is the foundation of care and the RN the catalyst. Health informatics can support this workflow in varying degrees. Each work process is repeatable, potentially rendering an outcome that changes the pathway of care and even the sequence of thought.

Group think (ideology) or shared collaborations meld thoughts and foster debates, which are essential for good decision making. The size for the body of knowledge in the health field is huge. Some knowledge is in raw data that the health industry is codifying to facilitate the assimilation process. Large data in multiple forms whether written, audio, video or text have been catalogued and stored in libraries around the world in different languages whether machine-readable or human language. The core to good healthcare through health informatics is to embrace systems. One size does not fit all. What has been done well for decades is enabling care and collecting data.

When you consider a system from an engineer's perspective, the precision of getting the right answer or to solve a problem or to control the speed of an elevator is not punching the button for you for a specific floor and looking at the lights. The "back end" process is what is critically important – initiating a cascading sequence of steps in response to the elevator occupant's selection of a floor, and ensuring that the steps all occur in that predetermined sequence, and providing feedback to the system if an issue arises. The feedback loop or the reporting of outcomes in a relevant and meaningful way as the control systems that start the lift, stop the lift and apply the braking on an elevator will support predictability, discovery through enabled research and the body of knowledge against which theorem datem can be tested.

Dialectic Learning is the RN's best source of knowledge to the future, social networking, and conversing with your peers through peer-to-peer centers of excellence. A rhetorical question has to be asked; when did we stop learning from others? The answer is never, however communications and collaborative nursing will change the medium and the methods but not the form unless a discovery leads to a better way of nursing. The story of the 15-year-old discovering a way to detect Pancreatic Cancer comes to mind. The head line is: "Jack Andraka invents a dipstick-type sensor for early and reliable detection of pancreatic, ovarian, and lung cancer" [2]. It is this type of innovation and pivotal discovery that has the yet unmapped potential to change that way nursing is delivered and communicated.

Mind Mapping, Visual Thinking

In this chapter, we have already discussed active thinking where the individual switches into a conscious cognitive processing mode or state of mind. Mind mapping or visual thinking is a method of storing, organizing, prioritizing, learning, reviewing and memorizing information. It presents an overview and summary of a body of knowledge that fuses words and pictures together. This fusion of critical thinking, words, and images helps simulate logic and creativity for proficient and effective thinking practices involving the five senses [3].

As the future unfolds, there is one guarantee. There will continue to be vast and ever growing reservoirs of data, information and knowledge. The capacity to handle this deluge of data and to critically think and visualize the small nuggets of extraordinary intelligence becomes more elusive. Harkening back to the body of work by Florence Nightingale, you find that as a statistician she was able to find ways to represent large quantities of written data from her log books in a visual depiction called a Rose Graph using polar coordinates Fig. 19.1. Nightingale had discovered that the majority of deaths in the Crimea were due to poor sanitation rather than

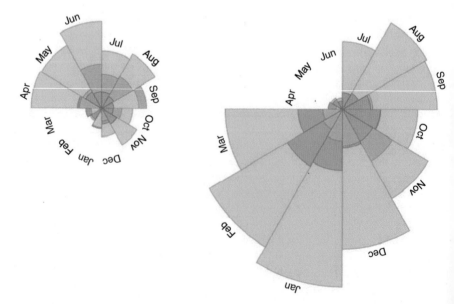

Fig. 19.1 Rose diagram. These diagrams are used to visualize data in multiple dimensions allows the human brain to think visually and solve complex problems

casualties in battle. She wanted to persuade government of the need for better hygiene in hospitals [4].

These same diagrams are used to visualize data in multiple dimensions allows the human brain to think visually and solve complex problems. Draw the right picture and you can literally transform the way we see the world. Figure 19.2, *Your Ideal Future*, is an illustration of a mind map that typifies your future.

The mind mapping technique can be applied to understanding a schema of care related to a specific drug therapy, refer to Fig. 19.3, Nurse Management for Dextoamphetamine Therapy. This drawing does not show a pathway, a road map or a sequence of related ideas; it is a schema of related elements organized in a meaningful way to describe nursing management for a particular therapy. This mind map suggests the key nursing management activities are: doing, assessing and decision making.

Ahn et al. [5] state that, "[...] mind mapping encourages the nurses to maintain a holistic view of the patient. A complementary approach to the traditional tabular and narrative based nursing care plan is referred to as mind mapping. A mind map [in the context of a nursing plan] is a graphical representation of the connection between concepts and ideas." Mind mapping is a very effective tool to visually think through large qualities of information and concepts in a framework that has relationship but not necessarily order, which in many ways emulates life itself. Nursing has to deal with many sources of information in many forms: assimilating, discerning and formulating a diagnosis and a nursing care treatment plan.

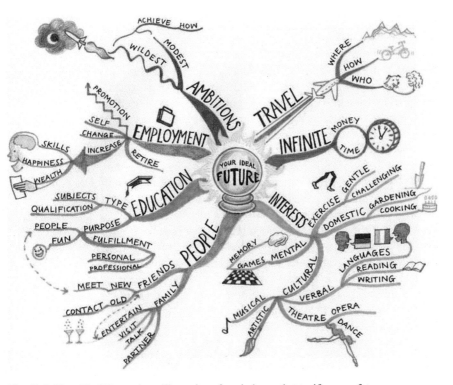

Fig. 19.2 Your Ideal Future, is an illustration of a mind map that typifies your future

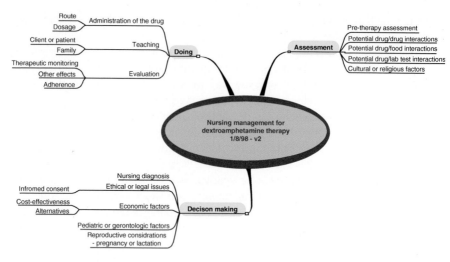

Fig. 19.3 Nurse management for dextoamphetamine therapy

Five Element Theory

A large organization or business (which healthcare is) takes on the characteristics of a lumbering giant. The view to business whether large or small, public or private, should consider the elemental interaction of the change dynamic formulated by the Ancient Chinese. The current and dominant focus of business function performance management tends to be based on measuring goals and objective within particular disciplines such as: clinical outcomes, financial measures, wait-times, service deliver, and learning and innovation. However, the five element theory formed the fundamental basis of systems thinking of the Ancient Chinese [6].

Figure 19.4 illustrates the five elements and the nourishing effect each element of a strategic balance scorecard category has on each other. The dotted lines illustrate the controlling relationships between the elements and the lines (1), (2) and (3) that govern those relationships related to business growth. Growth is a change to the business and as Wang indicated it is just as important to control the interactions of the five elements as it is the elements themselves [6].

The five element theory is one of the Chinese worldviews and methodologies which most Chinese scholars have recognized over the past millennia. Viewing the universe as revolving around the five basic elements of everyday life—Wood, Fire, Earth, Metal, and Water, [analogous to business functions] (see Fig. 19.4). The five element model reinforces two complimentary and opposite external cycles, one nourishing and the other controlling. Internally each of the five elements maintains harmony through balance, managing the positive and negative forces. Table 19.1 provides a summary and overview of the model.

The questions that arise are: "Why is this significant?" Why map a contemporary comprehensive management control system such as the balance scorecard [7; p277], to an ancient Chinese model? Wang's research paper [6] made a compelling case that

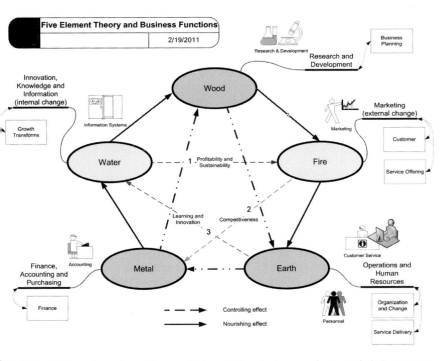

Fig. 19.4 The five elements and the nourishing effect each element of a strategic balance score-card category has on each other. Five elements: Wood, Fire, Earth, Metal, and Water, [analogous to business functions]

Table 19.1 Five element theory in a contemporary context

Basic element	Business function	Mind-map affinity	Balanced scorecard
Wood	Research and development	Business planning	Mission, strategy and goals
Water	Innovation, knowledge, information & growth	Information systems and growth transforms	Potential for learning and growth
Metal	Finance, accounting and purchasing	Finance and balance sheet	Financial performance
Earth	Operations and human Resources	Organization and change, service delivery	Internal business process indicators
Fire	Marketing (external change)	Customer/clinical relations and the patient service offering	External, patient service indicators

there is a correlation between present day management systems and the ancient Chinese model. The Chinese model does point out a variation on the balanced score-card and more recently Program Budgeting/Marginal Analysis in the healthcare field. That is the emphasis on the relationship system determining the impact that one basic element has on the other, essentially the ebb and flow caused by human interaction.

Table 19.2 Basic element inter-relationships

Element inter-relationship	Balance Scorecard	Figure 19.4	Business impacts	Life-cycle stage
Water–fire	Knowledge, innovation, growth External, customer service	Arrow (1)	Profitability and sustainability	Renewal or start-up
Fire–metal	External, customer service Financial performance	Arrow (2)	Competitiveness	Growth or Egress growth
Earth–water	Internal process indicators Potential learning and growth	Arrow (3)	Learning and innovation	Ingress growth

Referring to Fig. 19.4, the relationship that water has on fire [1] is one of profitability and sustainability. Without the ability of an organization to innovate, learn and grow [3] then the marketing or customers will not be satisfied with the product or service [2]. This can be stated affirmatively as well; if the organization has the ability to innovate, learn and grow then the marketing or customers will be more satisfied. Table 19.2, Basic Element Inter-relationships, summarizes the dynamic that exists in the ancient Chinese model that are associated with various lifecycle stages of a business.

While all the other elements, specifically wood, earth and metal, support the maintenance of a healthy organization, it is the dynamic between water, fire, earth and metal that shines the light on what needs to be in place to support transformational change or growth. These dynamics: (1) promote renewal; (2) promote egress change or stabilization; and (3) ingress growth or transformative growth (Table 19.2).

Why is the theory of the five elements significant to the healthcare industry and the characteristics that manifest the change dynamic? These five elements exist in all organizations big and small. Nursing Informatics contributes to the dynamic through facilitation, adaptation and renewal. Further, nursing informatics experts have strong roles in change management and as leaders in supporting information management for clinical data, and clinically-relevant data, they have much to contribute to organizational management and business processes.

Embrace the Change Dynamic: Positive or Negative

The different lifecycle stages include (a) initiation or start-up, (b) expansion with a significant rate of change, (c) maturity establishing consistency and predictability, (d) diversification where the organization develops strength through verity, and (e) decline. The lifecycle stages with their emphasis on control and feedback function as a closed system [similar to the elevator and the passenger and its control systems] that does not interact with the external factors or the environment [8].

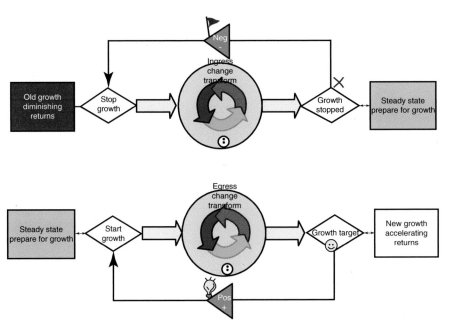

Fig. 19.5 Entrepreneurial Facilitator's Dilemma

The five element model features the relationships of all factors for an organization to survive and thrive.

Organizational change can be both adaptive and transformative. Sundarasaradula and Hasan [9] note that "major transformative change [...] involves profound reformulation of the organization's mission, vision, structure, management, and basic social, political and cultural aspects of the dynamic equilibrium". Healthcare organizations must be responsive to the need for transformative change, commit to becoming adaptive, and clearly contextualize their transformation within a business perspective to ensure that the implemented approach is proactive, incremental, measureable, and sustainable. Pre-transformation steps to make the environment conducive for transformation include: (a) workforce training, (b) cultural management, (c) strategy formation, (d) key performance indicators, and (e) feedback mechanisms for monitoring key indicators [10, 11]. From these lists, the elements that need to be monitored in healthcare are not just tangible measures but also measures that relate to knowledge, learning and organizational culture for the long term (Fig. 19.5) [12].

Inertial Conflict: Resistance to Change

The attitude or the way of thinking, whether it is the manager-director for the hospital or "group think" of the Board, has the most profound impact on the organization regardless of the level of maturity to which the business has evolved. Around this frame of reference are a number of psychological (psychogenic) and state-of-being

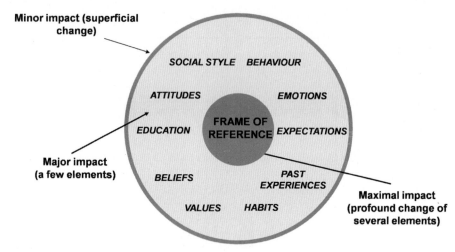

Fig. 19.6 Change and frame of reference

(ontological) factors that contribute to the organization change dynamic. These same factors are deeply embedded in the collective culture of the organization (see Fig. 19.6) [13].

There are a number of cultures that can influence the inner workings of an organization especially in the absence of strong leadership [14]. These include: (a) a process culture based on workflow with little feedback, (b) a power culture concentrating power among a few, (c) a role/hierarchy culture delegating authority in a structured organization, (d) a task culture solving a particular problem, (e) a person culture that exists within and individual, (f) a constructive culture encouraging interaction, (g) a market culture a competitive workplace external facing and controlled, and (h) an adhocracy culture a dynamic workplace with leaders that stimulate innovation [14].

Coping with Urgency and Rate of Change

When considering a change dynamic in the workplace, especially in healthcare informatics, the changes tend to vary from urgent with a high rate of change to passive with limited or prescriptive change relating to a specific scope of practice in a specialty, role or discipline. John Boyd, a fighter pilot for the US Air Force in Korea and Vietnam, was puzzled by the acts of war as was Florence Nightingale. Under fire, Colonel Boyd wished to understand the decision making process shaping operations. He developed the OODA Loop that served to explain the nature of surprise and shapes operations in a way that unifies Gestalt psychology, cognitive science and game theory in a comprehensive theory of strategy (Fig. 19.7).

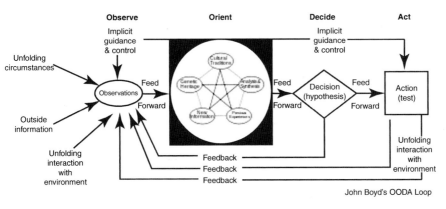

Fig. 19.7 The OODA Loop. The OODA Loop includes sequential activities including Observe (detecting information), Orient (interpret information), Decide (make a clear decision), and Act

The OODA Loop includes sequential activities including Observe (detecting information), Orient (interpret information), Decide (make a clear decision), and Act [15]. The underlying rationale of this model is the concept of agility, which enables rapid response, faster adjustments, and greater success [15]. This model is used by corporations, governments and the military today to cope with urgent and varying degrees of change and requires the organization to be both holistic in its view and tactical in its operations. This dualistic abstraction of the workflow process requires the decision maker to be ambidextrous in decision making.

What does this mean to the nurse and the healthcare workplace?

For a company – including a healthcare organization, to succeed over the long term, it needs to master both adaptability and alignment — an attribute that is sometimes referred to as *ambidexterity* [16; p50]. Birkinshaw and Gibson [16] developed a model where there exist two types of ambidexterity in business; structural and contextual. The characteristics of each are present in Table 19.3, Organizational Ambidexterity. These two types juxtaposed appear to be mutually exclusive. Herein lies the organizational challenge and the potential for conflict.

O'Reilly and Tushman [17]; p13] referred to Teece's tripartite taxonomy of sensing, seizing, and reconfiguring, where ambidexterity requires a coherent alignment of competencies, structures and cultures to engage in exploration, […]focused on exploitation. O'Reilly and Tushman [17] also identified the key factor to success for any organization is organizational discipline and efficiency, and a dedication to innovation and continuous improvement. They distinguish this approach as requiring a short-term approach rather than a longer-term approach, which is required for more research focused companies.

When considering any organization change, management team leadership is essential to showcase a compelling vision and strategic intent with a clear picture of the intra-organizational relationships to leverage skills and infrastructure. Considering this cultural paradox, the need for leadership and vision to shift the focus from the near term to longer term is essential.

Table 19.3 Organizational ambidexterity

	Structural ambidexterity	Contextual ambidexterity
How is ambidexterity achieved?	Alignment-focused and adaptability-focused activities are done in separate units or teams	Individual employees divide their time between alignment-focused and adaptability-focused activities
Where are decisions made about the split between alignment and adaptability?	At the top of the organization	On the front line – by salespeople, plant supervisors, office workers
Role of top management?	To define the structure, to make trade-offs between alignment and adaptability	To develop the organizational context in with individuals act
Nature of roles	Relatively clearly defined	Relatively flexible
Skills of employees	More specialists	More generalists

Consumerism, Service and Operations

There a number of competing forces impacting the delivery of consistent, high quality, cost effective healthcare. Currently and into the foreseeable future, consumerism will increasingly impact the demands on the system, change clinician roles, and necessitate efficiencies. This will all happen regardless of whether or not the patient perceives a satisfactory level of quality care. Escalating costs and demands on the healthcare systems are exacerbating tensions on available resources that are already stretched to the limit. Embracing health consumerism, being innovative, working within the system as an *intrapreneur* and showing leadership in the future will be key tenets of the nursing informatics professional.

Health Consumerism

Health consumerism is an interesting word as it relates to healthcare in general and nursing in particular. Commerce is simply the act of a buyer buying something that a seller has for sale. Consumerism is the ever-increasing demand to purchase goods or service or to take part in commerce. Robinson [18] described how consumerism places the needs or priority of the individual above those of the collective, driving decisions based on personal needs rather than the good of society. While the demand for transparency, accountability, and fiscal efficiency is served by individual choice, it concurrently drives the escalation of demand for greater consumption.

How does this apply to healthcare? Translating this concept to both the workplace and the delivery of healthcare services, the patient is encouraged to acquire healthcare service in ever-greater amounts, thus creating a paradox. The "consumer" patient is encouraged to take advantage of a system that is struggling with the demand and the quality of care the patients are getting. Cohen et al. [19] state that,

"In healthcare, consumerism is not a product or program. Instead, it is an orientation to new care delivery models that encourage and enable greater patient responsibility through the intelligent use of information technology."

With Cohen et al. [19], the consumerism definition has taken on the freedom of choice and an invitation to take advantage of alternative approaches to delivering healthcare. They go on to espouse four guiding principles to ensure that next-generation innovation yields the returns that providers, patients, and other stakeholders expect: (1) keep the consumer at the center of innovation, (2) keep it simple, (3) link products and services to a broader "ecosystem" of care, and (4) encourage health in addition to treating illness [19].

The advancements of technologies in mobility, visualization, intelligent databases and social network all contribute to the proliferation of patient centered delivery of healthcare in any location. This does sound like the panacea for all that ails the patient. The caution is that there are always trade-offs and both the informatics professional and digital age nursing practitioners need to understand not only the benefits, but the risks and challenges this emerging context brings to the patient, the providers, and the organizations charged with patient safety. Examples of current consumer health solutions are: mHealth, Personal Health Records, access to reputable online sources of information, life-line for the elderly and infirmed, and remote monitoring of heart rates and other key health indicators. Consumerism is not just for the patient, any participant providing health services can and are consumers.

Upon reflection, consumerism emphasizes the underlying realization that healthcare is actually a business and not an altruistic action. This realization prompts the need for leadership that is not just clinical in nature but understands the different facets of business that provide the framework of a healthy system for service delivery.

Service Management

Service management plans can take many different forms, from a specific problem that needs to be solved to a general strategy to improve service considering: (a) the service or product, (b) the people, (c) the technology, and (d) systems both workflow process related and technology supported [20]; p67]. The best way to illustrate the implementation of a service management plan in healthcare is to provide a good example [21].

The example is the surgical services area. This part of the delivery of health services tends to touch all aspects of acute care across the hospital and in some regards impacts primary care. Ambulatory services and the emergency service also have links to the surgical services area. As healthcare moves toward health consumerism, there will be demands for the system to act more like a business, demonstrating service value, which will require the key care providers and managers to understand service management consideration.

Service Management Case Study

Surgical Service Management

This service plan focuses primarily on the operating rooms and the core services in the surgical area. The other service areas such as: booking and scheduling, labs, diagnostic imaging, pharmacy, equipment and material supply, housekeeping, day surgery clinic, ambulatory care, and post-operative care units (PACU) are services units contributing to the overall delivery of operating room (OR) services.

The strategic goal of this service plan is primarily focused on improving the service quality to the operative patient. The operating room service is a job shop type of service with a high degree of judgement and customization. After assessing the services quality provided to the patients, two areas of variance were revealed. The responsiveness variance for resourcing is based on a lack of information regarding the work process performance measures, and the reliability variance is based on not knowing the reasons for delays, cancellations and inconsistent booking practices.

The surgical area support services blueprint considers: (a) the line of interaction between the customer (patient) and the onstage contact personnel (key contacts in the health care encounter), (b) the line of visibility between the onstage contact personnel and the backstage contact personnel, and (c) the line of internal interaction between the backstage contact personnel and the support processes.

The facility relationships and the process flows give a better understanding of the OR support services area for service planning. The Operating Room Services Context Diagram (Fig. 19.8), illustrates the high-level context of support services to the service plan target area, the OR services unit.

Facility Relationships

The running of a hospital is a complex environment. There are a number of disciplines, departments, and specialties all with a set of clinical standards and policies, procedures and best practices. The organizational relationship model (Fig. 19.9) depicts the relationships of the various service areas to each other and to the operating rooms. The diagram at a high level also shows the flow of information.

Process Flows

There are a number of steps required to prepare a patient and the OR for the surgical event. The core process areas include: (a) Booking and Pre-Admission, (b) Surgery Pre-diagnosis, (c) OR set-up, (d) Supply to the OR, (e) Pre-surgery, (f) Surgery, and (g) Post-Operative Care. Each of these process areas incorporates a number of processes and sub-processes as depicted by Work Breakdown Structure and Process Flow (Fig. 19.10). The key areas of potential service improvement are external support entities, exchange of information, or a hand-off of responsibility in the service delivery value chain.

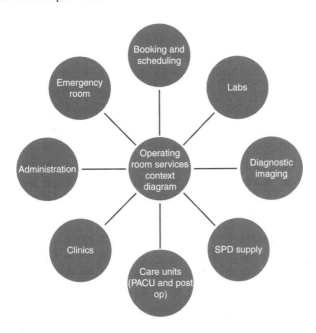

Fig. 19.8 Operating room
services context diagram

Organizational relationship model

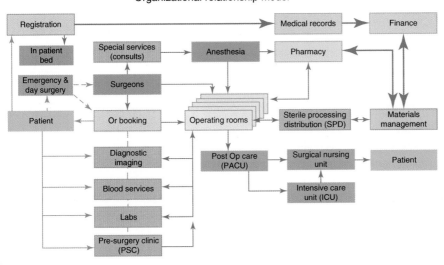

Fig. 19.9 Organizational relationship model

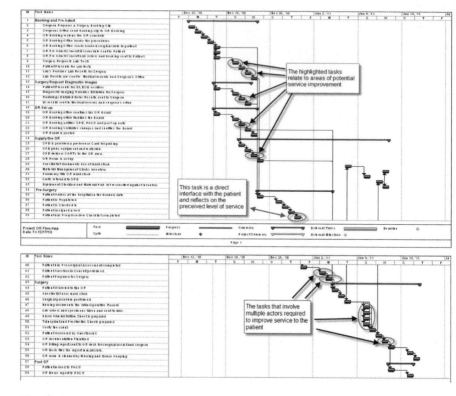

Fig. 19.10 Work breakdown structure and process flow

Strategic Goal and Objectives

The strategic goal of this service plan is primarily focused on improving the service quality to the operative patient. The top three objectives in order of importance are as follows:

1. Objective one: To maintain and gradually improve the flow of information and communication internal and external to the surgical operating room areas, eliminating redundant processes and excess paper processing and improving patient care by providing timely nursing documentation to the post-operative care areas, ER, ICU, PACU and the post-operative care units within 2 min of the patient out of room time;

2. Objective two: To minimize the time it takes to order, process and provide results to the operating rooms, reducing the resulting time for stat orders to the OR potentially reducing the time the patient is under anaesthesia;

3. Objective three: To optimize and systematically monitor, evaluate and act on changes that will improve the use of the operating rooms from 60 to 80 % occupancy during prime-time surgical hours of 7:30–16:30. This will be achieved by

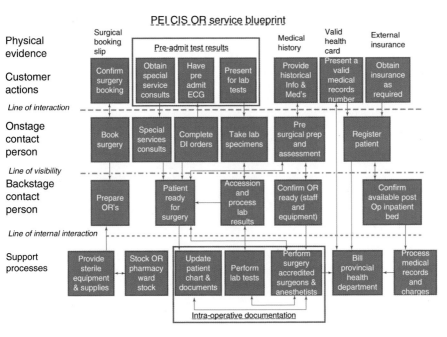

Fig. 19.11 OR service blueprint

effective use of an electronic scheduling application to assign, book, shuffle, cancel and confirm surgeries.

Surgical Area Support Services Blueprint

The surgical area support services blueprint considers: (a) the line of interaction between the customer and the onstage contact personnel, (b) the line of visibility between the onstage contact personnel and the backstage contact personnel, and (c) the line of internal interaction between the backstage contact personnel and the support processes, see (Fig. 19.11) [20]; p71].

Line of Interaction

The patient line of interaction from the surgical area perspective is with the booking office and the pre-surgical clinics in ambulatory care areas that perform the requested tests and provide the necessary consults. This process is not coordinated and is left to the patient to make sure the tests are performed prior to the date of surgery. The health card, extended health insurance and the validation of patient history and home medications are all points of intersection with the patient. None of these processes are time sensitive for scheduled surgeries but are very time sensitive for emergency surgery.

Line of Visibility

The line of visibility is the internal interface behind the patient contact person and the back stage personnel that prepare the facility, personnel, and the supplies for the

Service management model

Outside - in   Inside - out

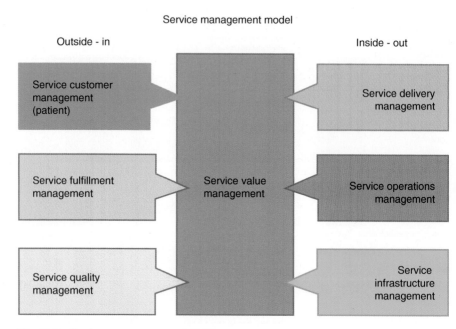

Service customer management (patient)		Service delivery management
Service fulfillment management	Service value management	Service operations management
Service quality management		Service infrastructure management

Fig. 19.12 Service management model [22]

surgery. This line of visibility is the highest candidate for process breakdown and slowness as outlined in the process flows. It is also the easiest area in the surgical support model to institute change without directly impacting the surgeons or the front-line patient contacts. The management of the case preparation in the line of visibility is high candidate to improve the service support quality in preparation for surgeries both booked and emergent. This area contributes to deficiencies in responsiveness quality assessment category.

Line of Internal Interaction

The line of internal interaction is the core of the operating room area, the supply and billing for services. The "Surgery" application currently being implemented satisfies the Intraoperative Documentation illustrated by Fig. 19.12. The key to improved service in this case is to ensure the appropriate data is collected, analyzed and reported. Steps are being taken to capture performance measures to understand the gaps related to the internal interaction. This should identify actions that can be taken to improve responsiveness and reliability.

Surgical Area Support Services Plan

The surgical support services plan provides a framework to take advantage of quality and/or productivity improvement opportunities. There are several opportunity areas in the front-line interaction, process flows and the management of the case readiness leading up to a surgical date. Data to interpret the internal interactions need to be evaluated on a regular basis to implement a continuous quality improvement program.

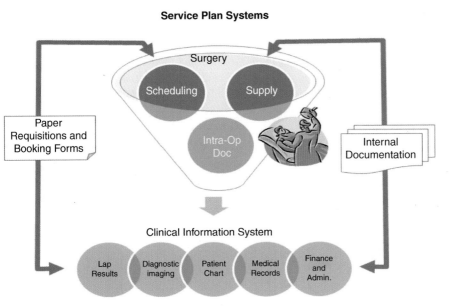

Fig. 19.13   Surgical services support systems

Service Management Model

The service management process in the past for the surgical areas has been process flow driven and the decision-making reactive and based on evidential data that was collected by the core operating services and not based on a holistic view of a service blueprint. No individual stakeholder contributes more or less to the overall performance of the surgical services.

The surgeons are certainly central to the surgical services; however there are a number of other stakeholders involved directly and indirectly in the quality service being provided. Figure 19.8 is a conceptual service management model developed as part of the Service Management Body of Knowledge (SMBOK) [22].

The service management model names three outside-in areas of service management and the three inside-out areas required to create service value. The two service management areas of interest for the surgery area are: the service quality management and service delivery management.

This does not mean that the other areas are not important, service quality management manages things such as capability and performance and delivery management manages continuity, capability and service levels. Both areas 'shine a light' on the factors influencing the quality of service in the surgical areas.

Service Support Systems

The service support systems depicted by Fig. 19.13 are delivered by several applications. The system supports the electronic exchange of internal documentation and supports sending lab results to the OR for the anaesthesiologists.

The patient service interface is primarily paper and telephone. There needs to be a system to monitor the readiness and the progress of the pre-admit patient, tracking lab tests, diagnostic imagining and specialty consultations. How will this happen?

The service management plan for the operating room areas is complex, but serves as an excellent illustration of the factors and the details that a health informatician needs to be aware of and to lead or positively influence in the healthcare setting. The health informatics intrapreneur will need to become knowledgeable in the workflow, the objectives, performance indicators, and able to analyze systems and the functionality to support the operational needs of the business.

Operational Management

Operations Management is central to delivering the services to the patient and it is a core aspect of daily activity in the healthcare system. Referring to the surgical services case study, there were a number of operational functions that needed to be taken into consideration. Inventory management in the sterile processing centre, financial management providing the equipment in the operating theatre, and the bed management are all part of the operational management of the surgical service unit.

Conceptually or the highest level of abstraction, operations management does not change. There are variations of processes and workflows depending on the service areas and the role and reporting in the overall operational landscape. Slack et al. [23] in Fig. 19.14 have illustrated functionally the relationships between the core operations functions and the support functions of an organization. This functional perspective applies to organizations delivering products and services which the healthcare system does. Strangely this chapter has looked at the future, how to prepare for change and understand the dynamics that technological advancements tend to create. Operations management is the opposite to change. It is the constant around which chaos and transformation find haven. This harbour in the sea of change is the place where management goes back to benchmark and consider the benefits of a particular change, innovation, or adaptation has afforded the organization.

Scenario Four

Nursing staff at the Gray Rock General Hospital have been instructed in their scope of practice methods to discard all medications that have been opened or the seal has been broken. A senior nurse in the Oncology treatment center was administrating drugs that were provided by the Hospital Pharmacy. As the drugs were being administered, a patient had an adverse reaction to the first medicine. Once the clinical emergency was averted, the nurse took the unused second vial of medication and disposed of it. The single vial of medication was worth $35,000. The Pharmacy could have returned the specialized medicine and was very upset that this medication was disposed of. The operational processes and workflow need to be changed. Who should initiate the request for change?

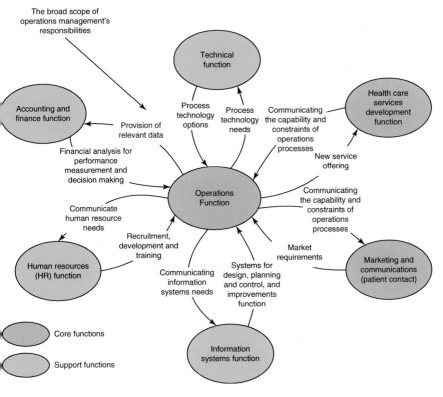

Fig. 19.14 Functional relationships between the core operations functions and the support functions of an organization [23]

First Generation Digital Workplace

The Net generation thinks visually and can multitask on many different levels. The Internet, videos, gaming, text messaging and social networking have honed the Net generation worker's visual thinking skills. The Net generation is "the first global generation ever; the Net Geners are smarter, quicker, and more tolerant of diversity than their predecessors. They care strongly about justice and the problems faced by their society and are typically engaged in some kind of civic activity at school" [24].

Nursing is not immune to this generational empowerment, which stems from ubiquitous information technology influencing all aspects of personal and professional life, including the future in Nursing Informatics. The "old guard" immigrated to the digital age and does not possess the digital literacy the Net Geners have accepted as their norm; the future of the old guard has now been realized in the present. The changing of the guard will be transformative and it has already started. Many of these changes can be introduced by the organizational Intrapreneurs.

Leadership and Intra-Preneurial Spirit

The leadership role is fundamental to support successful growth and transformation. Leadership from the intrapreneur is crucial [25].

Wilson et al. [26] describe the significant distinction between entrepreneur and intrapreneur in terms of health reform and the nursing roles supporting reform. The commonly recognized term 'entrepreneur' reflects the same independent business approach for nursing as is present in more traditional business ventures. Nurses are increasingly able to establish independent practice outside of healthcare organizations, and maintain self-employment through their professional innovation and service provision. On the other hand, nurse intrapreneurs are those nurses who develop and drive innovation from *within* an organization, and who consequently share the benefits and risks of such innovation. Wilson et al. note that innovations developed by intrapreneurs "often involve efforts to transform workplace climate or culture, improve processes, or develop new products or services".

The culture, the drive, service values and work ethic all emanate from the organizational leadership. The image, the motivations, and values held by the head of the leadership portray the soul of the organization. The key to the intrepreneurial role is not mainly to be an intrapreneur (Table 19.4) but be able to complement the [leadership] [27]. The key characteristics of an intrapreneur are outlined in Table 19.4.

Why is it important to consider intrapreneurial characteristic as it relates to nursing informatics? The simple answer to this question is adaptive leadership comes from the intrapreneurs who are buried deep in the operations of healthcare. Remember that innovation and an employee with intrepreneurial characteristics will be key orchestrators of transformative change. Innovation doesn't mean inventing a new practice. It can be as simple as asking that the layout of a screen in the information system will facilitate the workflow and reduce patient risk. These characteristics speak to two of the A's, Attitude and Aptitude, discussed in more detail below

Jacque Filion [28] states that the definition of an entrepreneur/intrapreneur includes at least six elements (Fig. 19.15). These elements if present in an individual or in the work place will facilitate adaptive change.

Table 19.4 Intrapreneurial characteristics

Risk adverse
Sensitive to the internal and external environments
Politically skilled
Adaptive
Knows the limits of what is acceptable
Perfectionist
Accountable
Uses resources wisely
Results oriented
Collaborative leadership

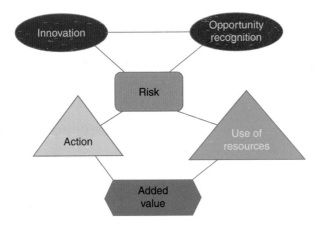

Fig. 19.15 Main elements describing an intrapreneur

DeJong and Wennekers [29]; p8] in their study to understand entrepreneurial employee behaviour defined an intrapreneur as:

> Previous work has proposed various definitions of intrapreneurship. These definitions share a number of features. First, intrapreneurs are proactive individuals with a strong desire for action. They are 'self-starters' who do not have to be asked to take an initiative. In fact, they usually do not even ask for permission, and may ignore disapproval and other negative reactions from their environment about their ideas. Second, their proactive behaviour is focussed on the pursuit of an opportunity without regard to the resources they currently control. Somehow intrapreneurs always seem to find a way. And third, intrapreneurs often pursue something that in some sense is 'new' or 'innovative', i.e. intrapreneurial behaviours and actions deviate from the status quo.

The future in health informatics will be a return to the historical roots where those nurses who, by nature, are entrepreneurial and embrace transformative changes that are underway in healthcare will tend to become leaders in their area of practice. This does not mean that best practice should be eliminated or subverted, however there are opportunities to expedite approved changes and room for visual active thinking. The nurse has the potential to be the center of the locus of change resulting from the synergistic advancement of technology and informatics.

Survivor's Kit Bag

The survivor's kit bag is quite simple. The four A's of success in health informatics and nursing include: (a) aptitude where the individual has the talent for informatics not just nursing, (b) attitude embracing change, exercising leadership, and fostering collaboration, (c) ability to assess, make an informed critical decision and take action, and (d) abstraction knowing when to actively think visually and holistically and when to think autonomically without critical thinking and based on prescriptive process and workflow.

Table 19.5 Strategic potential assessment criteria

Assessment area (wood)	Required stage two growth key performance criterion	Internal consideration
Strategic potential		Related references
Business growth	Strategy to create and grow the business	[20, 30; p90, 31–33]
Strategic options	Create multiple options for strategy and exit	[20, 30; p90, 31–33]
Value creation	High value creation from high profit margins & cash generation	[20, 30; p90, 31–33]
Innovation value business model	Open superior business model that matched the service offering	[20, 30; p90, 31–33]
Goals & objectives	The goals and objectives are clear and communicated	[20, 30; p90, 31–33]

Every decision a nurse needs to make includes: Scientific method, Problem Solving, Decision Making, Diagnostic Reasoning and Inferences. Health informatics facilitates these processes but does not act as a substitute for good well thought out decision making.

What do you put in your survivor kit bag: (a) a flashlight to visually see your way, (b) an axe and hammer so you can build shelter by knowing the technological tools, (c) a mirror to hold court with yourself fostering your inner judgement and intuition, letting your deep personal knowing and sub-conscious speak to you, (d) actively listen and charging your knowledge batteries, (e) embracing the unknown and mapping your future. Your survivor kit is a new mindset!

Internal Modality

Internal modality items are items that the nursing informatics professional can influence and control. Internal actions are a response to external forces. These are a reflection of organizational goals and objectives and the measures established at the beginning of a planning cycle. These values will be skewed if the organization sets goals and objectives that are not specific, measurable, achievable, realistic, and timely.

Strategic Potential (Table 19.5) is the category that provides the outline for the business. How is the business going to change or evolve to deliver on its goals? What is the organization going to do to create value for the stakeholders? What goals and objectives will the business need to achieve to consider success? Finally, is the organization a match for the service offering? There is no definitive answer to these questions. The degree to which the healthcare organization achieves or exceeds these measures is important. Conversely it is important to understand if the healthcare system is underachieving.

Internal Resource (Table 19.6) is the category that looks at the people from a leadership, roles and responsibilities, capacity, and organizational culture

Table 19.6 Internal resources assessment criteria

Assessment area (earth)	Required stage two growth key performance criterion	Internal consideration
Internal resources		Related references
Leadership	CEO able to show leadership & innovation	[20, 30; p90, 32–34]
Management team effectiveness	Management team skilled compatible & motivated to achieve	[30, 33]
Delegation of roles and responsibilities	The leadership able to delegate responsibility and authority	[30; p91, 33, 35]
Contextual experience	Able to use prior experience and knowledge of the services industry	[30; p91 31, 33, 35]
Staff capability	Able to recruit experienced people from within the industry	[30; p90, 31, 35, 36]
Adaptive and flexible organization	The staff are adaptive and flexible to accommodate change	[30; p91, 20, 33, 35]
Collaborative culture	The organization is collaborative	[20; p91, 20, 37]
Ambidextrous growth orientation	The organization is able to accommodate adaptive and disruptive change, entrepreneurial team	[9, 35, 37]

perspective. The ability of the organization to deliver a quality service, to be adaptive and able to accommodate change both planned and disruptive is core to getting to the future state and the business transformation through with the organization will need to transition. This starts at the top.

Learning and Innovation (Table 19.7) is the category that prepares the business its people, the infrastructure, the market and the stakeholders for a change in direction. Learning and innovation is the unique character trait that sets organizations apart. A learning organization is adaptive, creative, and finds opportunity from every corner of the market creating services that are differentiated from their competitors. This category is the first step to re-energizing or re-tooling a business. If an organization invests in its people and innovation before a current product or service life-cycle starts to reach maturity, the organization will be able to catch the next wave of growth. This re-vitalization is typically characterized but the plateau or 'steadying the ship'.

External Modality

The external factors are elements that an organization can attempt to influence but cannot be controlled. The reference to market relates to patients and in the context of consumerism in healthcare and the patient as a customer of health services external factors start to have relative importance. A healthcare system that is not dictated by the healthcare professionals but influenced by the perceived value provide to the patient is a notion that will turn the healthcare system up-side-down. The patient and their needs and how well these needs are met will become the most important external factor.

Table 19.7 Learning and innovation assessment criteria

Assessment area (water)	Required stage two growth key performance criterion	Internal consideration
Learning and innovation		Related references
Innovation leadership	Able to lead the market using prior experience	[9, 20, 30; p89]
Innovation related to customers' needs	Application solves a problem derived from customers' needs	[20; p89, 30, 37]
Technology differentiation	Differentiated technology with optimal performance & cost benefits, with limited obsolescence	[20, 30; p84, 89, 34]
Intellectual property	IP protection with clear ownership & control	[30; p89, 34]
Speed to market	First to market	[30; p89, 34]
Feasibility of implementation	Challenges can be over-come	[30; p89, 34, 37]
Emphasis on self-development and learning	Staff with initiative and current knowledge	[34, 37, 38]

Table 19.8 Market opportunity assessment criteria

Assessment area (fire)	Required Stage Two Growth Key Performance Criterion	External consideration
Market opportunity		Related references
Market demand growth rate	Able to provide service to an aging changing demographic	[30; p89, 34]
Market cost structure	Low or high-cost/declining inclining costs, Competition–cost provider	[34, 39]
Patient base	Known, identified patients, chronic or acute, local or remote	[30; p89, 31]
Patient interaction	Trust & open relationships with patients and the healthcare reputation	[30; p89, 33]
Partnerships & networks	Long-term partnerships within strong suppliers and technology networks	[30; p89, 33]
Competition	Differentiated service in relation to the competition, funded and non-funded	[30; p89, 33, 34]
Distribution	Established service channels	[34, 40]

Market Opportunity (Table 19.8) is the category that assesses the market and how well the organization is achieving market reach, customer retention, and more importantly reputation through relationships and customer engagement. Table 19.8 is framed in opportunity but just as well can be considered risks if the patient is not viewed in the center of the mind-map of the care plan. Service firms are only as good as their last job and how they handle issues and deal with objections shape their earned reputation. Health services are no different.

Investment, Risk and Return (Table 19.9) is the category that delivers to the stakeholders and investors. This category measures the more traditional

Table 19.9 Investment, risk & return assessment criteria

Assessment area (metal)	Required stage two growth key performance criterion	External consideration
Investment, risk & return		Related references
Investment reward	High return & profitability in relation to investment	[30; p89, 34, 41]
Investor attraction	Attractive to potential investors such as insurance companies with growing equity	[30; p89, [34]
Risk	Acceptable risk of loss in worst-case scenario	[30; p89, 33]
External stakeholders	Meet expectations of major external stakeholder groups	[7, 34]
Viability & cash-flow	Viable with predictable break-even & cash-flow	[30; p89, 34, 41]
Timescale	Long-term opportunity & income funding streams	[30; p89, 34]
Manage capital needs	Minimum investment required to support growth (operating and equity)	[30, 34]

performance indicators. Solid business fundamentals are still required to act as the foundation for transformative change. Good financial statement grants permission for the business to seek financing that is required to advance the quality of care and the deployment and implementation of health informatics.

Cross-Over Crisis

In every organization there are internal and external forces impacting the stakeholders. The cross-over crisis arises from trying to determine which master the organization serves? Is it the management team requiring results and the business objectives being met – or is it the patients and the services they require? This is a rhetorical question, as there is no correct answer, and patient care is largely the business objective of any healthcare system. Offering another perspective however, is the concept of "Service value". This occurs when the service organization consistently exceeds the customer's expectations. Value to the organization occurs when the organization exceeds productivity expectations of the senior management team. These two types of value, the former being external and the latter internal to the organization both contribute to the success or failure of the business (Fig. 19.16).

Emerging Technologies

The term emerging technologies is a bit of an oxymoron. Technologies do not emerge! Technological ideas emerge from ingenuity, adaptation and creativity. With significant investment, hard work and a little luck, a technology may garner market

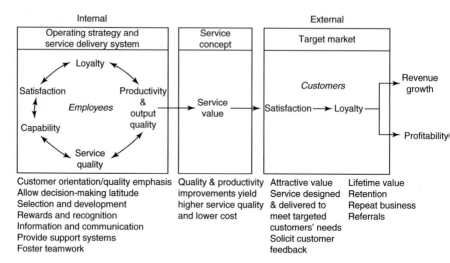

Fig. 19.16 Service profit chain

favor that generates the investment interest to overcome regulatory requirements, market testing, and eventually acceptance in a healthcare setting.

Some technologies come from the "grassroots" where a nurse or user decides to put forward a change in process or technique leading to better outcomes – as was the case with Florence Nightingale when she promoted cleaning and sterilization. Some technologies, especially in the pharmaceutical areas, can take years to get to market following many millions of dollars in research and development. This section provides a context for technologies now in the healthcare setting either by ongoing discovery or simple adaptation. This list of technologies is not exhaustive but a chronicle of their relevance in the healthcare setting.

Social Networking

Social media is a platform that can assist nursing faculty to help students gain greater understanding of communication, professionalism, healthcare policy, and ethics [42]. Social Networking is at the center of dialectic learning or learning while working together. Schmitt et al. [42] conclude that the future applications of technology in nursing education continue to expand, nurse educators must become early adopters and disseminators of the feasibility, acceptability, and outcomes of technology integration. The sole purpose of social networking sites is to engage others through electronic means. One of the challenges of improving the health of the population and patients is education. Using this very popular medium, nurses can assist in public education and act as the knowledge brokers to patients, interest groups, families and communities. This first digital generation views the integration and use of technology into their lives a defining characteristic. Finding employment, advancing their social lives, becoming knowledgeable on a topic, keeping track of news events and letting others know what you stand for and who are your friends and what are they doing represent a profile of yourself which can be pretty revealing. The caution with this technology is to respect what you are intentionally using it for, the privacy of others and contribute in a knowledgeable way.

Non-repudiation of Identification Technologies

Security in health informatics and healthcare systems is a significant concern. Non-repudiation of identification is when the system, and by extension the users, are assured that you are who you say you are. Martz [43] quotes from John Barkley, "Non-repudiation of origin protects against any attempt by a message originator to deny sending a message." She goes on to state:

> Non-repudiation of Origin (NRO) provides the recipient of a message with evidence of origin of the message, which will protect against any attempt by the originator to falsely deny having sent the message.
>   *Authentication + Integrity = Non-Repudiation of Origin (NRO)*
>   Non-repudiation of origin defines requirements to provide evidence to users/subjects about the identity of the originator of some information [43].

Computing systems can encrypt data on the storage medium as data and information transit communications networks all over the world. Operational procedures such as down-time and system back-ups maintain the integrity of the data at a systems level, however the biggest challenges in health informatics is at the end-user interface. The end-user interface refers to the appliances the end-users employ to access the various systems. Tablets, workstations, iPad's, mobile phones and their applications and data loggers such as portable glucose monitoring devices are considered end user devices. These devices require (1) security that can accommodate handoff from one staff member to the other, (2) integrity of the data so that it is backed up and does not get transmitted to users and accounts that might compromise the privacy of an individual, and (3) the continuity of service relating to patient care and critical data required to treat the patient.

The NRO is a combination of technologies, protocols and third party auditability. The concept of giving information to a third party to verify the sender of information is indeed who they say they are is a little more challenging to implement. The rudimentary precursor to the protocol and the information exchange is how do you uniquely identify a user in a reliable way?

A wide variety of approaches and technologies exist for identity management, such as retinal scans, RFID's (radio frequency identification), swipe cards, chips, finger prints, voice signature, facial recognition and even DNA. These tools to prove your identity are new in some cases and widely used in other such as the chip on your debt card. There is still a need for trust and to exercise vigilance to protect your PIN (Personal Identification Number) as an example.

Case Study

A nurse was on the floor dispensing medication using the electronic medication cart. It is an organizational policy and best practice for nurses to sign off the computer or lock the computer screen and keyboard before leaving the cart. It was Thursday on the medical-surgical unit and the nurse was verifying the Doctor's post-operative orders when a Code Blue (cardiac arrest) was called. In his haste to attend the emergency code, the nurse left the medication cart without locking the screen or signing out of the eMAR (electronic Medication Administration Record). The nurse became pre-occupied with the acute state of the patient and forgot the cart had not been locked. The Shift Supervisor directed a new nurse at shift change to complete the rounds of dispensing the meds.

The second nurse continued to use the screen with the open session and started to document nursing progress notes, dispense medications (some of the medications were controlled substances), obtain vitals on the patients and document results. By the end of a 12 hr shift, the second nurse started to log off the computer according to policy and practice guidelines and realized that she had spent the entire shift documenting and dispensing medications under her colleague's credentials.

If an adverse event were to happen to any of the patients the second nurse tended, whose license would be in jeopardy and who would be the subject of legal and/or disciplinary action? What does the second nurse do to correct the fact that she spent a complete shift cross-credentialed with her colleague who was on the previous shift? Do nothing and shutdown the computer? Notify the Shift Supervisor and then shut down the computer? Or notify the Shift Supervisor and seek advice? Or open all the charts under her own credentials, place a nursing note on every chart and notify the Shift Supervisor about what happened. Should the second nurse get the Shift Supervisor to notify the chart auditor, to report the cross credentials and to confirm there is a progress notes on every impacted chart? Which nurse would be affected or subject to professional sanctions if these changes were not made and something catastrophic happened to one of the patients?

This case illustrates the potential consequences and impact if the wrong person accidentally forgot to log-off or log-on properly. But what would happen if someone *knowingly* logged in under someone else's credentials and started to order narcotics, and dispense them to themselves, and the system could not explicitly validate the identity of the new user? The boundary between the end-user and the health information system is a trusted one. It is critically important now and into the future that this is honoured. It does not matter how sophisticated the technologies are at the point of care if the trusted access bound is broken. Your patients, their safety, and their information are at risk.

Hands-Free Technologies

Hands-free technologies in healthcare start to push the boundaries of what we consider to be "hands on" nursing. Hands-free can mean robotic surgery, remote consultations, using a head-sets or hands free microphone for documenting cases while still in the sterile field and voice activated searching of clinical information, to an iPad or Smart Phone, Siri-like voice or animated avatar providing advice based on a questions and answer sequence leading to suggested diagnosis and treatment. What is wrong with this picture? Readers might assume that a hands-free approach equates with a "hands off" approach to patients and a step away from the caring aspect of their professional role. Not so – but it is imperative that nurses understand how the hands free trend fits within the scope of caring and patient care.

How would a nurse informatician participate in the brave new world of touchless care? The first thing is touch the patient and facilitate the caring process. Someone needs to have their hands in play. As a care provider, and a facilitator of care, it is important not to forget the basic tenets of care. These being connect, observe, analyze, assimilate, decide and act. Is there any reason at all why these should change? NO, NO, NO.

Clarity and Quality

Clinical documentation is one of the first topics in nursing education, and attention to this professional and legal requirement. The abbreviations, units of measure, time intervals, interventions, and other elements of care need to be precisely documented to meet standards of practice, comply with legislative and organizational requirements, and ensure patient safety and continuity of care. Significant work has been undertaken to systematize care through the development of clinical pathways. The danger of frameworks and prescriptive healthcare behaviour is that the clinician could start to rely on the system as the primary mechanism to determine clinical appropriateness and blindly following the clinical pathway rather than thinking critically.

Healthcare information systems have evolved, often to a high degree of sophistication. Documentation is codified for pathologies, especially when it comes to documenting cancers. Emergency rooms have questions and answer computing to facilitate the care but to also provide consistent documentation and terminology. Terminology resources such as SNOMED CT used to document clinical care and ICD-10 to document diagnosis and coding for treatment plans provide the clinician with a means to document consistent information that can be extracted, analyzed and reported. The higher the quality of the data captured in the system, the better the analysis and the higher the probability the analysts might be able to tease knowledge and value from the data to help provide better and safer clinical care in the future.

Healthcare Anywhere

Healthcare anywhere addresses the mobility of the patient, the provider, and the service delivery organizations. Abbott [44] states that clinical environments are complex, stressful and safety critical, heightening the demand for technology solutions that will help clinicians manage health information efficiently and safely.

These challenges are exacerbated by the escalation of consumerism in health where patient are taking an increasingly active role in their own care and the quality of care that the system provides. This democratization of health information is cultivating a new dynamic and introduces another dimension to the work and the knowledge a health professional needs to sift through to act as a mediator or more correctly moderator in the patient plan of ONE. The patient plan of one refers to one complete electronic medical record and treatment plan that is complete and refers to a single record that reflects labs, diagnostic imaging, all hospital visits whether ambulatory outpatient or acute care. It should also have a wellness profile which reflects the lifestyle and steps to prevent disease. One plan, one patient, one record will require interfaces between systems, patient access legislation, and dialogue as to whose data is the patient record and how is it accessed and for what purpose. If a patient is on vacation and needs to visit a health centre, the patient's record should be accessible by the patient to assist the attending health care providers.

There is enormous diversity of highly portable, increasingly compact, and powerful information and communication technology devices on the market which is evidence of industry response to the growing demand [44]. Abbott goes on to describe the clinical expectations of such devices [44]:

> Un-tethering a provider [and/or patient] from a physical "place" with mobile technology and delivering the right information at the right time and at the right location are expectations for effective and safe clinical practice. [The usability of mobile device need to address], (1) input ease, (2) portability, (3) security/safety, (4) efficiency gains, and (5) general ease/intuitiveness.

This area of future consideration will call on the ingenuity of a practice that tends to thrive in stability and lumbering change. The demands from the patient and the 1st Generation Digital Care worker will force evolution of existing processes into a new perspective and paradigm. The key to acting as a change agent in this shifting environment is to consider your role as an intrapreneur, looking for ways to foster efficiencies and have the courage to bring these ideas forward in a way that is grounded in service value to the patient and the healthcare organization.

Heads-Up Computing

Heads-up computing refers to providing information, communication, and processing to the user without interrupting the field of vision or involvement in the sterile field. Heads-up computing allows the user to engage with the system without having to use a keyboard or turn from a line of sight. Hands-free phones with voice recognition were first developed in the mid 1980's for the operating room to allow the surgeon or others to answer the phone while still in the sterile field. The application of this technology was quite rudimentary but did address a specific problem.

Today we have voice recognition, audio avatars answering questions, and have controlled dialogue with the user to get a task complete. A good example of this technology is the use of GPS in cars. On-Star© developed by General Motors can provide information from inside the car, alert an operator and in the event of an accident, mobilize EMS and 911. These applications are starting to emerge in cell phones giving patients the potential to be very mobile but tethered to some very sophisticated monitoring equipment.

Heads-up displays (HUD) applied to the healthcare setting can enable the practitioner to focus and organize information in a way that facilitates clinical safety and optimizes workflow. This technology was originally developed in World War II by the German air force to provide better accuracy on their gun sights [36]. HUD has been used in commercial aircraft, sunglasses and video games. Heads-up displays allow users to receive data on a screen in front of them, so they don't have to look elsewhere, thus disrupting what they're concentrating on.

Application of this technology to the healthcare setting offers endless possibilities. Surgeons could monitor vital signs on their protective visors or overlaid on a laparoscopic monitor. Nurses could monitor a patient down the hall while dispensing medications to other patients. This technology could also be included in learning strategies where a tutorial can be viewed on a heads-up display, allowing users to actually imitate the instructor on a real system. It is possibly that the tablet or input device could communicate with the heads-up technology providing tips and tricks or suggested navigation or corrective action.

Nanorobotics

Nanorobotics are expected to be one of the game-changing technologies in healthcare. Paracha [45] reports that:

> Scientists throughout the world are working to develop novel and potent therapeutic strategies for cancer and in this field scientists [...] have successfully treated the cancer with the help of "DNA nanorobots". Researchers are of the opinion that due to the aptamers' ability to identify proteins responsible for different diseases, this method can be used in a number of diseases.

Atherton [46] published an article on magnetic microbots that can carry a payload of medication to any part of the body. Wikipedia [47] records:

> Potential applications for nanorobotics in medicine include early diagnosis and targeted drug-delivery for cancer, biomedical instrumentation, surgery, pharmacokinetics monitoring of diabetes, and health care.
> In such plans, future medical nanotechnology is expected to employ nanorobots injected into the patient to perform work at a cellular level. Such nanorobots intended for use in medicine should be non-replicating [where the nanorobots cannot reproduce themselves], as replication would needlessly increase device complexity, reduce reliability, and interfere with the medical mission. Nanotechnology provides a wide range of new technologies for developing customized solutions that optimize the delivery of pharmaceutical products.

Significant research and investment is currently being directed to nanorobotic technology for medical advances. It is still too early to determine how significant the emergence of nanorobotic will be in medicine and control or treatment of cellular level diseases such as cancer, leukemia, Alzheimer's, blood disorders and genetic abnormalities.

Will these technologies have an impact on nursing informaticians? The response to this question is another question. What role does the nurse have in observing, assimilating and deciding whether the treatment is benefiting the patient? Are there patterns of adverse effects or patterns of improvement? Are you the next Jack Andraka [48]?

Jack Andraka used what he found through Google searches and free online science journals to develop a plan and a budget. Jack contacted about 200 people including researchers at Johns Hopkins University and the National Institutes of Health with a proposal to work in their labs. He got 199 rejections before he finally got an acceptance from Dr. Anirban Maitra, Professor of Pathology, Oncology and Chemical and Biomolecular Engineering at Johns Hopkins School of Medicine. Jack worked after school every day, on weekends and over holidays at Maitra's lab until he developed his test [48].

Autonomic Information Systems

As health informatics systems have evolved, they have become more integrated and the data being retained is exploding concurrently with the accelerated need for computing capacity. Health information systems are distributed all over the globe. Adamczyk et al. [31] describe the rationale and how autonomic information systems work:

> For decades, system components and software have been evolving to deal with the increased complexity of system control, resource sharing and operations management. [...] A challenging problem is how to construct a system able to discover new resources during runtime [while the programs are running] automatically generate an intermediate management layer and apply selected policies with limited human intervention.

This advancement is a very technical one but illustrates how technology firms identify the problem and go to work to solve the problem. This technology takes on the role of system control by applying rules and activating resources on demand to ensure large complex systems remain operational.

In the human body, the autonomic systems are those which are involuntary in the computing systems context, the adaptation of the system to the user is transparent and appears to behave involuntarily without human intervention. The difference is that the autonomic health information systems have been designed to behave in a predictive way based on rules and a rules engine that supervises the available resources and applies them as required based on these rules. This functionality is usually connected to a database and system resources and not the applications that are using the resources.

Silver Lining Clouds: Big Data Synthesis, Cognitive Crawler

Is there a silver lining in all the hype around cloud computing? To answer this question, you must first undertake a brief tutorial on cloud computing. Cloud computing is the processing, storage and connectivity over the Internet to run your applications in a shared online environment where the computing capacity and storage can grow on demand. This is an over simplification but it does reflect the essence of the technologies.

The silver lining is that there is now a place to store the copious quantities of documentation generated by the health care system. Nursing notes, clinical progress notes, incident reports, drug interactions, provider orders, doctors' notes, and patients' lab results all comprise a part of an electronic health record. This data being available in a shared computing environment somewhere in the network and protected with proper security, minimizes the capital investment required to create and sustain a complex electronic infrastructure, and delegates operational support to an environment that grows and shrinks based on demand.

Big data is currently a buzzword or popular phrase used to describe the massive volume of both structured and unstructured data, that is so large that it's difficult to process using traditional database and software techniques. The technologies in development by database software vendors will enable organization and researchers to access and utilize the huge datasets that are being created by the electronic health record systems [49].

Making sense of all this data is the "cognitive crawler", which is a design methodology and tool that provides the parameters for a search engine that makes seek decisions based on thought process algorithms for exploration. The cognitive crawler is based on the ability to recognize structured patterns and it can drill down in a database, a cloud presence or websites, optimizing search and computing, reducing costs, and increasing search performance. Describing the relationships of data, their characteristics and their co-relationships produce new predictive patterns leading to a better understanding of a disease. This might sound a little farfetched but these systems are being used to search seismic data to locate oil and gas and in its simplest application predict search topics on Google.

To satisfy the inquisitive mind, why is this important for nurses and healthcare? Quite simply, at no time in human history has so much data been available with the tools and the computing capacity to observe, assimilate and render new ground breaking original thought. Combined with the demands for fiscally accountable, outcome optimization, and client centred care, and there is a strong imperative to generate new knowledge from the existing data and to use it to transform processes, programs, and approaches to health, health care delivery, and healthcare management.

Patient Command Centre

The first consideration when you read the phrase "Patient Command Centre", you might think of a call center or a center that receives alerts from patients that have transponders attached to them. That would be true in most cases but that thinking would be in the current or in the present state, not the future state.

The Patient Command Centre is the first component to supporting the patient plan of one. Imagine if the patient was carrying a medical card or similar device, which could be presented, scanned, or grant access to a health professional/provider where all pertinent information is presented similar to an electronic health alter. Can a patient be their own advocate for their own patient care data? The individual becomes their own command center regardless of jurisdiction or provider.

Consider the previous discussion on consumerism and now apply your active thinking skills from the patients' perspective. The patient should be able to remotely select the services she or his wishes to participate in and the set up "My Home Command Centre". Who do I wish to connect with? What services do I need? How frequently do I want to receive the service?

What alerts does the patient wish to transmit and to whom? Is there a sequence of events that will determine which command paths are followed to activate or dismiss interventions? Will the patient hold a Personal Health Record (PHR) that potentially will decide on outcomes? Does this PHR contain a digitally signed Advanced Directive or Do Not Resuscitate declaration? Can the patient upload performance data such as heart rate standing and active heart rate during an exercise routine? Based on the patient's health and activity, a living coach similar to iPad's Siri could motivate the most sedentary of patent. What role does the nursing informatician play? Nothing is pre-determined at this point. Nursing has an opportunity to become an active designer in future scenarios and further define nursing roles in support of innovative patient care, patient autonomy and ways in which evolving technologies can be harnessed to support efficient and effective health care.

Connecting the Dots

The musing of what will happen in the future has been the subject of dreamers and profits since the beginning of time. What kinds of things will help you navigate change? Being attuned to your surroundings, recording data accurately, and identify trends as was the case with Florence Nightingale. Looking into the future and making prognostications is folly. There are so many things that can happen that will change the course of history. There are no precise algorithms that will provide a clear or quantifiable roadmap.

The trick to getting to the future is not to *predict* it but to *prepare* for the future and to be open to everything that comes your way. The tenets to seeing your way forward in the future are:

- Visualization: see, observe and create. Think actively with all your senses.
- Self-Actualization: motivation and plan. Do not sit and do nothing. Be motivated by your passion for caring and giving care and plan you path or mind-map your future.
- Information Synthesis: assimilate and decide. Take the information you have been given, look for patterns and understand what they mean and then decide to do something with your newfound knowledge.

The last task to prepare for time travel into the future is getting the feel for "Digital Caring". Figure 19.17 is a mind-map to the future in Nursing Informatics.

Nursing informatics mind map to the future

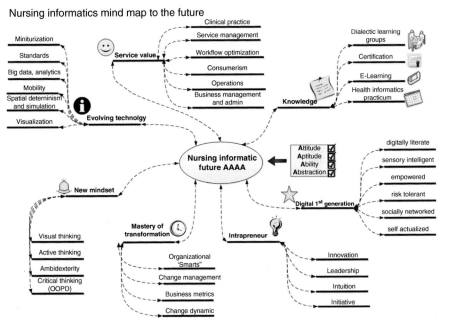

Fig. 19.17 Digital caring

This map summarizes all that you have learned in this chapter and positions you for "Digital Caring". As the first generation digital care workers enter the system the future has no bounds, it is a continuum of change and transformation in the context of the real business work where money, service value, operational methods and intrepreneurship become part of your journey.

Downloads

Available from extras.springer.com:

Educational Template (PDF 89 kb)
Educational Template (PPTX 120 kb)

References

1. Louis M, Sutton R. Switching cognitive gears: from habits of mind to active thinking, human relations [The Tavistock Institute of Human Relations]. 1991. From website: http://hum.sage-pub.com/content/44/1/55. Retrieved 29 Sept 2013.
2. Mercola J. 15-year-old invents new test for early, reliable detection of pancreatic cancer. 2013. From website: http://www.stonekingdom.org/. Retrieved 15 Aug 2013.

3. Sicinski A. Visual thinking magic: the evolutions of extraordinary intelligence Melbourne, Australia. 2013. From website: http://blog.iqmatrix.com/how-to-mind-map/. Retrieved 1 Oct 2013.
4. Nightingale F. Diagram of the causes of mortality in the army of the east. 1858. From website: BBC.The.Beauty.of.Diagrams.4of6.Florence.Nightingale.PDTV.Xvid.AC3.MVGroup.org. avi. Retrieved 3 Oct 2103.
5. Ahn H, Yeon E, Ham E, Paik W. Patient modeling using mind mapping representation as a part of Nursing Care Plan [Dept. of Nursing Science, Eulji University; Dept of Computer Science, Konkuk University] Korea. 2003. From website: http://link.springer.com/static-content/. Retrieved 18 Sept 2013.
6. Wang K. Business life cycles and five elements theory National Taipei University Taipei, Taiwan. 2005. From website: http://systemicbusiness.org/. Retrieved 28 Jan 2011.
7. Daft RL, Armstrong A. Organization theory & design 1st Canadian ed. Toronto: Nelson Education Ltd; 2009.
8. Hanks S, Watson C, Jansen E, Chandler G. Tightening the life-cycle construct: a taxonomic study of growth stage configurations in high-technology organizations, Entrepreneurship Theory and Practice. 1993. From website: https: http://www.allbusiness.com/management/change-management/. Retrieved 25 Jan 2011.
9. Sundarasaradula D, Hasan H. A unified open systems model for explaining organizational change Chapter 11 University of Wollongong. 2005. From website: http://epress.anu.edu.au/. Retrieved 5 Jan 2011.
10. Perumal S, Pandey N. Process-based business transformation through services computing Tech Mahindra Ltd. Pune, India. 2008. From website: http://www.waset.org/journals/waset/. Retrieved 3 Feb 2011.
11. Sniukas M. A 5-step process for business transformation and organizational stability Innovation 360 Institute. 2009. From website: https://i360insight.com/. Retrieved 15 Feb 2011.
12. Melenovsky M, Sinur J. Having a BPM maturity model is important for long lasting BPM Success Business Rules Journal. 2006;7(12). From website: http://www.BRCommunity.com/a2006/b325.html. Retrieved 16 Feb 2011.
13. DMR Group. Fundamentals of change [presentation]. Montreal; 1996.
14. Wikipedia. Organizational culture. 2011. From website: http://en.wikipedia.org/wiki/Organizational_culture/. Retrieved 4 Feb 2011.
15. Enck RE. The OODA Loop. Home health care management. 2012;24(3), 123. From website: http://hhc.sagepub.com/content/24/3/123.full.pdf+html. Retrieved 1 Dec 2013.
16. Birkinshaw J, Gibson C. Building ambidexterity into an organization MIT Sloan Management Review. 2004. From website: http://faculty.london.edu. Retrieved 20 Mar 2011.
17. O'Reilly CA, Tushman ML. Ambidexterity as a dynamic capability: resolving the Innovator's dilemma Graduate School of Business [Stanford University]. 2007. From website: www.hbs.edu/research/pdf/07-088WP.pdf. Retrieved 20 Mar 2011.
18. Robinson JC. Managed consumerism in health care. Health Affairs. 2013;32(12). From website: http://content.healthaffairs.org/content/24/6/1478.full. Retrieved 30 Nov 2013.
19. Cohen SB, Grote KD, Pietraszek WE, Laflamme F. Increasing consumerism in health-care through intelligent information technology [Am J Manag Care] McKinsey and Company, San Francisco. 2010. From website: http://www.ncbi.nlm.nih.gov/. Retrieved 2 Oct 2013.
20. Fitzsimmons JA, Fitzsimmons MJ. Service management operations, strategy, information technology. 6th ed. New York: McGraw-Hill/Irwin; 2008.
21. Murray SP. Prince Edward Island (PEI) Clinic Information System (CIS) surgical areas support services [Athabasca University] Charlottetown; 2010.
22. USMBOK. The universal service management body of knowledge (USMBOK™) Service management 101 and IMC. 2008. From website: http://www.usmbok.org/usmbok_ip_guidelines.html. Retrieved 18 Dec 2010.
23. Slack N, Chambers S, Johnson R. Operations management. 5th ed. Prentice Hall, Pearson Education Saffron House, London, UK; 2007.

24. Tapscott D. Growing up digital. The Tapscott Group [Martin Prosperity Institute, Rotman School of Management] Toronto. 2008. From website: http://www.growingupdigital.com/. Retrieved 31 Sept 2013.
25. Murray SP. Entrepreneurial Facilitator's Dilemma: surviving stage two business growth "portage or shoot the rapids" [Athabasca University], Charlottetown; 2011.
26. Wilson A, Whitaker N, Whitford D. Rising to the challenge of health care reform with entrepreneurial and intrapreneurial nursing initiatives. Online J Issues Nurs. 2012;17(2), Manuscript 5. From website: http://nursingworld.org/MainMenuCategories/ANAMarketplace/ANAPeriodicals/OJIN/TableofContents/Vol-17-2012/No2-May-2012/Rising-to-the-Challenge-of-Reform.html. Retrieved 6 Dec 2013.
27. Normand RA. Growing from entrepreneur to manager. 2007. From website: http://www.isbminc.com. Retrieved 29 Dec 2010.
28. Filion LJ. Defining the entrepreneur complexity and multi-dimensional systems, some reflections [Working Paper# 2008–03] HEC Montreal; 2008.
29. De Jong J, Wennekers S. H200802 Intrapreneurship: conceptualizing entrepreneurial employee behaviour [SCALES-initiative (SCientific AnaLysis of Entrepreneurship and SMEs)], Zoetermeer, The Netherlands (NL); 2008.
30. Good WS. Building a dream seventh edition, a Canadian guide to starting your own business. Toronto: McGraw-Hill Ryerson; 2008.
31. Adamczyk J, Chojnacki R, Jarzab M, Zielinski K. Rule engine based lightweight framework for adaptive and autonomic computing [Institute of Computing Science, AGH- University of Science and Technology] Heidelberg\Berlin: Springer; 2008. From website: http://www.ics.agh.edu.pl. Retrieved 25 Sept 2013.
32. Bhide AV. The origin and evolution of new businesses New York: Oxford University Press; 2000. From website: www.bhide.net. Retrieved 8 Dec 2010.
33. Norton B. Managing an early-stage business for rapid growth C-Level Enterprises. 2004. From website: http://www.managingforgrowth.com. Retrieved 18 Dec 2010.
34. Timmons JA, Spinelli S. The opportunity: creating, shaping, recognizing, seizing. Chapter 3: [Athabasca University RVET-651 Reading] New venture creation. McGraw-Hill/Irwin; 2003. pp. 79–117.
35. Cook LS, et al. Human issues in service design. Journal of Operations Management Elsevier Science B. V. [Athabasca University ESMT-614 Service Management]. 2002. Retrieved 15 Nov 2010 from AU Digital Library.
36. Stark C. The long and winding road to personal heads-up displays. 2012. From website: http://mashable.com/2012/02/26/heads-up-displays/. Retrieved 22 Oct 2013.
37. Jones N. SME's lifecycle: steps to failure or success? [Assumption University, Graduate School of Business]. 2011. From website: http://www.moyak.com/papers/small-mediumenterprises. Pdf. Retrieved 8 Jan 2011.
38. Morgen SD. Organizational change, training and development, and motivation. 2009. From website: http://www.businessballs.com/. Retrieved 20 Feb 2011.
39. Anantadjaya S, Mulawarman S. Influencing factors on project overrun: is it intrapreneurship School of Business, Faculty of Business Administration, Swiss German University, BSD City. 2010. From website: http://www.globalresearch.com.my. Retrieved 14 Dec 2010.
40. Kotler P, Keller KL. Marketing management. 13th ed. Upper Saddle River: Prentice-Hall; 2009.
41. Fraser LM, Ormiston A. Understanding financial statements. 8th ed. Upper Saddle River: Pearson-Prentice Hall, NY; 2007.
42. Schmitt T, Sims-Giddens S, Booth R. Social Media Use in Nursing Education American Nurses Association Silver Spring. 2012. From website: http://www.nursingworld.org/. Retrieved 15 Sept 2013.
43. Martz C. NRO – Non Repudiation of Origination birds-eye.Net. 2013. From website: http://www.birds-eye.net/. Retrieved 21 Oct 2013.
44. Abbott PA. The effectiveness and clinical usability of handheld information appliance [Health Systems & Outcomes Department, John Hopkins University School of Nursing], Hindawi Publishing Corporation, Nursing Research and Practice. 2012;2012, Article ID 307258.

45. Paracha UZ. "DNA Nanorobots" have successfully been used for cancer treatment [Wyss Institute at Harvard University]. 2012. From website: http://technorati.com/. Retrieved 22 Oct 2013.

46. Atherton KD. These magnetic nanobots could carry drugs into your brain: the robots are coming from INSIDE the blood! 2013. From website: http://www.popsci.com/technology/. Retrieved 22 Oct 2013.

47. Wikipedia. Nanorobotics. 2013. From website: http://en.wikipedia.org/wiki/Nanorobotics. Retrieved 23 Oct 2013.

48. Aronson B. Jack Andraka — 15-year-old invents cancer test 100 times more sensitive & 26,000 times cheaper than current tests. 2013. From website: http://www.bradaronson.com/jack-andraka/. Retrieved 23 Oct 2013.

49. Webopedia. Big data. 2013. From website: http://www.webopedia.com/. Retrieved 20 Oct 2013.

Part V
Education

Chapter 20
Nursing Education

Paula M. Procter

Abstract It is acknowledged that the whole of this text is about advancing your understanding of nursing informatics which is education, this chapter focusses upon the key message that education must take on the mantle of preparing future generations of nurses to be active participants in information and communications technology (ICT) developments across healthcare rather than just teaching 'computer skills'. A humanistic model of information is offered to try to explore ways of moving away from a mechanistic approach to health ICT and this is linked to progressive development from inactivity to wisdom. In conclusion some key learning outcomes are presented for consideration.

Keywords Learning • Information • Humanistic information model • Driving information change through curricula • Information wisdom • Educators

Key Concepts

Learning
Information
Humanistic information model
Driving information change through curricula
Information wisdom
Educators

Opening

Society in general has coped with the first few years of the twenty-first Century and in most cases coped well. However, recent events have clearly awakened a more

---

The online version of this chapter (doi:10.1007/978-1-4471-2999-8_20) contains supplementary material, which is available to authorized users.

P.M. Procter, RN, MSc, FBCS, FIMIANI
Department of Nursing and Midwifery, Sheffield Hallam University,
Mercury house, 38 Collegiate Crescent, Sheffield S10 2BP, UK
e-mail: p.procter@shu.ac.uk

© Springer-Verlag London 2015
K.J. Hannah et al. (eds.), *Introduction to Nursing Informatics*,
Health Informatics, DOI 10.1007/978-1-4471-2999-8_20

415

cautious outlook, particularly in the light of expenditure on all areas of commerce, industry and government, with a call to account in all areas including that of health-care. Instead of the expected down turn in healthcare cost, with a push towards preventative rather than curative (or acute care) provision, the cost of healthcare is rising each year.

The question must be what can nursing education do in relation to the development and use of information and communications technology to advance nursing in meeting societal challenges? The direct answer is that education is the key to the future of nursing's continued use and leadership role in information and communications technology across health and social care. We have seen examples of where this is effective in earlier chapters and in the next chapter you are offered examples of key learning technologies.

The use of information and communications technology (ICT) in the commissioning, delivery and audit of health and social care is now 'normal'. Nursing pioneers around the world drove the development of this "new normal"; some from the United States are featured by AMIA (2013) see nursing pioneers [1]. Now more than ever the "new normal" is being driven by patients and population demand. In many countries patients are able to access and control their care records, they are able to choose their care provider and they are able to leave their evaluative comments for all to read through on-line technologies, such abilities are changing the face of health and social care provision.

In past years there has been a significant need for ICT skills development amongst nursing students and qualified practitioners. ICT skills education is no longer such a cause for concern with the ubiquitous availability and use of digital devices. It is finally time to separate prerequisite technological skills from the nursing knowledge. This chapter will consider the ways in which nurse education can support information developments in health and social care for the benefit of patients and the public at large.

Education in nursing extends from pre-University/College through undergraduate to post graduate and beyond, what is considered in this chapter should be relevant at all levels. It is not our purpose to concentrate on specific courses for nursing informatics in isolation but to see education of nursing to be inclusive of all that is information significant. It is the intention to direct attention toward information and not technology in this chapter and visit the technology in Chap. 17.

There has been an exponential growth in the access to information through personal communication devices such as smart cell phones, tablets, television and game consoles to name but a few. Many of those entering nursing education, do so as 'digital natives' [2] with high expectation that not only will their education be inclusive of course material exchanged through technology but also their professional careers will be supported through information and communication technologies appropriate to their area of work. Nevertheless, there is still a difference between mere transference of skills and the understanding within a professional practice base. This difference needs to hold value in order to be accepted by the target audience, i.e. nursing students.

Learning About Information

We appear to be moving towards a belief that there are three elements that connect together to form twenty-first Century learning and these are personal value, content and environment [3] as they affect the student and the lecturer. We must not forget that behind all ICT enabled learning is a concept best embodied in a statement by Stonier:

> An educated workforce learns how to exploit new technology, an ignorant one becomes its victim [4].

Are nurses exploiting information and communications technology through education or are we merely using the technology in a mechanistic fashion so that we are becoming disillusioned slaves to the technology? Are we developing understanding of the governance and information generation, storage, retrieval, flows and use in order that we as nurses can ensure the systems implemented do not conflict with practice; or, are we just transferring words to a file downloadable by students?

It would seem appropriate to start with some thoughts around what we mean by information within a human context and linked to the personal value element suggested above. A review of a humanistic information model [5] will help form a basis from which we can generate further thoughts. The model uses engaging cog wheels as shown in Fig. 20.1 and demonstrates two significant features of humanistic information management, the first being that cogs turning generate power, we know that information is power; equally we can adjust the power requirement depending upon the value set we attribute to the information. The second is an attempt to reduce the

Fig. 20.1 Humanistic information model

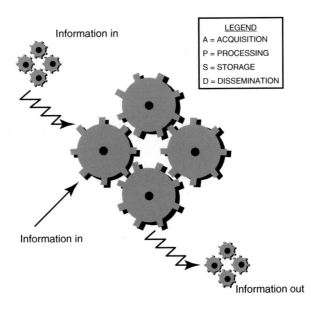

Information in

LEGEND
A = ACQUISITION
P = PROCESSING
S = STORAGE
D = DISSEMINATION

Information in

Information out

traditional linearity of information models and acknowledge that we deal with huge amounts of information every waking minute of the day.

Each cogwheel has a core function and yet, each cogwheel cannot act independently of the ones to which it is attached. To start with the 'Acquisition' cog, all our senses acquire information all of the time whether we want it or not, some of this information is bland but most information we acquire is value-laden, either with the senders' values, or our own. For example, national news will have different slants depending upon the target audience, the editor will determine the story to feature and we can see the result through comparing different news providers. We are dependent upon the considered values of the editor.

The cogs next to acquisition are to the right of the processing or filtering cog and to the left of the dissemination cog. The processing cog is where filtering of information takes place; here the conscious and subconscious decisions about information and how to manage information are considered. The processing cog is linked to the storage cog for it is here that intrinsic and extrinsic self exists [6] and the extrinsic self is a result of life experiences. Each person will filter (or value) information differently based upon his or her life and experiences. Decisions are made upon a matrix of previous such situations and outcomes. An example of filtering could occur when we pass into and out of rooms, offices, cars, or trains; how often do we consciously think about how to enter a room with a closed door, very rarely, for we have learned how to 'do doors'. However, if we have been standing at the door for some time and nothing happens then we might raise 'doors' into conscious thought and while we have been pushing at the door, we read 'pull' and act accordingly. The same could be said of a registered nurse approaching a patient; is it conscious or unconscious thought as we near the patient resulting in an action of some kind. We can see that the processing cog links back with the acquisition cog; this allows for 'enquiry' to help complete a process requiring new or additional knowledge, connecting self with out-sourced information.

The storage cog is a mass of information. If the model is being used to consider an individual and their information 'self', then the storage cog represents all the activities, experiences, thoughts, ideas and dreams of that individual. If the model is being used to consider an organisation then the storage cog represents all the previous work documented and/or experienced of that organisation. If the model is being used to consider a profession, for example nursing, then the storage cog represents the history of the profession along with all the standards and processes to the present. Some of the stored information may be immediately retrievable for most of us, but a lot of it is lost until an appropriate gateway is opened, for example for an individual a photograph bringing back memories or someone saying something which triggers a remembrance, or a file or document for an organisation or profession. The 'tip of the tongue' experience classically identifies something we know we know but the gateway is not completely open to the item. If the new information reaching the storage cog is incomplete we may feel the need to actively acquire further information. This can be at either a conscious or subconscious level in order to give both complete meaning and a gateway through which to connect to the new information so it can be found again when needed.

The dissemination cog is where we demonstrate our values to others and to our-selves be this associated with an individual, organisation or profession. Every action we make as an individual has a value, for example the way we use words and the very words themselves have a value. We decide what is of value and what is not. We can only operate on the information we have at the time, disseminated decisions are based upon known information. If after a decision has been made a new piece of information is obtained the decision may be different. Our filtering system can only operate in real-time however long that real-time might be. There is an automatic knock-on effect to dissemination; this too is in real-time whenever we communicate with others, either in person or through technology, for example the telephone, video calls or email.

What is required in nursing and health care generally, is a re-definition of healthcare roles and a definition of our 'value-sets'. We need to decide what is important for health care in this information intensive era. In addition, we also must determine how to prepare those starting, returning or continuing education who will practice further into this new millennium with the plethora of digital devices expected, the emergence of pharmacogenomics, nano technologies and medical innovation. We need to know how we filter information to meet the needs of our value-sets. What we do not need are replacements for clinicians and teach-ers by mechanistic computer systems/packages, which have neither the humanis-tic understanding nor the flexibility to respond to patients' needs in a supportive human way.

Nurse Education Driving Information Change

Within healthcare there are expected to be major information implications as we move further into becoming an information society [7]. Nursing education must be fully able to prepare practitioners to be ready to act as information management advocates for patients and clients, in order to help patients and clients navigate the masses of accessible information in a safe and effective way. Moreover, nurses also need to be prepared to act as custodians of health and social care information within a governance framework.

Nursing faces new opportunities and challenges, from both the society around us and the increasing demands to work effectively in an information intensive environ-ment. Nursing must look both to the past and to the future in order to prepare nurses to cope at the highest level with the demands placed upon them.

Taking the information model described, do we rely upon stored tradition or do we travel a less trodden path? Tradition in nursing is a strong influencer, which may be more in the minds of those who uphold it rather than in fact. We have seen poor tradition in action in both nursing education and in practice settings. In the world of health information technology, the plethora of computer systems introduced over the past 20 years has done little more than mechanize traditional processes; forms have been replicated on a computer screen under the guise of computerization. Similarly in nursing education, lecture notes have been loaded onto the Web under the guise of using the Web for teaching. Neither of these is helpful or effective for the purpose for which it was intended.

If we move away from tradition, life becomes considerably more uncomfortable. No longer can we rely upon previously safe methods in nursing education. It is easily understood why tradition plays such an important part in the nursing education of today. However, let us examine another possible area of consideration, that of developing curriculum that accepts the argument of conscious and subconscious thought. With the potential of reducing the currently crammed curriculum with one that has a clear mission of separating conscious and subconscious nursing.

We, in nursing education must get our act together and undertake the role of education within today's and tomorrow's information society or we are disadvantaging our students. We, in nursing education must take the lead as opposed to catching up around nursing/health informatics. As discussed in an earlier chapter the unique role nursing has is that of being the only health professional with 24/7 patient contact.

There is an information and communications technology continuum upon which we should all position ourselves. At the one end is information, where those positioned understand personal and professional value sets of information, its acquisition, its filtering (conscious and unconscious), its storage, its dissemination, and its use. At the other end is technology, where those positioned are fully versed with all manner of technology and are able to affect its use with competence. In the middle, are those positioned with the ability to have insight into information management and an insight into the possibilities of technology probably without the skills to affect such possibilities. At all times, while positioning ourselves on the continuum, we must be aware of the professional needs of nursing education and prepare ourselves to meet and surpass those needs.

Does Mrs Smith, admitted yesterday for a hip replacement operation expect a nurse to be skilled in word-processing, or does she expect a nurse to be skilled in information management? I would suggest the latter, although the words used by Mrs Smith may not be as above, more likely she will ask questions such as, *'This will help my walking won't it nurse?'*, *'I won't have too much pain after the operation, will I?'*, *'It is only two years since I was last in this hospital but everything seems to have changed.'* And *'I have no family who can come and collect me when I'm ready for discharge, how will I get home?'* The nurse must know how to obtain answers to these and similar questions and how to record any information outcomes from her answers.

In the next chapter we examine some ways in which nursing education has exploited technology to provide solutions now embedded into nursing courses by moving away from using the technology in a mechanistic fashion.

It is clear that there is growing reliance upon health based information from computer systems to inform local, State (or regional) and National decision making, *"Throughout many western national healthcare services, extensive e-Health infrastructures and systems are now viewed as central to the future provision of safe, efficient, high quality, citizen-centred health care"* [8]. The information generated will guide choices for provision of healthcare. As key informaticians, nurses need to understand why the information used must be accurate, timely and appropriate for us to be able to move forward with confidence in the healthcare provision choices made. Such confidence will be achieved through nursing education.

Nursing has been slow to embrace new technologies unless they have a direct relationship with the delivery of patient care, for example, a vital signs monitor, infusion pump or computerised patient medication orders/records. Nursing education has to consider the changing nature of nursing as influenced by information and communications technology. Similarly nursing education must also recognize the activities needed to retain a positive balance between nursing need found through patient care demand and the emerging information and communication technologies (eHealth).

Many working in the health industry consider the development of computer technology to support the delivery and evaluation of healthcare to be a very recent issue but this is very far from the truth and indeed in bygone years nursing was leading the way in clinical, managerial and educational use of computer technology. Whilst Chap. 4 deals with historical aspects of nursing informatics this short historical piece is included in this chapter as a critique on strategic educational decisions made in regard to nursing education. Decisions taken have had a direct impact on preparing nurses for informatics leadership roles within the health care domain.

In 1982, the first world congress for nursing and information and communications technology was held in London and attracted delegates from all over the world. It was this conference that resulted in the International Medical Informatics Association (IMIA) opening a Working Group specifically for nursing, this working group continues to be at the forefront of nursing informatics today.

At the 1982 conference Barber [9] stated '*Nursing is too big and too important to be left free-wheeling within the system [Health Services Computing] and the more effectively nurses grasp these systems, the more effectively will they be able to participate knowledgeably in the managerial and planning discussions.*' But overall nursing has been left outside the key discussions and system development and this is regrettable both for the profession and for patient care.

A paper from the 1982 conference by Constance M Berg entitled 'The Importance of Nurses' Input for the Selection of Computerized Systems' [10] offered nursing a choice, but in most cases this fell upon deaf ears. Sadly we didn't follow Berg's call to make the right choice '*The choice is there and the time to make the choice is now. The decision must be whether to act traditionally and have change thrust upon the profession [nursing] from the outside or to anticipate this revolution in nursing practice, familiarise nurses with it, and prepare them to take an active part in the introduction of computers into the nursing community*' [11]. In general, nursing has covered its head and hoped that this new development would go away, we are now paying for the take up of this choice.

Today, history seems to be repeating itself, for it was in the early 1960s that the WHO arranged international seminars on automatic data processing in health care but nurses were not invited until 1971 [12]. The last 10–15 years, as we entered the twenty-first Century, there has been paucity of champions taking forward the nursing agenda in information and communications technology (eHealth), even in the

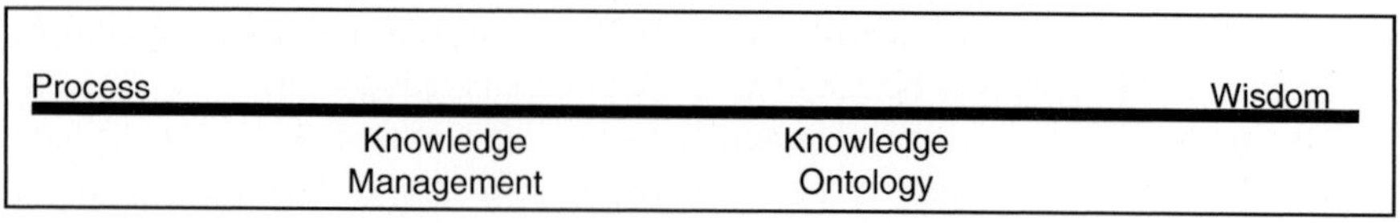

Process		Wisdom
Knowledge	Knowledge	
Management	Ontology	

Fig. 20.2 The basic education continuum that may help understanding around professional involvement with new technologies

preparation of the next generation of nurses in some countries the number of undergraduate curricula which include modules on eHealth can be counted on one hand.

There is a basic education continuum that may help understanding around professional involvement with new technologies (Fig. 20.2). At the start is **process**, which is where a series of actions, changes, or functions bring about a result; simple activity, which is grounded in day-to-day activities to attain a satisfactory outcome. Next is **knowledge management** where a range of practices are used by organisations to identify, create, represent, and distribute knowledge for reuse, awareness and learning. Here learning is taking place and this learning is iterative. **Knowledge ontology** could be described as sorting things into groups to form meaning. Ontology deals with questions concerning what entities exist or can be said to exist, and how such entities can be grouped, related within a hierarchy, and subdivided according to similarities and differences, along the lines of care classification, this higher level thinking/cognition works in theory but rarely in nursing clinical practice. Finally there is a state of **wisdom** which is an ideal that has been celebrated since antiquity as the knowledge needed to live a good life and to be at peace in our understanding of what we do and have the confidence to make new connections that add to our professional existence. In general, scholars have emphasised that wisdom includes various combinations of the following: knowledge, understanding, experience, discretion, and intuitive understanding, along with a capacity to apply these qualities well towards finding solutions to problems.

As mentioned earlier, nursing has embraced new information and communications technologies where they have a direct positive value in patient care but this could be described as the process of patient care, an advanced practitioner has raised their knowledge and practice to wisdom level.

As cited in earlier chapters the American Nurses Association (AMIA, 2008; Cited in Slider maintain that 3, HIMMS (http://www.himss.org/files/HIMSSorg/handouts/NI101.pdf, 2012) *"Nursing informatics (NI) integrates nursing science, computer and information science, and cognitive science to manage, communicate, and expand the data, information, knowledge, and wisdom of nursing practice"* [13].

Although the technology today is light years ahead of that used to be, there is still considerable evidence of mechanised use rather than true use of the power the technology offers. Frequently we see lecture notes on the web, PowerPoint presentations, and documents for students to access [14] this is using the web as a storage device, which is fine as long as it is recognised as such. But the technology can offer nursing students and lecturers/instructors so much more. The development of virtual learning environments has widened the horizon to some degree, but through informal observations it would appear that very few teachers use powerful ICT tools for much more than a text page-turner with a few web links and graphics.

Record keeping is one of the key requirements of nursing and is within the standards of conduct, performance and ethics for nurses and midwives in most countries (e.g. NMC, http://www.nmc-uk.org/Documents/NMC-Publications/NMC-Record-Keeping-Guidance.pdf 2008) [15] and yet in a recent project [16] where some 200 de-identified, full patient case notes were obtained it was clear that the nursing documentation was poor. Maybe this could be a reason why nursing is reluctant to move forward in terms of information and communications technology implementation. It is a known fact that a poor manual system will become a poor or inappropriately used technically supported system [17].

It seems as though there is something preventing nursing education embracing informatics across curricula. the barriers preventing nursing education moving forward with purpose in informatics curricula inclusion include the financial attitude. where informatics is seen as a cost rather than an investment; the applications being tactical rather than strategic; limited impact to a few showing an interest rather than creating a pervasive approach; seeing the technology as computers rather than considering multiple technologies; and finally, management tending towards delegation rather than taking a leadership role. Nursing education must overcome these barriers so that nurses of tomorrow will be fully involved in the design, development, implementation and evaluation [18] of clinical ICT systems and sadly this hasn't happened ubiqitously, so where does nursing education go from here?

There is a choice, but now our choice is more urgent than previously and the choice is either to continue to shy away from getting involved in the development, implementation, evaluation and leadership it is already too late to advise on the basic design and let nursing quietly disappear; or, to get involved through building our knowledge base and educating towards adding informatics wisdom to our professional knowledge in order that we can:

- understand and improve, influence and use new technologies and informatics, including remote care;
- find the most reliable sources of information to support evidence based practice;
- guide patients through publicly available information sources;
- incorporate ICT into patient consultations;
- manage the nurse patient relationship when the nurse is not physically in the same place as the patient;
- perform a quick and accurate data entry at the point of care;
- understand the legal and ethical issues associated with managing and sharing patient information;
- extract data to support decisions and monitor the outcomes of practice;
- understand the role of technology in the delivery and organisation of care
- train other users such as patients and carers how to use relevant ICTs

The final resolution around nurses and information and communications technology will depend upon nursing itself. There are ever increasing complex technologies which will require of us to use these correctly for our patients' safety and care such as nano technology, biotechnology, pharmacogenomics, radio frequency identity, and remote home monitoring to name but a few. Educators must play a significant role in generating knowledge in information and communications technologies in order the nursing can be at the forefront of future innovations and developments.

Downloads

Available from extras.springer.com:

Educational Template (PDF 97 kb)
Educational Template (PPTX 123 kb)

References

1. American Medical Informatics Association. Nursing informatics pioneers. Web site: http://www.amia.org/programs/working-groups/nursing-informatics/history-project/video-library-1 (2013). Last Accessed 16 Apr 2013.
2. Technopedia. Available from: http://www.techopedia.com/definition/28094/digital-native. Accessed 12 Sept 2013.
3. Brindley JE, Walti C, Blaschke LM. Creating effective collaborative learning groups in an online environment. Int Rev Res Open Distance Learn. 2009;10(3). Web link: http://www.irrodl.org/index.php/irrodl/article/view/675/1271. Last Accessed 16 Apr 2013.
4. Stonier T. Changes in western society: educational implications. In: Sculler T et al., editors. Recurrent education and lifelong learning. London: Kogan Page; 1981.
5. Procter P. Keynote address 'Apocalypse Shortly!'. In: Saba V, Carr R, Sermeus W, Rocha P, editors. One Step Beyond: The Evolution of Technology and Nursing. Auckland: Proceedings of the 7th IMIA International Conference on Nursing Use of Computers and Informatics Science NI 2000; 2000. pp 39–44.
6. Bryan RM, Deci EL. Intrinsic and extrinsic motivations: classic definitions and new directions. Contemp Educ Psychol. 2000;25:54–67.
7. OECD. Guide to measuring the information society 2011. Web link: http://www.oecd.org/internet/ieconomy/oecdguidetomeasuringtheinformationsociety2011.htm (2011). Last Accessed 16 Apr 2013.
8. Open Clinical. eHealth. 2011. http://www.openclinical.org/e-Health.html. Last Accessed 16 Apr 2013.
9. Barber B. Computers need nursing. In: Scholes M, Bryant Y, Barber B, editors. The impact of computers on nursing: an international review. North-Holland, Amsterdam, New York: Oxford; 1983. p. 25.
10. Berg CM. The importance of nurses' input for the selection of computerized systems. In: Scholes M, Bryant Y, Barber B, editors. The impact of computers on nursing: an international review. North-Holland, Amsterdam, New York: Oxford; 1983. p. 42–58.
11. Berg CM. The importance of nurses' input for the selection of computerized systems. In: Scholes M, Bryant Y, Barber B, editors. The impact of computers on nursing: an international review. Amsterdam: North-Holland; 1983. p. 58.
12. Tallberg M, Saba VK, Carr RL, et al. The international emergence of nursing informatics. In: Weaver CA, editor. Nursing and informatics for the 21st century: an international look at practice trends and the future. Chicago: Health Information and Management Systems Society; 2006.

13. American Nurses Association. Nursing informatics: scope and standards for nursing informatics practice. 2008. http://www.amia.org/programs/working-groups/nursing-informatics. Last Accessed 16 Apr 2013.
14. Toyama K. There are no technology shortcuts to good education. Educational Technology Debate. 2011. Web link: https://edutechdebate.org/ict-in-schools/there-are-no-technology-shortcuts-to-good-education. Last Accessed 16 Apr 2013.
15. Nursing & Midwifery Council. The code: standards of conduct, performance and ethics for nurses and midwives. NMC Publication. 2008.
16. In: Context. Web site: http://incontext.intrica.net/index.pl?dc=51. Last Accessed 16 Apr 2013.
17. Urquhart C, Currell R. Reviewing the evidence on nursing record systems. Health Inform J. 2005;11(1):33–44.
18. Ting-Ting L. Nurses' experiences using a nursing information system: early stage of technology implementation. Comput Inform Nurs. 2007;25(5):294–300.

Additional Reading

Donne J. Devotions Upon Emergent Occasions, and several steps in my sickness, 17th devotion, Meditation XVII, Printed by the Stationers' Company. 1624.

Nursing & Midwifery Council. Record keeping: guidance for nurses and midwives. Web link: http://www.nmc-uk.org/Documents/NMC-Publications/NMC-Record-Keeping-Guidance.pdf (2009). Last Accessed 16 Apr 2013.

Procter P. Use of a national/international telecommunications network for distance learning in an adult environment. In: Hovenga EJS et al., editors. Nursing informatics '91. Amsterdam: Springer; 1991. p. 710–20.

Procter PM. The development of an asset based model for postgraduate education on-line. In: Park H-A, et al. (editors). Consumer-centered computer-supported care for healthy people. Amsterdam, The Netherlands: IOS Press; 2006. pp. 167–171.

Scholes M, Bryant Y, Barber B. The impact of computers on nursing: an international review. North-Holland, Amsterdam, New York: Oxford; 1983.

Siemens G. Learning ecology, communities, and networks extending the classroom, elearnspace. 2003. http://www.elearnspace.org/Articles/learning_communities.htm. Accessed 20 Feb 2013.

World Health Organisation. eHealth definition. 2013. http://www.who.int/ehealth/about/en/index.html. Accessed 16 Apr 2013.

World Health Organisation. mHealth; new horizons for health through mobile technologies: second global survey on eHealth. Web link: http://www.who.int/goe/publications/goe_mhealth_web.pdf. (2011). Last Accessed 16 Apr 2013.

Chapter 21
Knowledge Networks in Nursing

Anne Spencer and Pamela Hussey

> *Education is not the filling of a pail ..... but the lighting of a fire.*
>
> *W B Yeats*

Abstract In the final chapter of this fourth edition Knowledge Networks in Nursing are discussed and presented. Building on discussions in Chap. 16 examples from various nursing practice domains are included using specific cases. This chapter demonstrates how nursing as a profession is tackling specific societal challenges by using communities of practice as a potential solution. Participants in the communities of practice are using their knowledge to collectively construct online resources that hold potential to positively impact on citizens' outcomes in society whilst concurrently advancing the profession of nursing.

Keywords Communities of Practice • Web 2.0 Technology • Knowledge networks in nursing • Health and social care • Education

Key Concepts
Communities of Practice
Web 2.0 Technology
Knowledge Networks in Nursing
Health and Social Care

In Chap. 15 of this text the use of information and communications technology within nurse education was explored. Questions relating to nurse education and the role of nurse educationalists in the use of information and communications technology to advance the profession in meeting societal challenges were considered.

The online version of this chapter (Doi:10.1007/978-1-4471-2999-8_21) contains supplementary material, which is available to authorized users.

A. Spencer, RN, BA (Hons), MSc
PETAL (Partners in Education, Teaching and Learning), Educational Technologist,
Dublin, Ireland
e-mail: aspencer@petal.ie

P. Hussey, RN, RCN, MEd, MSc, PhD (✉)
Lecturer in Health Informatics and Nursing, School of Nursing and Human Sciences,
Dublin City University, Dublin, Ireland
e-mail: pamela.hussey@dcu.ie

© Springer-Verlag London 2015
K.J. Hannah et al. (eds.), *Introduction to Nursing Informatics*,
Health Informatics, DOI 10.1007/978-1-4471-2999-8_21

In this chapter it is suggested that the answer for advancing the profession o nursing lies in education particularly in the use of emerging technologies in nurse education. Such an approach can advance nursing's' adoption and use of informa tion and communications technology within the broader context of health and socia care. This chapter focusses on 'real life' examples of how education is supporting nursing practitioners to become leaders, innovators and educators. It presents a brie summary of four established communities of practice that are successfully evolving whilst educating various stakeholders on specific health related topics.

Communities of Practice are increasingly demonstrating their effectiveness as edu cational frameworks. As an organic structure, Communities of Practice present oppor tunities for informal knowledge exchange and development of social networks [1] Formally recognised by WHO as effective network and partnership activities, com munities of practice also afford a collaborative approach, which in the current eco nomic downturn is pragmatic and purposeful. From a nursing informatics perspective perhaps one of the most significant COP which has evolved in recent years is TIGER [2]. The TIGER community which is discussed in detail in Chap. 14 has created a number of COP's which are using the TIGER VLE to inform and educate nurses globally on topics relating to nursing informatics. A core attribute of COP's is to use software platforms for social networks whilst harnessing the potential of enabling technologies. Cloud computing for example, can be used by nursing communities to come together to share expertise, experience and knowledge in both a synchronous and asynchronous manner. This sharing of expertise offers a greater potential for knowledge innovations to be cultivated to address society's health and social care needs across and between services on local, national and international platforms.

The Communities of Practice (COP) discussed in this Chapter have been selected as they offer a variety of differing approaches in design and are quite distinct in their subject areas. They relate to nursing informatics (PARTNERS) [3], Electronic Health Record education and training (EHRInsight) [4], mental health service user involvement and health promotion activity (Mental Health Trialogue) [5], and bone health education and falls prevention (Bone Health in the Park) [6]. The nursing leads for each of the COP's are from differing clinical and academic backgrounds.

An English philosopher Herbert Spencer (1820–1903), many years ago sug gested that the great aim of education is not knowledge but action. One form of action that is formally recognised within the World Health Organisation Strategic Directions Plan for Nursing and Midwifery for 2011–15 is the development of Communities of Practice (COP) [7]. Identified as an innovative approach for the uptake of new knowledge, Communities of Practice are increasingly demonstrating their effectiveness as agents of change.

The 4th edition of this text is an eBook and this chapter also includes a number of resources on the supporting website entitled www.intro2nursinginformatics.com. The material on the website can be classified into two groupings. Firstly *educational resources* to support the book as a space for supporting resources for the various chapters in this 4th edition, and secondly an *educational toolkit* which will help the reader to develop and present work in a professional portfolio for future continuing educational opportunities as they arise. Both of these resources are expanded upon in the associated website www.intro2nursinginformatics.com [8].

REALITY OF OUR WORLD TODAY

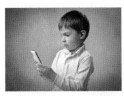
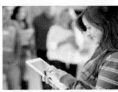
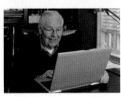
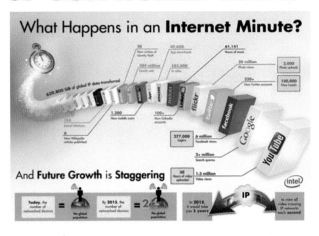

Fig. 21.1 Digital uptake in reality 2 (http://www.intel.com/content/www/us/en/communications/internet-minute-infographic.html) [9]

The Reality of Learning in the Twenty-First Century

Web 2.0 technologies offer practitioners a vehicle to develop and sustain Communities of Practice and increasingly can act as an enabler for the delivery of education and training of nurses. Earlier chapters in this edition explained the generations of computing developed since the 1940s and how fourth and fifth generation computing is increasingly shaping how we communicate and how we deliver health and social care. Nurse education is no exception to this approach as lecturers delivering nursing and midwifery undergraduate and postgraduate programmes exploit emerging technology to move beyond traditional didactic teaching modes to more constructivist learning approaches [9]. Learning is increasingly becoming a participatory process and Web 2.0 technologies can positively influence how we teach, communicate, collaborate, learn and create knowledge. A critical success factor that influences communities of practice development within the profession of nursing is the opportunity to co-construct and share knowledge in both formal and informal ways (Fig. 21.1).

Health as an Ecosystem

New terms to describe the impact of the global economic downturn include the creation of health ecosystems which can be linked in structure and form to communities of practice – a common denominator being sharing of expertise and action

Fig. 21.2 Nursing - An Eco
System

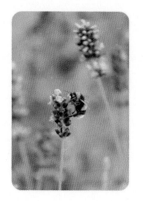

We need to effectively
use our environment,
and our skills and
professional 'know how
to navigate through the
current global 'climate
change' to strengthen
our future.

to address current health issues, such as chronic illness. There is an increasin
realisation that action must be taken to ensure provision of robust structures t
protect the healthcare system, which as a consequence of increasing fiscal cost
and an increasing and aging population is under threat. Chapter 15 noted the
nurses hold a unique function as they are the only healthcare professionals to inter
act with individuals, carers and families on a 24 h, 7 days a week basis. When on
considers the scale of skill hours and the overall projected costs of nursing ski
mix within healthcare, it is reasonable to suggest that within this emerging healt
ecosystem nursing as a profession is potentially vulnerable and so too are recipi
ents of health care. The profession as it is today faces a global challenge, similar i
nature to bees. The deliberate analogy to bees is drawn as there are distinct simi
larities to nursing 'communities' as both possess certain attributes as social group
Nurses are excellent communicators, structurally they are highly organised and ca
offer front line resilience to defend their specific community and respective popu
lations. How can nursing adopt and adapt to use informatics to ensure sustainabil
ity for the future of the profession is now a question that requires carefu
consideration.

The remainder of this chapter offers some examples of differing communities c
practice which strive to address this question (Fig. 21.2). Figure 21.3 offers an illus
trative overview of some of the communities of practice which are discussed in th
following sections.

Partners CT Community of Practice

PARTNERSCT is a community of practice devised as part of a nursing informatic
study completed in Ireland in 2010. The purpose of this study was to develop, wit
nurses, a shared assessment tool for older persons for use across and between si
differing health service providers. The project was entitled PARTNERSCT. Th
term was adopted as an acronym for *Participatory Action Research To develo
Nursing Electronic Resources* and the initials *CT* related to *Concepts and Term*

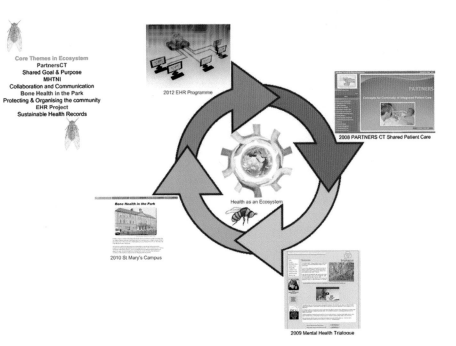

Fig. 21.3 Communities of practice in action

The community of practice has evolved since this date and is now entitled PARTNERS. The PARTNERSCT study sought to examine the complex process of patient referral across acute, primary and continuing care sectors as well as ongoing assessment data collection processes on individual patients over an extended time interval. The process involved six health service providers and 18 patients over a 6 month time frame, and the tool was devised from a patient centred perspective. A key output from the study was to understand the complexity of connected health from a nursing practice perspective i.e. sharing nursing records across more than one health service provider. To achieve interoperability health informatics standards were used to guide the development process. Interoperability in this context is described as achieving communication between different technologies and software applications for efficient, accurate, and sound sharing and of data. This communication process included two components (1) the data is understood at a computing level and can be transmitted across different service providers – computer science (2) Once data is received it is legible and fit for purpose – information science. To deliver on both of these components health informatics standards are required.

Health informatics standards which are discussed in detail in Chap. 7 offer a set of rules, regulations, guidelines, and definitions with technical specifications to make the integrated management of health systems viable at the computer and information science levels [10].

Health informatics standards were therefore viewed within the PARTNERS study as a set of guidelines to direct the development work. The PARTNERS team

considered the standards as *Models of Thought* created by health informatics expe
to assist practitioners engaged in such studies to steer through the developme
process in an incremental and co-ordinated fashion. These Models of Thoug
offered the practitioners a set of labels to reference their ideas, increase understan
ing whilst informing the discussion. As this project was part of a PhD study,
action research design was adopted. Dymek's Action and Sense Making Moc
(2008) was used to assist the group to develop a shared *Model of Meaning*. Th
resulted in a set of agreed concepts and terms to be used by the nurses in the prot
type patient assessment and referral tool which was agreed to be piloted over
6-month duration [11], argues that adapting existing frames with new emergii
work practices is the first step of an action cycle. In many instances this approa
requires a fundamental change in organisation's thinking and the implementati
process requires change at a schemata level. By linking this course of action wi
informatics, Dymek (2008), provides a key component for the development ai
implementation of information systems [11; p. 576].

In this study, the participating nurses from different services agreed upon a set
specific concepts and terms to enable shared care of elderly patients using a shar
assessment which was evaluated as fit for purpose. Using a mixed methods approa
the study integrated a Community of Practice to address local challenges whi
were experienced by the participating nurses. The resources were published on
dedicated website and subsequently used within nursing informatics education
Ireland. Examples of this project are available to view from PARTNERSCOP we
site [3].

The process of developing the PARTNERs tool included capturing practi
workflow activities with group participants, and mapping the process for simila
ties and differences in the existing respective health service providers to each oth
A detailed analysis of the existing assessment documentation in each service w
carried out. Early recognition that there was a great deal of overlap in the concep
and terms collected across the service was evident, however the order in which da
was collected and the qualifiers used in the measurement of concepts were dissin
lar, and a revised structure was agreed and piloted by all participants.

Specific educational sessions were offered on language construction using Ogd
and Richards Semiotic Triangle [12], and consideration was given to using langua
that was referenced and standardised. The semiotic triangle which was original
conceived by Ogden and Richards in 1923 is considered a seminal thesis which h
influenced the development of language upon thought particularly in regard to t
science of symbolism [12]. The semiotic triangle and Freirks semantic stack [1
offered the team clarity on decision making and were used to make sense, locai
and build the assessment tool within the context of the participant's clinical pra
tice. Figure 21.4 offers a summary of the PARTNER's activity as a process.

A key finding from the study in regard to data analysis was identifying potenti
health issues (Level 3 data) and one health issue identified as significant by partic
pants was in relation to medication management. It emerged that in one speci
case a number of hospital readmissions could be avoided if communications acro
and between services could be timelier using specific data on patient transfer. Oth

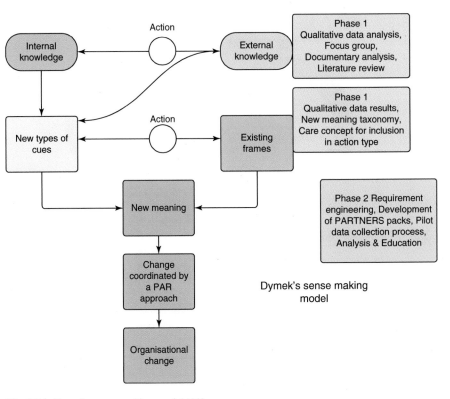

Fig. 21.4 Dymeks sense making model [11]

issues that arose related to the importance of documenting social care needs and the direct bearing such data can have on maintaining outcomes at their current status as opposed to individuals deteriorating on discharge home to the community. Figure 21.5 offers a summary illustration of the devised conceptual framework created by the participants.

Mental Health Trialogue Network

The notion of Trialogue COP is a difficult to define or gain consensus on; however, within the Mental Health Trialogue Programme (Fig. 21.6) Ireland it is described as:

> A conversation between three or more people or groups using a form of open communication known as Open Dialogue. The Trialogue uses open dialogue as a means to allow everyone to participate in the conversation [14]. Open Dialogue enables the creation of a common language and a mutual understanding around the given topic. There is no exclusivity or expert knowledge or power, with the diverse experiences and expressions carrying equal weight. The combined expertise is taken on board by all in the Trialogue and together they create a shared reality that is mutually acceptable and accessible to all.

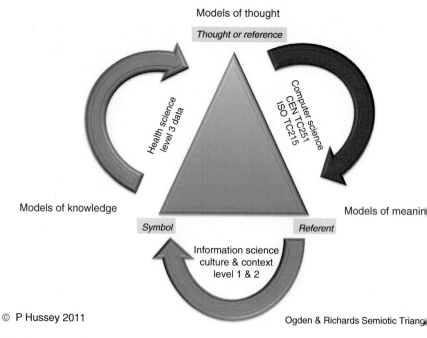

© P Hussey 2011

Ogden & Richards Semiotic Triangle

Fig. 21.5 PARTNERS conceptual framework

MENTAL HEALTH TRIALOGUE NETWORK

trialogue

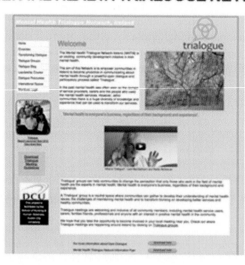

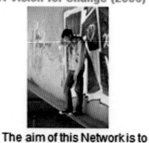

A Vision for Change (2006)

The aim of this Network is to empower communities in Ireland to become proactive in communicating about mental health through a powerful open dialogue and participatory process called 'Trialogue'.

Fig. 21.6 Mental Health Trialogue

Led by Dr Liam MacGabhann, a practicing mental health nurse and lecturer from Dublin City University, Ireland, the core purpose of this community of practice is to empower local communities within Ireland to become more proactive in Open Dialogue and a participatory process. The focus to date has been to examine national policy in relation to mental health service delivery and to discuss the issues that impact directly on local communities within Ireland. Trialogue relates to three differing perspectives in this instance the perspectives of the service user, the community and the health care professional. Since its inception this community of practice has evolved to have a number of European and International partners. The web site URL is accessible from http://www.trialogue.co [5]. Recent statistics from the website indicate over 35,000 hits since February 2012.

Bone Health in the Park

The second community of practice is Bone Health in the Park (http://www.bone-health.co) [6] and is situated in St Mary's Campus, Dublin, Ireland – this care facility is the largest care provider for older persons in Ireland (Fig. 21.7). This COP is led by Daragh Rodger an Advanced Nurse Practitioner in care of the older adult and health promotion. There are currently two care initiatives emanating

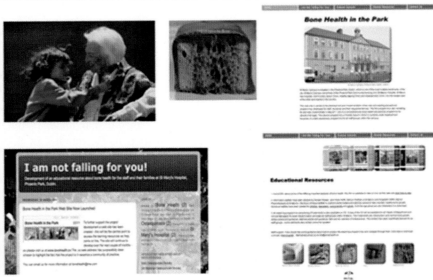

Fig. 21.7 Bone Health in the Park

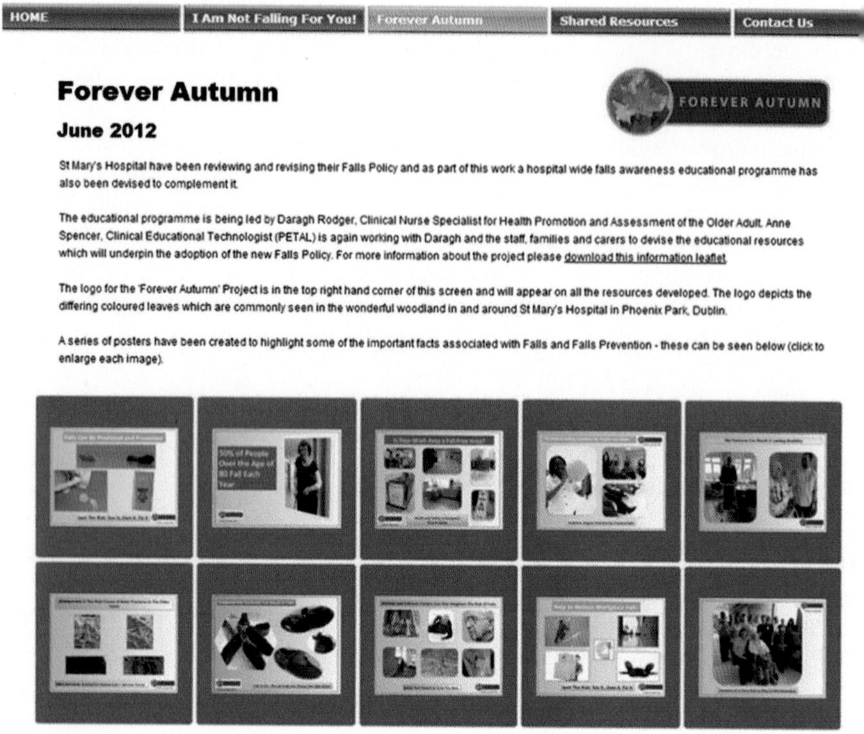

Fig. 21.8 Forever autumn

from this COP. The first is entitled 'I am not falling for you!' and is a proactive approach involving key stakeholders to advocate and promote the importance of maintaining bone health throughout life (with a particular focus on osteoporosis). The principle objective is to ensure that all patients, caregivers, staff, and their families are better informed about the importance of maintaining general bone health throughout life from a toddler to old age; this includes differing lifestyle choices in relation to both diet and exercise. It is envisaged that an understanding and appreciation of these will contribute to a reduction in the number of falls related bone injuries.

The second element to Bone Health in the Park is 'Forever Autumn' an initiative to increase falls risk awareness amongst all clinical and non-clinical staff in St Mary's and to introduce a new falls risk assessment tool whilst informing staff about the revised Hospital Falls Policy.

In the last year the web site has received 28,000 hits (Fig. 21.8). In March 2014, both I am not falling for you! and Forever Autumn have been recommended for deployment nationally.

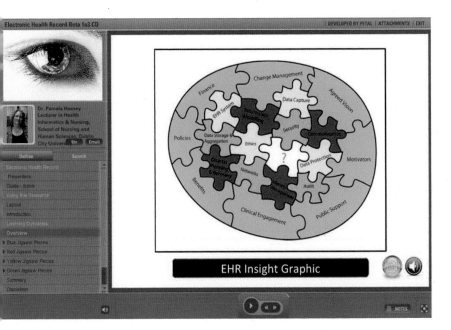

Fig. 21.9 EHRInsight

EHRInsight

The EHRInsight Community of Practice (more information about this COP is available at http://www.petal.ie [4] was devised in 2013 by academics across a number of institutions in Dublin. This open source resource has been designed specifically for the education and training of student nurses, engineers and computer science students and is intended to be used as a primer for understanding electronic health records in context (Fig. 21.9).

The Electronic Health Record often described as the heart of any health ecosystem is at varying degrees of implementation globally. In many OECD countries significant investment has been made on national deployment of electronic health records but the vision for clinicians has yet to be fully understood or indeed embedded into the practice setting. Recent evidence suggests that there is a move away from large monolithic centralised EHR delivery to a more localised development approach. Localised development programmes can be implemented in an incremental way with more focussed clinical engagement based on service needs to achieve meaningful use.

In 2012 a group of academics from Dublin Institute of Technology in Kevin Street (Dublin), Trinity College Dublin and Dublin City University opted to create a resource for students on electronic health record. The resource was designed specifically for use with both undergraduate and postgraduate students from across a number of disciplines including health informatics, nursing and computer science and engineering. Key design principles were to devise an introduction to EHR and its variants and to make evident to the viewer EHR scope purpose and function. The resource is intended as an introductory piece and includes critical factors identified from the literature, which are considered important for future national or regional implementation of EHR. Some of the sections of this resource are at differing stages of development as is the knowledge base on EHR implementation nationally and internationally.

Discussion

Nursing and its future use of technology within the scope of healthcare needs to be managed carefully and strong leadership is now required. In this edition Chaps. 16 and 17 have identified the importance of education on informatics, and the training of nurses on information and communication skills. Delivery of such skills and understanding will enable nurses to protect not only the profession of nursing but also the health Ecosystem which is increasingly under threat and the individuals who use this ecosystem. Much is written reporting nurses as knowledge workers in eHealth care who through a process of assimilation convert data to information – information to knowledge and with experience, convert knowledge in context to progress the profession [15]. By considering health as an ecosystem and comparing health to the natural ecosystems of bees offers for instance presents us with a space to reflect and consider ourselves as knowledge workers in a dynamic global environment. Experiences discussed in this chapter and the evidence reviewed would suggest that communities of practice are a sensible approach to adopt [17].

Education, particularly in nursing informatics is a key requirement and should underpin all undergraduate and postgraduate programmes. It is for this reason that this chapter and other chapters in this book have integrated differing multimedia and interactive resources including screen casts and web sites that may be used as a springboard for further education and training in informatics competencies.

Two other emerging communities of practice for 2014 which are still within their relative infancy are firstly ENS4Care – this European project is a thematic network comprising of six work packages with the main aim of developing evidence based guidelines for the implementation of ehealth services in nursing and social care (http://www.ens4care.eu/) [18]. Secondly ISHCA is being developed by a team of practitioners in St Mary's Hospital, Dublin this is an acronym for Implementing and Supporting Holistic Continence Awareness and more information is available from the web site at http://www.ishca.net [19].

Downloads

Available from extras.springer.com:

Educational Template (PDF 90 kb)
Educational Template (PPTX 127 kb)

References

1. MacPhee M, Suryaprakash N, Jackson C. Online knowledge networking: what leaders need to know. J Nurs Adm. 2009;39(10):415–22.
2. TIGER. Available from: http://www.thetigerinitiative.org/. Accessed 29 May.
3. PARTNERS Community of Practice. Available from: www.partnerscop.com. Accessed 29 May.
4. EHRinsight.. Available from: http://www.petal.ie. Accessed 29 May 2013.
5. Mental Health Trialogue Ireland. Available from: http://www.trialogue.co/. Accessed 29 May 2013.
6. Bone Health in the Park. Available from: http://www.bonehealth.co/. Accessed 29 May 2013.
7. World Health Organisation nursing and midwifery services strategic direction 2011–2015 report. Available at: http://www.who.int/hrh/nursing_midwifery/en/. Accessed 2 Feb 2011.
8. Introduction to nursing informatics. Available from: www.intro2nursinginformatics.com. Accessed 29 May 2013.
9. What happens in an internet minute. Available from: http://www.intel.com/content/www/us/en/communications/internet-minute-infographic.html. Accessed 26 Mar 2014.
10. Pan American Health Organisation (PAHO) eHealth Strategy and Plan of Action (2012–2017). Available at: http://new.paho.org/ict4health/. Accessed 17 Nov 2012.
11. Dymek C. I.T and action sensemaking: making sense of new technology. In: Reason P, Bradbury H. The Sage book of action research. 1st ed. Sage: Thousand Oakes; 2008. p. 573–79.
12. Ogden CK, Richards IA. The meaning of meaning. 8th ed. Orlando: Harcourt Brace Jovanovich; 1989. First edition published 1923.
13. Freriks G. The rise of two level model EHR systems EHRland workshop presentation, Dublin Institute of Technology, Dublin, Ireland, June 2010.
14. Mac Gabhann L, McGowan P, Ni Cheirin L, Amering M, Spencer A. Mental Health Trialogue Network Ireland, transforming dialogue in mental health communities, DCU. ISBN: 978-1-873769-15-7. Available from: http://www.trialogue.co/.
15. Matney S, Brewster P, Sward K, Cloynes K, Staggers N. Philosophical approaches to nursing informatics data- information-knowledge-wisdom framework. ANS Adv Nurs Sci. 2010; 34(1):6–18.
16. Li LC, Grimshaw JM, Nielsen C, Judd M, Coyte PC, Graham ID. Evolution of Wenger's concept of community of practice. Available at: http://www.implementationscience.com/content/4/1/11. Accessed 6 June 2010.
17. Wenger E, Traynor B. Available from intro to communities of practice. http://wenger-trayner.com/theory/. Accessed 23 Aug 2013.
18. ENS4Care. Available from: http://www.ens4care.eu/. Accessed 25 Mar 2014.
19. ISHCA. Available from: http://www.ishca.net/. Accessed 25 Mar 2014.

Appendix 1
International Nursing Informatics Associations

1. ACENDIO Association Common European Nursing Diagnosis Interventions and Outcomes http://www.acendio.net/.
2. AMIA American Nursing Informatics Association http://www.amia.org/programs/working-groups/nursing-informatics.
3. BCS British Computer Society Nursing Specialist Group http://www.bcs.org/category/10013.
4. CNIA Canadian Nursing Informatics Association http://cnia.ca/index.html.
5. HISINM Health Informatics Society of Ireland Nursing and Midwifery Group http://hisinm.ie/.
6. TIGER International Initiative http://www.tigersummit.com/.
7. Australia Nursing Informatics NIN http://www.hisa.org.au/members/group.aspx?id=85335.
8. ASIA HIMSS http://www.himssasiapac.org/development/committee.aspx.
9. Sweden http://www.swenurse.se/.

© Springer-Verlag London 2015
K.J. Hannah et al. (eds.), *Introduction to Nursing Informatics*,
Health Informatics, DOI 10.1007/978-1-4471-2999-8

Index

© Springer-Verlag London 2015
K.J. Hannah et al. (eds.), *Introduction to Nursing Informatics*,
Health Informatics, DOI 10.1007/978-1-4471-2999-8